Third Edition

Body Massage

Mo Rosser

updated and edited by

Greta Couldridge & Sue Rosser

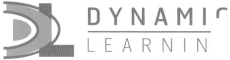

HODDER
EDUCATION
AN HACHETTE UK COMPANY

Photo credits: p. xiv ©R Sheridan/Ancient Art & Architecture Collection Ltd; p. xv ©The British Library Board, Or.6810,f.27v; Figure 1.2 Science Photo Library/Alamy; Figure 2.10 DR M.A. ANSARY/SCIENCE PHOTO LIBRARY; Figure 2.11 Medical-on-Line/Alamy; Figure 2.12 MIKE DEVLIN/SCIENCE PHOTO LIBRARY; Figure 2.13 Vasili Yurkevitch/photographersdirect.com; Figure 2.14 DR P. MARAZZI/SCIENCE PHOTO LIBRARY; Figure 2.15 DR P. MARAZZI/SCIENCE PHOTO LIBRARY; acne vulgaris on p. 120 Medical-on-Line/Alamy; basal cell carcinoma on p. 121 DR P. MARAZZI/SCIENCE PHOTO LIBRARY; carbuncle on p. 122 Wellcome Photo Library; dermatitis on p. 122 Libby Welch/Alamy; eczema on p. 123 JOTI/SCIENCE PHOTO LIBRARY; furuncle or boil on p.124 Getty Images/Science Faction; herpes simplex (cold sore) on p. 125 Science VU/Visuals Unlimited, Inc.; impetigo on p. 126 DR P. MARAZZI/SCIENCE PHOTO LIBRARY; melanoma on p. 127 Scott Camazine/Alamy; oedema on p. 128 DR P. MARAZZI/SCIENCE PHOTO LIBRARY; pediculosis capitis on p. 129 Medical-on-Line/Alamy; pediculosis corporis on p. 129 Wellcome Photo Library; psoriasis on p. 130 BIOPHOTO ASSOCIATES/SCIENCE PHOTO LIBRARY; pustule on p. 131 JANE SHEMILT/SCIENCE PHOTO LIBRARY; tinea capitis on p. 131 SCIENCE PHOTO LIBRARY; tinea corporis on p. 131 Arterra Picture Library/Alamy; tinea pedis (Athlete's foot) on p. 131 DR P. MARAZZI/SCIENCE PHOTO LIBRARY; rosacea on p. 131 DR P. MARAZZI/SCIENCE PHOTO LIBRARY; scabies on p. 131 Medical-on-Line/Alamy; sebaceous cyst on p. 132 DR P. MARAZZI/ SCIENCE PHOTO LIBRARY; herpes zoster (shingles) on p. 132 CUSTOM MEDICAL STOCK PHOTO/SCIENCE PHOTO LIBRARY; skin tags on p. 133 PATRICK G./SCIENCE PHOTO LIBRARY; squamous cell carcinoma on p. 133 DR P. MARAZZI/SCIENCE PHOTO LIBRARY; urticaria on p. 134 DR P. MARAZZI/SCIENCE PHOTO LIBRARY; p. 230 UpperCut Images/Alamy; p. 231 Kurhan – Fotolia; p. 232 Image Source; p. 234 Solaria – Fotolia; p. 237 iofoto – Fotolia; p. 240 i love images/Alamy; Figures 8.1–8.3© The Carlton Group.

Every effort has been made to trace and acknowledge the ownership of copyright material. If any have inadvertently remain unacknowledged the publishers will be glad to make suitable arrangements at the earliest opportunity.

Orders: please contact Bookpoint Ltd, 130 Milton Park, Abingdon, Oxon OX14 4SB.

Telephone: +44 (0)1235 827720, Fax: +44 (0)1235 400454. Lines are open from 9.00 a.m. to 6.00 p.m., Monday to Saturday, with a 24-hour message-answering service. You can also order through our website www.hoddereducation.co.uk

British Library Cataloguing in Publication Data
A catalogue record for this title is available from the British Library

ISBN 978 1 444 13711 8

First Edition published 1996
Second Edition published 2004
This edition published 2012
Impression number   10   9   8   7   6   5   4   3   2   1
Year   2016 2015 2014 2013 2012

Hachette UK's policy is to use papers that are natural, renewable and recyclable products and made from wood grown in sustainable forests. The logging and manufacturing processes are expected to conform to the environmental regulations of the country of origin.

Cover photo © Carl Drury

Illustrations by Barking Dog Art and Simon Tegg Illustration

Photos of massage movements in Chapter 7 © Greta Couldridge. All other photos of massage routines and movements © Andrew Callaghan

Typeset by Integra

Printed in Italy for Hodder Education, an Hachette UK company, 338 Euston Road, London NW1 3BH

Contents

Acknowledgements

Before her death in 2006, Mo asked Greta and me to work together on rewrites and new editions of her books. Mo was an extremely conscientious and diligent person who dedicated herself to the pursuit of excellence in everything she did. Her thorough knowledge of the subject and her long experience as a physiotherapist all contributed to the enormous success of these textbooks. It was therefore a very daunting task when we were approached by Hodder to collaborate on this third edition of *Body Massage*.

I have been fortunate to have in Greta a co-writer whose knowledge of the subject, the methods of assessment, and the business is equal to Mo's and whose diligent and painstaking approach has ensured that this edition is as good as it can be. Mo is a hard act to follow, greatly respected by colleagues and students and we were at pains to produce a new edition that lived up to its original. We hope that we have achieved this.

I am indebted to my father, Gwyn, and my partner, John, for their love and support and especially to my daughter, Izzy who has put up with my long absences with good humour and patience.

Sue Rosser

Having agreed to work with Sue on this new edition, neither of us imagined what a challenge it would turn out to be. I knew Mo for very many years as a friend and colleague and had proofread earlier editions of her books for her. She was a wonderful lady who taught me a lot, and knowing that she believed in my ability gave me the confidence to embark on this project. One of the best things to come out of this collaborative process is the forming of a strong bond with her daughter, Sue. We have spent a lot of time together this year and have laughed and cried and reminisced as well as working hard on the book.

I would like to thank my partner, Peter, a very special person, for his patience and encouragement as I have immersed myself in working on this book. Thank you also to my close friend, Kay Treby, for contributing her time and expertise in helping to develop the face and scalp massage routines.

Special thanks to Stuart Turner, BSc (Hons) MSST, Sports Therapist, for his invaluable advice and contribution in updating Chapter 7, Additional massage techniques.

Greta Couldridge

We are indebted to Angela Barbagelata-Fabes, Chairman of The Carlton Group, and Janice Brown, Director of HoF Beauty, House of Famuir, for their expertise and advice about mechanical massage and infra-red equipment and its use.

We would also like to thank Pauline Coyle, Principal Examiner for VTCT, for being so free with her time and advice and Jane Wilson, Debbie Paul and Anne Paton for contributing their experiences in the industry; and Kip Ward and Emily Murphy for being such great models.

A special thank you goes to Alison Smales and the team at the Arena Hair & Beauty Salon at Kingston College, for helping us with the photo shoot for this book. Thanks to our wonderful models, Dominica Mimma Deufemia and Janet Hargreaves, and to Deborah Carrington for make-up.

We are grateful to Gemma Parsons at Hodder Education for her support and patience.

SR and GC

Introduction

This book has been revised and updated to meet the National Occupational Standards (**NOS**) set by Hairdressing and Beauty Industry Authority (**Habia**) and Skills for Health (**SfH**). It meets the new requirements of the various awarding bodies in the beauty and complementary therapies industries.

It will provide you with a comprehensive and in-depth knowledge and understanding of massage techniques and enable you to develop your practical skills in order to become a competent therapist. Moreover, it will encourage you to develop an enquiring and self-critical approach to your work, which will enhance your studies and your working practices. The book will also be of value to those already qualified in this field, particularly the chapter on Additional Massage Techniques, which will broaden your knowledge and skills further, as part of your continuing professional development (**CPD**).

The information provided will guide you towards safe and effective practice. Great emphasis is placed on the responsibility carried by you, as an employee, or employer, to be well informed and to maintain the highest standards of safety and hygiene. Relevant information regarding the regulations and legal requirements is provided.

The text provides an overview of anatomy and physiology, and explains the application and the effects of massage on body systems, as well as its psychological effects. Underlying structures are clearly described and explained. The systematic approach will greatly aid your learning and provide a useful quick reference guide in the workplace.

The text is full of helpful suggestions and ideas for applying your knowledge in a variety of practical situations, as well as vital reminders of hazards and points to consider. Guidance is provided for dealing with, and caring for, each client on an individual basis. Contra-indications are carefully explained and advice given on the appropriate action to be taken.

The importance of consultation and accurate assessment is discussed, with guidance on meeting the needs of each client. Advice is given on planning effective treatments, selecting appropriate techniques and setting realistic targets using specific examples of client profiles. Consideration is also given to the timing and costing of treatments, together with post-treatment observations and feedback.

Emphasis is placed throughout on high standards of client care and all the factors that will contribute to the success and effectiveness of the treatment. The book gives you a method of evaluating your performance and reflecting on your practice in order to maintain these high standards and with a view to continuing professional development, which is so vital a part of today's competitive world.

Multiple-choice questions are included at the end of most chapters, with answers given at the end of the book. This will help to consolidate your knowledge and prepare you for theory assessments. Other chapters include different methods of self-assessment, such as activities or short-answer questions where these are more appropriate to the subject matter.

The aim of the book is to help you to become a caring, competent and successful therapist. It will emphasise that you will require an understanding of biological principles, an appreciation of the technique and effects of all massage manipulations, together with highly developed motor skills, sensitivity, integrity and dedication.

Therapeutic techniques are once again recognised in mainstream medicine, for the relief of pain, improving the circulation and in general health care. Basic massage and other more advanced techniques are now carried out in hospitals, health centres, clinics etc, by therapists, nurses, and other health staff who have received training in these specialised areas. Athletes, sportsmen and women, dancers and actors include massage in their training schedules to aid recovery, promote relaxation and to prevent or treat soft tissue injuries.

A qualification in massage offers numerous opportunities for employment in a variety of establishments, worldwide. These include beauty salons, spas, clinics, sports and leisure centres, large department stores, luxury cruise liners or working as a self-employed therapist.

Massage continues to be practised throughout the world and we have much to learn from other cultures. It is hoped that this book will provide you with a sound foundation on which to build, and encourage you to explore and evaluate other techniques and theories. Expertise and excellence will develop through constant practice, self-assessment and evaluation of results. Massage offers an extremely rewarding and fulfilling career for those seeking a caring role in society.

Here are some examples of career paths taken after qualifying.

In the workplace

Anne recommends keeping two diaries if you are working as a mobile therapist; one to take with you and one at home with all the details of where you are going. This is important from a personal safety point of view, so that there is a record of where you are. It is also useful if you mislay one diary or if you are taking bookings on the move.

Be aware !

Anne advises that you always make it particularly clear to male clients what the treatment entails, and doesn't entail, in order to avoid unfortunate and embarrassing misunderstandings.

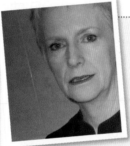

Anne Paton

Career path

Anne Paton trained initially at a Sports Injury Clinic and obtained qualifications in: Remedial Massage Therapy and Sports Massage. She undertook many other courses while working and qualified in Indian Head Massage; On-Site Chair Massage; Thermal Auricular Therapy; Rejuvanessence Facial Massage and No Hands Massage.

She decided to train as a massage therapist because:

'I was always my family's massage therapist and had often thought that if more people had massage then the doctors' waiting rooms would not be so full. Following a whiplash injury, I went to the osteopath and found that the pre-treatment massage he gave me was every bit as effective as all the bone crunching he gave me later, and so I decided to train professionally and buy my own equipment. During training, the clinic had the contract for treating the injuries of the Warrington Rugby Team. Practising on them was a good grounding as those boys had muscles like iron!'

She built up her massage business during the evenings and weekends while working part time in an office. Following a house move, Anne wrote to the local paper. They sent a reporter for a massage, who wrote a follow-up article. The business grew from there, highlighting the importance of personal recommendation. One of the best things that Anne found was being able to fit her business around bringing up her young children.

Of the skills required to be a good therapist, Anne says:

'Massage Therapy is a caring profession and if you don't care about your clients then you won't enjoy it; each session will become mechanical and unsatisfying for you and the client. To be a successful massage therapist you have to be able to listen and to respond sympathetically to your client. You have to really love your job and not just be in it for the money. As a mobile therapist you have to be prepared to work long and sometimes irregular hours.'

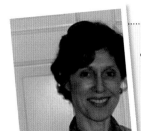

Jane Wilson

Jane Wilson trained at a College of Further Education and has qualifications in Swedish Remedial Massage, Reflexology, Aromatherapy and Indian Head Massage. She decided to train formally as a massage therapist after taking an evening class that introduced her to body massage and reflexology.

She says of her training:

'Working at college on members of the public was very useful as a way of developing my approach and professionalism, but still with the tutors support as back-up if necessary.'

Jane recommends considering different places of work and types of career within the industry, and suggests:

'Working for an organisation may suit you more than working alone, so I'd recommend trying both if you can.'

In terms of the skills necessary for being a successful therapist, Jane feels that if you love your work, the client will feel it! She stresses that the ability to engage with a client, will help them to relax and trust you.

'Listening carefully to what they have to say about themselves shows the client you are interested in them and want to give them a treatment that is right for them: be observant and read body language to assess for muscle tension or mobility problems.'

Be aware

Jane advises to always be aware that you are touching someone's body, so you must be alert to boundary issues; you must also pay attention to your own personal care, especially of your hands, the main contact point with your client – skin needs to be smooth and nails need to be short.

Learning point

Jane makes the point that giving a massage can be physically quite draining, so you will need to check that you eat well most of the time and try to lead a healthy lifestyle.

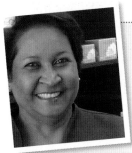

Debbie Paul

Debbie Paul works as a holistic massage therapist. She qualified comparatively late in life at the age of 49. Following a career in accountancy, she pursued her interest in massage therapy and enrolled at a central London college. On graduating she began work at a hotel and spa.

Of the skills required to be a good massage therapist, Debbie says:

'The most important thing is to ensure that the person you are massaging is relaxed and comfortable first. I found also that the first contact with the person is very important.'

Debbie's enthusiasm for her new career is clear. She gives some excellent advice:

* 'It's never too late. I did it at the age of 49 and I am going from strength to strength.
* Get experience. Try lower paid jobs at first if necessary, to build up your expertise.
* The feedback from your clients is very important.
* Keep up to date with different techniques.
* Add to your continuing professional development (CPD) with different massage courses.
* Keep your mind open to changes in the industry.
* Join support groups, perhaps through your training school.
* Always be professional in your approach to what you do.'

In the workplace

Jane gives the following advice: 'Like everything now, the massage industry is very competitive, so giving your clients a good value service will benefit everyone.'

Remember

Debbie advises: 'A positive feeling can affect your work. Any negative attitude can be transferred to your client.'

Best practice

Debbie adds: 'If I feel I haven't used a technique for some time I practise on my friends and family.'

Guidance for learning and development of skills

This book provides information and direction for those interested in studying body massage treatments.

The material has been selected and organised to meet the requirements set by the various awarding bodies in line with NOS. The text includes the main components, namely *underpinning knowledge, understanding* and *skill instruction.*

When you pursue this course of study and practice, you will acquire:

- the underpinning knowledge and understanding to make you a safe and competent therapist
- the skills necessary to perform all the massage manipulations on the various parts of the body and on different types of client.

Learning

Skills learning

Learning how to massage is the same as learning any other skill, such as playing an instrument. You may find it difficult at the beginning but it will become easier with practice and experience. The more you practise, the faster you will improve. Watch carefully when manipulations are demonstrated by your tutor, then practise them yourself to develop the correct techniques immediately.

Before you start practising, learn the names of the main massage groups and the type of movement involved, e.g. those in the *effleurage* group are stroking movements; those in the *petrissage* group are kneading or pressure movements. Then learn the names of each manipulation and the movement involved.

Massage manipulations vary greatly in the dexterity required to perform them – some are very much easier than others.

Each time you practise a new manipulation, try to break the movement down into small steps. Practise each step on a model until you are satisfied that you are performing them correctly, then link them together to perform the complete movement. The text has been organised to help you follow this step-by-step approach. Follow the technique section for every manipulation. Once you have mastered the movement you can then move on and concentrate on improving coordination of speed, depth and rhythm.

Knowledge and understanding

You will require background knowledge and clear understanding to be competent in your work and to be able to explain the effects and benefits of the treatment to your clients.

Remember
Regular practice of hand exercises will improve strength and dexterity.

Best practice
Use your time in training to consolidate your knowledge and clarify any areas of confusion. *Always ask* for further explanation if you are unclear about anything.

Health and safety legislation

You must understand the health, safety and welfare requirements related to your work. These will enable you to practise safely and protect yourself, colleagues and clients from harm. The relevant health, safety and welfare issues are discussed in the next chapter together with Local Authority regulations. These are legal requirements for all people in the workplace and are concerned with the hazards and risks in your place of work. They cover important emergency procedures including fire drill and first aid.

They include safety issues related to equipment and practices, and stress the importance of high standards of hygiene, which must be practised at all times to prevent the spread of diseases. Staff, clients and others must be protected from cross-infection and infestation. Hygiene relates to your own personal appearance and hygiene practices, e.g. clean uniform, short nails, frequent bathing, hand washing before touching the client and after each treatment etc. It also includes salon hygiene, e.g. clean linen and towels for each client, prompt and safe disposal of waste into appropriate waste bins, according to legislation.

Communication

You must be able to communicate effectively and pleasantly with all types of people. You must recognise the importance of carrying out and recording a detailed client consultation and obtaining a signed consent form before starting the treatment. You must be able to create the right conditions and prepare the room and the client for treatment. Appropriate body language, tone of voice and a friendly manner are vital for developing a rapport with clients. It is this rapport that will ensure repeat business and recommendation.

Best practice
Establishing client trust through good communication also helps with aftercare sales of products to maximise the benefit of the treatment.

Anatomy and physiology

Knowledge of the structure and function of the body is necessary, as this will enable you to identify the structures you are working over and understand the effects produced on the body systems.

It will help you to learn this subject if you try to visualise the tissues underneath your hands as they move over a part when massaging.

- Your hands are in contact with the skin: what is the skin composed of? Could you label a section through the skin?
- Under the skin is the subcutaneous layer: what is it made of?
- Under this lie the muscles: can you name these muscles and give their action?
- Under the muscles lie the bones connected at joints: can you name the bones and the joints?

As well as the overview of each body system in Chapter 2, in Chapter 5 you will find the anatomy of each body part immediately before the massage routine for that area. For example; the anatomy of the leg is immediately before the leg massage routine. As you massage the leg, think of the structures underneath your hands and mentally do the following:

- Name the bones and the joints that lie underneath.
- Name the muscles and note the fleshy parts, which can take heavier manipulations and are easier to knead, wring, pick up and roll than the more tendinous parts.
- Name the lymph nodes and their location.

Remember that arteries are deep, and blood flow through the arteries is governed by the contractions of the heart. You are not likely to affect this arterial blood flow with massage. Veins lie towards the surface, therefore massage will increase blood flow in the superficial veins.

Lymphatic vessels lie throughout the tissues and the flow of lymph will be increased by massage.

Revise the relevant anatomy both before and after the massage lesson. It becomes easier to remember when you relate it to practical work.

Learning point

Prepare cards to remind you of the structure (on one side of the card) and its function (on the other). These can be used in games and quizzes to reinforce your learning.

Learning styles

Familiarise yourself with the diagrams and photographs, write lists, test yourself and each other at every opportunity. Different people favour different styles of learning. Try to find out your own preferred style and develop methods of helping yourself to remember key facts. This book contains a variety of learning features to help you develop knowledge and skills. These include boxes in the margin to highlight:

- best practice
- learning points
- things to be aware of
- workplace practices
- key points to remember
- activities for self-evaluation.

As well as diagrams and photographs, flow charts and other visual learning tools are used to show procedures and other information. Make sure that you understand them – ask your tutor for guidance.

Assessment

Different awarding bodies have different ways of assessing whether you are competent to practice. Any assessment is an opportunity for you to show how able you are. You will provide evidence of your ability to the assessor or examiner, who will judge your performance against the requirements of the awarding body.

Do not be apprehensive when you come to be assessed. Providing you have worked consistently you will have gained the skills and knowledge required to succeed. This book has been designed to help you achieve your goals.

During training, develop the habit of reflecting on:

- what you have learnt
- your performance of techniques
- feedback from others about your skills.

Following this reflection, establish a plan for self-development. Chapter 9 'Reflection, evaluation and continuing professional development' explains the importance of this for your career and gives suggestions of activities that will enhance this life skill.

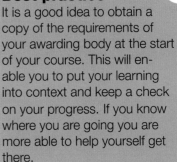

Best practice
It is a good idea to obtain a copy of the requirements of your awarding body at the start of your course. This will enable you to put your learning into context and keep a check on your progress. If you know where you are going you are more able to help yourself get there.

A brief history of massage

Massage has been practised throughout the centuries since the earliest civilisations. It has been used medically as a therapeutic healing treatment and also for invigorating, soothing and beautifying the body. Massage or rubbing is an instinctive act for relieving pain and discomfort, and for soothing and calming. The use of fats and aromatic oils for anointing and lubricating the body is referred to in the Bible and in the Koran.

The word 'massage' has its origin in the Arabic word *mass* or *mass'h*, which means 'to press gently'. The Greek word *massage* means 'to knead' and the French word *masser* means 'to massage'.

Massage in ancient times

The earliest evidence of massage being used is found in the cave paintings of ancient cave dwellers. These wall drawings and paintings show people massaging each other. Various artefacts also found contain traces of fats and oils mixed with herbs. These indicate that lubricants may have been used, perhaps for healing, soothing or beautifying purposes.

As early as 3000 BC, the Chinese practised massage to cure ailments and improve general health. Records of this can be found in the British Museum. Ancient Chinese books record lists of massage movements with descriptions of their technique. One of these books, *The Cong Fau of Tao-Tse*, also contains lists of exercises and massage used to improve general health and well-being. The Chinese found that pressure techniques were very effective on specific points and they developed special techniques called *amma*. This was the beginning of the development of acupressure and acupuncture. Around this time, the Yellow Emperor, Huang Di, wrote a book, the Neijing Suwen, which has been translated as *The Essential Text of Chinese Health and Healing*. This took the form of a dialogue between the Emperor and his acupuncturist, Qi Bo. The treatise dealt with the need for balance in the body and includes reference to massage movements.

These massage techniques spread to Japan, where they were further developed. The Japanese used similar pressure techniques on specific points, which they called *tsubo*. This form of massage has been practised over the centuries; it has recently regained recognition and popularity and is now known as *shiatsu*. Many therapists have studied these techniques, which they combine with other forms of treatment for the benefit of their clients.

Records show that the Hindus practised massage as part of their hygiene routines. A sacred book called the *Ayur-Veda* (The Art of Life), which was written around 1800 BC, describes how shampooing and rubbing were used to reduce fatigue and promote well-being and cleanliness.

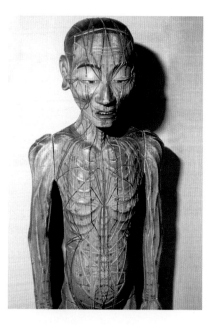

An ancient Chinese acupuncture and massage study figure, showing treatment points.

The Egyptians and Persians used massage for cosmetic as well as therapeutic effects. They mixed fats, oils, herbs and resins for care of the skin and beautifying the body and face. Pots and jars containing these creams have been found in Egyptian tombs. Cleopatra is said to have bathed in milk and then to have been massaged with aromatic oils and creams by her handmaidens.

The practice of massage spread from the east into Europe, where it was well established by 500 BC.

Massage in classical Greece and Rome

The Greeks believed in the cultivation of a healthy mind and body, which is similar to the 'holistic approach' practised by many people today. Rituals of bathing, massage, exercise or dancing were practised by men and women. They encouraged the pursuit of physical fitness and organised regular sporting, gymnastic and athletic competitions. Massage was used before events to improve performance and after events to relieve fatigue and aid recovery. Gladiators and soldiers were massaged before battle to give vigour and promote fitness and health, and afterwards to aid recovery, healing and relaxation. Homer writes in the poem *The Odyssey* of Greek soldiers being rubbed with oils and anointed by beautiful women to aid their recovery and regain strength on return from battle.

Around 500 BC the Greek physician **Herodicus** used massage with oils and herbs to treat medical conditions and diseases. **Hippocrates**, who is now thought of as the father of medicine, was a pupil of Herodicus. He began to study the effects of massage on his patients. He concluded and recorded that 'hard rubbing binds, soft rubbing loosens, much rubbing causes parts to waste but moderate rubbing makes them grow'. Hippocrates also concluded that it was more beneficial to apply pressure in an upward direction, i.e. towards the heart, as we practise today. In Hippocrates' day, the function of the heart and the circulation of the blood were not known. It is therefore remarkable that he reached this conclusion only by observing the effect on the tissues of different strokes. With our knowledge of the heart and circulating blood we understand why pressure upwards is more beneficial: the condition of the tissues improves because deoxygenated blood and waste products are removed quickly as massage speeds up blood and lymph flow. Even without the benefit of this knowledge, Hippocrates taught his pupils that massage movements should be performed with pressure upwards to promote healing.

The Romans followed similar routines to the Greeks. They practised bathing, exercise and massage for health and social relaxation. Large private and public baths were built. These included water baths and steam rooms, gymnasium and massage areas. The baths were maintained at different temperatures and progress was made

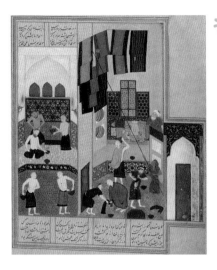

This ancient Persian document shows bathing and massage in a Turkish bath.

from cold to hot baths. Wealthy Romans would use these daily for cleansing, exercising, relaxing and socialising. Servants were always in attendance, with oils and creams to massage their masters when required. The Romans built similar baths in the countries that were conquered by their armies. Many such baths were built after the Roman conquest of Britain in 55 BC, and their ruins can be seen in Britain today in towns and cities such as Bath, Caerleon and St Albans.

Galen (130–201 CE), a Roman of Greek birth, further developed some of Hippocrates' ideas on massage, including the variety of possible strokes and directions. He wrote '... the rubbings should be of many sorts, with strokes and circuits of the hands, carrying them not only from above down and from below up, but also subvertically, obliquely, transversely and subtransversely ... But I direct that the strokes and circuits of the hands should be made of many sorts, in order that so far as possible all the muscle fibres should be rubbed in every direction.' Galen also wrote about the effect of massage on the digestive system and as an aid to ridding the body of waste products.

A little later, another Roman, **Aulus Cornelius Celsus** (25 BC–57 CE) wrote about the use of 'frictions' to aid recovery from disease and to promote healing. He too, saw the value of such massage as lying in its ability to rid the body of 'noxious' substances.

Massage techniques recorded from these times include manipulations known as squeezing, pinching or pummelling. They relate to the petrissage and percussion movements used today.

The Dark Ages to the Renaissance

Little is known about massage or health and beauty practices throughout the Dark and Middle Ages, i.e. from the decline of the Roman Empire around 500 CE until the Middle Ages around 1400 CE. Few records remain from those days of wars, strict religions, superstition and persecution. Little value was placed on education, the arts, physical health and fitness.

Following this period came the Renaissance (rebirth) in 1450 CE. Interest in the arts and sciences flourished and there was renewed interest in health practices. Once again we see massage advocated and practised for therapeutic purposes.

In the sixteenth century, the French surgeon **Ambroise Paré** (1517–90) promoted and developed the use of massage. He was the personal physician to four French kings. He is reputed to have successfully treated Mary Queen of Scots with massage. Paré graded massage into gentle, medium and vigorous. We use similar categories today, namely soothing or relaxing, general, and stimulating. Many other physicians copied his methods and massage was established medically.

The development of modern massage techniques

Modern massage techniques have evolved mainly from a system developed by a Swedish physiologist called **Per Henrik Ling** (1776–1839). He developed a system of passive and active exercises known as 'Swedish Remedial Gymnastics' and also a system of massage movements. Ling used the terms 'effleurage', 'petrissage', 'vibration', 'friction', 'rolling' and 'slapping'. Most of these terms are still used today, but some changes and modifications have been made in the groupings and names of manipulations.

In England, the eminent surgeon **John Grosvenor** (1742–1823) used massage to treat joints. He recommended massage for the treatment of rheumatism, gout and stiffness of joints.

Dr Johann Mezgner (1839–1909), a Dutch physician, developed massage for use in rehabilitation and used it successfully to treat many diseases and disorders. He adapted massage techniques in the light of his knowledge of anatomy and physiology. His theories, based on sound scientific principles, became accepted as medical practice and gained him many followers, particularly in Germany and America.

In America, **John Harvey Kellogg** (1852–1943) a medical doctor, who ran a sanitarium using a holistic approach, wrote a book called *The Art of Massage,* which discussed the physiological effects of massage, the underlying structures, joint movements and procedures for massage. Kellogg had several unusual views on healthy living and is perhaps most well known for inventing cornflakes!

In Germany, **Professor Albert Hoffa** (1859–1907) published a book on massage, *Technik der Massage,* which is still considered by many to be one of the most fundamental of texts on massage. Again, it describes how to execute the strokes and the most appropriate procedures, and includes many techniques that are still adhered to today.

The work of Ling and Mezgner established massage as an effective therapeutic treatment. Techniques were taught in medical schools and the beneficial effects became widely recognised and accepted in the medical field.

British surgeon, **Sir William Henry Bennett** (1852–1931) introduced London doctors to massage as a method of treatment and he established a department of massage at St George's Hospital.

Nurses were encouraged to train and use massage for the treatment of patients, under the guidance of doctors. In 1894 a group of women founded the Society of Trained Masseuses. Rules and regulations for training and examinations for qualifying were established. These women raised standards and fought to establish massage therapy as a reputable profession.

Twentieth-century developments

During the First World War the demand for massage to treat the injured grew and many more massage therapists were trained. Membership of the Society of Trained Masseuses grew and in 1920 it amalgamated with the Institute of Massage and Remedial Exercise. In recognition of the valuable work contributed by its members during the war, a Royal Charter was granted and the title was changed to the Chartered Society of Massage and Medical Gymnastics. The title was changed again in 1943 and became the Chartered Society of Physiotherapy. In 1964 its members became state registered. This protected and gave status to those qualified therapists who were practising in clinics and hospitals, and made it impossible for those without a recognised qualification to practise in hospitals.

With the development of alternative electrical-based treatments, the use of massage to treat medical conditions declined. There was rapid growth in electrotherapy and eventually massage ceased to be part of physiotherapy training. It became little used as a therapeutic treatment in hospitals. There was, however, a continuing demand for massage in clinics, health farms, fitness and leisure centres.

In 1966 the City and Guilds of London Institute explored the possibility of establishing a course in beauty therapy to include massage. This course would provide thorough training, background knowledge and a recognised professional qualification that ensured a high standard of practice. In 1968 the first full-time course was offered in colleges of further education. The British Association of Beauty Therapists and Cosmetologists, the International Health and Beauty Council and other organisations also developed courses and offered certificates and diplomas.

The growth in complementary medicine and the holistic approach to health has increased the demands for well-qualified practitioners, not only in massage but also in aromatherapy, reflexology, shiatsu etc. Qualifications are now developed in line with National Occupational Standards (NOS) which are regulated by Habia and Skills for Health.

Learning point

Habia (Hairdressing and Beauty Industry Authority) is a government-approved organisation responsible for setting and maintaining standards in the hair and beauty industry in the UK. The GCMT (General Council for Massage Therapies) is the governing body for massage therapies in the UK, established with a view to setting and maintaining standards of professional conduct within the massage therapy industry. SfH (Skills for Health) is a body licensed by the UK Commission for Employment and Skills. It is responsible for setting and maintaining standards in all health-related industries in the UK. All three organisations work together to develop National Occupational Standards for these industries and to regulate and approve the relevant qualifications.

Health, safety and hygiene

After you have studied this chapter you will be able to:

1. explain the legal requirements under the Health and Safety at Work Act
2. distinguish between hazard and risk
3. explain the safety considerations related to electrical equipment
4. describe the correct techniques for lifting
5. explain your responsibilities according to Fire Regulations
6. carry out risk assessments for fire, hazardous substances and general risks in the workplace
7. differentiate between bacteria, viruses, fungi and parasites
8. distinguish between natural immunity and artificial immunity
9. explain the importance of maintaining high standards of personal hygiene and hygiene in the workplace and describe the factors to be considered.

Health and safety is about preventing any person sustaining injury, being harmed in any way or becoming ill at work. It involves following correct, safe procedures and taking every possible precaution to protect everyone in the workplace.

Health and safety laws and regulations apply to everyone, whether they are employers, managers, employees, self-employed, full- or part-time, paid or unpaid workers and visitors. Health and safety issues refer to hazards and risks in the workplace and how to eliminate them.

Hazard means anything that can cause harm.
Risk is the chance, great or small, that someone will be harmed by the hazard.

Health and Safety at Work Act 1974

This is the main legislation covering health and safety in the workplace. Other safety regulations and codes of practice come under this main Act.

The Act states that employers and employees have a legal duty to ensure, so far as is reasonably practicable, the health, safety and welfare of all persons at work, i.e. all employees and other persons on the premises, such as clients and visitors.

The Health and Safety Executive (HSE) provides information and publications on all aspects of health and safety regulations, implementing directives from the European Commission. (There is more on the HSE in the next section.) These cover a wide range of health, safety and welfare issues. The directives included here are those most relevant to you.

The Act of 1974 and the new regulations mean that employers must, by law, provide a safe working environment for all members of the workforce, including those with disabilities and other persons using their premises.

Maintaining health and safety in the workplace

Requirements for employers

As an *employer* you are required to:

- provide a safe working environment; you must recognise hazards or problems, and take the appropriate actions to minimise or eliminate them
- have a written health and safety policy that sets out how these issues are managed
- assess the risks that may arise from work activities
- record the findings of the risk assessment
- consult with employees regarding health and safety issues
- provide health and safety information, training and supervision for all employees
- keep a record of any problems that have been identified and rectified.

The Health and Safety Executive (HSE)

This is a body of people appointed to enforce health and safety law. Inspectors from the HSE or from your Local Authority have the statutory right to inspect your workplace at any time, with or without prior notice. During the visit the inspector will be looking at the premises, the working environment and the work practices. They will check that you are complying with health and safety law and will assess whether there are any hazards or risks to the health, safety or welfare of anyone on the premises.

The inspector can:

- inspect all aspects relating to health, safety and welfare
- take photographs
- ask questions or talk to anyone in the workplace
- investigate any complaint
- offer guidance and advice.

The inspector will ensure that you, as an employer have arrangements in place for consulting with, training and informing all staff on all matters relating to health, safety and welfare. All staff will be given the opportunity to speak to the inspector privately should they wish to do so. The inspector will provide you with information and highlight areas of concern. They will also explain why enforcement action is to be taken.

If a breach of the law is found, the inspector will decide what action to take. The action will depend on the severity of the problem.

Actions that may be taken by HSE inspectors

- Informal notice: If the problem is a minor one, the inspector may simply explain what must be done to comply with the law. If asked, they will confirm any advice in writing.

- Improvement notice: If the problem is more serious, the inspector may issue an improvement notice. This will state what needs to be done and the time limit by which it must be done. At least 21 days must be allowed for corrective action to be taken.

- Prohibition notice: If the problem poses a serious risk, the inspector may give notice to stop the activity immediately and not allow it to be resumed until corrective action is taken. The notice will explain why such action is necessary.

- Prosecution: A failure to act upon an improvement or prohibition notice may result in prosecution. The courts have the power to impose unlimited fines and, in some severe cases, imprisonment.

As an employer, you have the right of appeal to an industrial tribunal when an improvement or prohibition notice is served should you disagree with it, or feel that it is unjust. The instructions on how to appeal appear on the back of the notice.

Requirements for employees

As an *employee* you are required to:

- take reasonable care to avoid harm to yourself or to others by your behaviour or working practices

- cooperate with, and help your employer to meet the statutory requirements

- refrain from misusing or interfering with anything provided to protect the health, safety and welfare of all persons as required by the Act.

To comply with these requirements you must:

- not put yourself or others at risk by your actions

- abide by the rules and regulations of the workplace

- know who is responsible for what in the workplace and to whom you should report problems

- adopt good working practices and follow correct procedures

- be alert to any hazard that may pose a risk to yourself or to others and promptly take the appropriate action to minimise or eliminate the risk

- be competent in selecting appropriate treatments and in administering them correctly and safely to the clients

In the workplace
If you are unable or unsure how to deal quickly with a hazard, then you must report the situation to someone else immediately. Seek advice from a supervisor or someone qualified to deal with the situation.

- follow the correct technique for all treatments, understand the effects, and be alert to contra-indications and contra-actions
- adopt high professional standards of dress and appearance
- maintain the highest standards of personal and workplace hygiene
- report faulty equipment to the person responsible for dealing with these issues
- not ignore any hazard or risk; make sure that corrective action is taken
- report any problems that you have identified and rectified.

Health, safety and welfare

The Workplace (Health, Safety and Welfare) Regulations (1992) (as amended)

This regulation covers health, safety and welfare in the workplace. A 'workplace' means any place where people are employed or are self-employed. It includes outdoor areas, such as paths.

Health issues under these regulations

Adequate ventilation

Premises must be well ventilated: removing stale air and drawing in fresh clean air without draughts.

Comfortable working temperature

It is difficult to select the temperature to suit everybody: around 16°C is recommended. The temperature should be comfortable for working but the client will usually be inactive and may feel cold: make sure that they are also warm enough.

Adequate lighting

Lighting must be adequate to enable people to work and move around safely. It should be suitable for the treatment in progress. Low, soft lighting is desirable for the majority of massage routines.

Cleanliness and hygiene

Premises must be cleaned regularly to the highest standard. Floors, furniture and fittings should be washed and disinfected where possible. Walls and ceilings should be kept free from dust and cobwebs. All towels and linen used should be washed after each client.

Hygiene is discussed later in this chapter.

Waste

Waste must be stored in suitable, covered bins and disposed of in accordance with regulations.

In the workplace

At staff meetings, be prepared to discuss issues of health and safety with all other workers. Shared knowledge makes for a safer working environment.

In the workplace

Towels and linen should be washed at a temperature of at least 60°C, although there are now environmentally friendly products available that claim to reduce the need for high temperatures. They contain stain-removing enzymes. However, if a client has an infectious condition like head lice or scabies, boil washing will be necessary.

In the workplace

Under the Environmental Protection Act 1990 and the Controlled Waste Regulations 1992, materials contaminated by body fluids are categorised as Group A clinical waste. Such waste must be disposed of in yellow refuse sacks, which must be sealed when they are three-quarters full. A registered waste carrier will then collect these sacks.

Adequate space for working

The working area, containing a couch, trolley, chair, stools and waste bin should be large enough for you and the client to move around in easily, without having to negotiate obstacles.

Safety issues under these regulations

Maintenance of equipment

Everything in the workplace, the equipment and systems, should be maintained in efficient working order. If a fault occurs in any machine or other equipment, it must be taken out of use immediately. It must be clearly labelled 'FAULTY – OUT OF USE' and stored away from the working area. The fault must be reported and the appropriate action taken to repair it.

Floors and traffic routes

Floors should be sound and even, with a non-slippery surface, and they must be kept free of obstacles. Any spillages, such as water, oil and powder should be wiped up immediately because they will make the floor slippery, which may result in someone slipping and falling. Doors should be wide enough for easy access and exit. Stairs should be sound and well lit. A handrail should be provided on at least one side of the stairs.

Falls and falling objects

Every effort must be made to prevent anyone falling on the premises. Stable, even, non-slip floors will help. Leads should not trail across the floor but should lie along the wall. Stools and bins should be stored under couches. Other equipment must not be left around but must be stored correctly.

Every effort must be made to prevent objects falling and injuring people. Storage shelves must be checked regularly and examined for any damage that may weaken them. Objects should be stored and stacked safely in such a way that they are not likely to fall. Shelves should not be overloaded and should have maximum load notices.

Windows

These should be clean, and open easily. Ensure that they can be seen clearly, so that people will not walk into them.

Sanitary conveniences

Toilets and washing facilities should be available to all persons. These rooms should be cleaned and disinfected regularly, well lit and ventilated. There should be hot and cold running water; soap, preferably in a dispenser; and drying facilities such as paper towels, or dry air machines to prevent the spread of micro-organisms.

Best practice
In order to maintain the highest standards of hygiene and to avoid contamination from micro-organisms, you should avoid travelling to and from work in your uniform.

Welfare issues under these regulations

Drinking water

An adequate supply of fresh drinking water must be provided, either direct mains water, a chilled water dispenser or bottled water.

Changing rooms

These rooms must be clean, suitable and secure, where outer garments can be removed and uniforms put on. Changing rooms are also desirable for clients although the treatment area may also be used if privacy for the user can be ensured.

Facilities for resting and eating

Food and drink should not be consumed in the treatment areas. A suitable room should be allocated for eating, and furnished appropriately.

Safety considerations when dealing with hazardous substances

The Control of Substances Hazardous to Health (COSHH) Regulations (2002) (as amended)

This law requires you, as an employer, to control exposure to hazardous substances to prevent ill health. It protects everyone in the workplace from exposure to hazardous substances.

Hazardous substances found in the workplace include:

- cleaning agents
- disinfectants
- massage products – oils, creams, lotions, gels and talcum powder.

Hazardous substances can enter the body via many routes, for example:

- broken or damaged skin
- eyes and ears
- nose and mouth
- hair follicles.

Substances hazardous to health may cause the following:

- skin burn
- skin allergic reaction, such as dermatitis
- skin irritation
- irritation of nasal passages and lungs or allergies to products, especially fine powder or dust, resulting in the development of asthma
- breathing difficulties

- nausea and vomiting if swallowed
- eye damage.

COSHH requires you to:

- *assess* the risk from exposure to hazardous substances to anyone using your workplace. You will need to examine all the substances stored and used in your place of work and identify the ones that could cause damage or injury. You will need to consider any risks that these substances present to people's health.

- *decide* what precautions need to be taken. Check the manufacturer's advice on use, storage and disposal. Read the information carefully. Consider whether the substance can enter the body or damage any part of the body.

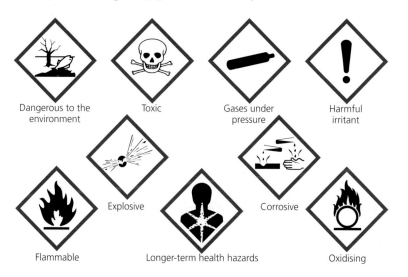

Dangerous to the environment   Toxic   Gases under pressure   Harmful irritant

Explosive   Corrosive

Flammable   Longer-term health hazards   Oxidising

Figure 1.1 The eight hazard symbols

- *control* or reduce the exposure to hazardous substances. Consider the use of other, safer, products. Store all products safely and label them clearly to reduce any errors in handling. Wear gloves when handling cleaning agents. Take care when handling and using fine powders such as talc; avoid releasing the fine particles into the air and avoid inhaling any powders; also protect your client.

- *ensure* that control measures are in place and regularly monitored for effectiveness. Keep records of all control measures and any tests or problems arising.

- *prepare* procedures to deal with accidents, incidents and emergencies. Immediate steps must be taken to minimise the harmful effects and damage. These procedures should be clearly written and placed in a prominent and accessible place.

- *train* and supervise all staff. Ensure that all employees understand the risks from all the hazardous substances they have to deal with. Inform them of the rules and regulations for using, storing and transporting or disposing of hazardous substances.

- *ensure* that all employees understand the importance of reporting any problems or shortcomings when dealing with hazardous substances.

In the workplace

After completing a risk assessment you are required to label containers of hazardous substances with warning symbols. This is particularly applicable if you decant substances from their original container.

Learning point

All manufacturers/suppliers are legally required to provide guidelines in the form of material safety data sheets (MSDSs) with details of use and storage and disposal.

Best practice

Health and safety of staff and clients should underlie everything in the workplace. A regular meeting should always include an agenda item allowing all staff to report and discuss health and safety issues, and matters arising should be dealt with swiftly.

In the workplace

Compile a file containing all MSDSs and COSHH assessments and store where everyone can access the information.

Organisation:

Recorded by:
Date:

What is the hazard?	Indicate the people at risk	Describe the possible risk	Assessment of the level of risk: High Med Low	What controls do you have in place?	What further actions need to be taken?	By whom	By when (agree specific date)	Review date (agree specific date)	Comments
Disinfectant	Therapist and other staff	Skin irritation	Medium	Use of gloves	Training in correct usage and procedure in case of accidental spillage				
	Therapist and other staff	Eye irritation	Low	First-aid box equipped with eye bath	Training in emergency procedure				
	Therapist and client	Loss of effectiveness if stored for a long time/incorrectly, leading to contamination and cross infection.	Medium	MSDS forms Appropriate labelling and dating of decanted solution including hazard symbols	Training in handling of hazardous substances including appropriate dilutions				

Table 1.1 Sample COSHH risk assessment

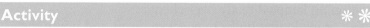
Activity

Consider any hazardous substances in the workplace. These will include any fine powders such as talcum powder, oils, creams or lotions, cleaning agents etc. Fill in a COSHH risk assessment, including all possible risks from each substance.

Safety considerations when using electrical equipment

Provision and Use of Work Equipment Regulations (PUWER) (1998) (as amended)

Together with the Electricity at Work Regulations 1989, the PUWER regulations require that all equipment provided for use at work is:

- suitable and safe for the intended use
- inspected regularly by a competent person and maintained in a safe condition
- used only by those who are fully informed, trained and competent in their use.

You may use several different types of electrical equipment in the workplace. It is therefore very important that you understand, and are able to assess, the hazards and risks associated with their use and know what action to take to eliminate or minimise them.

The main hazards and risks are:

H. exposed parts of the leads, wiring or cables
R. contact with these will result in shock or/and burns, which may prove fatal
H. faulty equipment
R. contact will cause electric shock
H. faults in the wiring or overloading the circuit
R. may cause fires resulting in injury, or even death if the fire is severe
H. water in the area where electrical equipment is used or working with wet hands
R. will result in electric shock
H. trailing leads and cables across the floor
R. will trip people up and may result in injury
H. loose-fitting bulbs
R. may fall on clients, causing burns, or fall on linen and towels, causing fires
H. loose angle-poise joints on lamps
R. lamp may fall onto client, causing burns, or fall on linen and towels, causing a fire

Learning point

Many organisations, including the HSE, use a formula to calculate the level of risk. This involves comparing the likelihood of the risk occurring with the impact of the risk. You can find useful tools on the internet or by contacting the HSE.

Learning point

Portable appliance testing (PAT testing) should be carried out by suitably competent individuals who are able to use and interpret the findings of the specialised testing equipment. Faulty equipment is best dealt with through the manufacturers.

In the workplace

How regularly PAT testing is done is dependent on a variety of factors, such as how frequently equipment is used, the type of equipment and the construction of the equipment. Refer to the manufacturers' guidelines.

Be aware

The checking of equipment should never be overlooked. It is a requirement of Public Liability Insurance that equipment used is fit for purpose. Failure to notice faulty equipment could result in a claim against you for negligence.

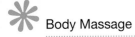
H. positioning lamps directly over clients

R. falling or exploding bulbs may cause burns and injure the client

Precautions and responsibilities when using electrical equipment

- Arrange regular testing of electrical equipment – this is required by law.
- Ensure that people using electrical equipment are trained and competent to do so.
- Follow the correct procedures when using electrical equipment.
- Purchase equipment from a reputable dealer who will provide an after-sales service.
- Ensure that all equipment is regularly maintained and in a safe condition for use.
- Examine leads and cables regularly to ensure that they are without splits or breaks that may expose bare wires.
- Use proper connectors to join wire and flexes; do not use insulating tape.
- Examine all connections making sure that they are secure.
- Ensure that the cable is firmly clamped into the plug to make certain that the wires, particularly the earth wire, cannot be pulled out of the terminal.
- Do not overload the circuit by using multiple adaptors. Report any overloading of the circuit, to appropriate person.
- Plug the machine into a near and accessible identified socket so that it can be switched off or disconnected easily in an emergency.
- Keep electrical equipment away from water. Do not touch any electrical part with wet hands.
- Ensure that flexes and cables do not trail over the working area but are fixed along the wall.
- Examine all equipment regularly, especially portable machines, as they are subjected to wear and tear.
- Remove faulty equipment from the working area and label clearly FAULTY: DO NOT USE and inform appropriate person.
- Keep a dated record of when checks were carried out, including all findings and maintenance.

Reporting

Reporting of Injuries, Diseases and Dangerous Occurrences Regulations (RIDDOR) (1995)

RIDDOR places a legal duty on employers, the self-employed and those in control of premises to report work-related incidents.

These incidents must be reported to the Health and Safety Executive (HSE) or your Local Authority (LA).

If you inform the Incident Contact Centre (ICC), they will report and forward the information to the correct enforcing authority on your behalf.

See website for more information: www.riddor.gov.uk

By law, the following incidents must be reported:

- deaths
- major injuries or poisonings
- any accident where the person injured is away from work for more than three days
- injuries where members of the public are taken to hospital
- diseases contracted at work
- dangerous occurrences that did not result in reportable injury but might have done.

First aid at work

The Health and Safety (First Aid) Regulations (1981) (as amended)

These regulations require you, as an employer, to provide adequate and appropriate equipment, facilities and personnel to enable first aid to be given to employees and others if they are injured or become ill at work.

First aid is the immediate treatment administered when any person suffers an injury or becomes ill at work. The minimum first-aid provision at any workplace includes:

- a suitably stocked first-aid box placed in a precise, easily accessible and clearly labelled site
- an appointed person to take charge of first aid arrangements.

Be aware

An *appointed person* is not the same as a *designated first-aider*. There is no requirement for the appointed person to be trained in first aid, whereas the designated first-aider must have an up-to-date first-aid qualification recognised by the HSE. An appointed person must not, therefore administer first aid.

In the workplace

First-aid provision must be available at all times to people at work. It may therefore be necessary to appoint more than one person to be in charge, depending on the size and structure of your workplace.

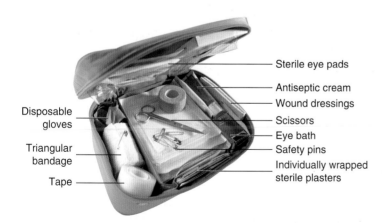

Disposable gloves

Triangular bandage

Tape

Sterile eye pads

Antiseptic cream

Wound dressings

Scissors

Eye bath

Safety pins

Individually wrapped sterile plasters

Figure 1.2 First-aid box

Learning point
The HSE states that the contents of a first-aid box will depend on what you assess your needs to be.

Best practice
Check the contents of the first-aid box regularly. Write a list of the items in the box when it is new and use as your checklist.

The duties of the designated first-aider include:
- taking charge and administering appropriate treatment, if able, when someone is injured or falls ill
- calling an ambulance if required, depending on the seriousness of the injury
- taking responsibility for the contents of the first-aid box and restocking as required.

The duties of the appointed person are limited to:
- calling an ambulance if required, depending on the seriousness of the injury
- taking responsibility for the contents of the first-aid box and restocking as required.

All employees must be informed of the arrangements for first aid. Notices situated in clearly visible places must inform them of who the appointed person and/or the designated first-aider is, where they can be found, and where the first-aid box is located.

Manual handling

The Manual Handling Operations Regulations (1992) (as amended)

This regulation requires you, as an employer, to assess the risk to employees when lifting or handling heavy goods and to provide training in safe techniques.

Many of the injuries reported each year to the HSE and LAs are the result of manual handling, i.e. lifting, transporting or supporting loads by hand or bodily force. The accidents primarily cause back injuries but hands, arms and feet may also be injured. These injuries may build up over time as a result of repetitive movements, or may be caused by a single instance of poor-lifting technique or an attempt to manage too heavy a load. You may be required to receive, check and handle deliveries and transport them to the stock room, or to move couches in the workplace. It is therefore essential that you are able to assess the risk and protect yourself from injury.

Before lifting or moving anything, assess the risk as follows:
- How heavy is the load?
- Can you reduce the load?
- Do you have to lift it off the floor? This produces the greatest risk.
- Can you get assistance from another person?
- How far do you have to move it?
- Can you rest it halfway on a chair or table to ease the effort?

Lifting techniques

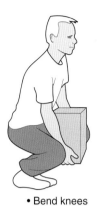 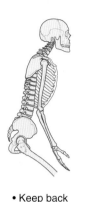

• Bend knees   • Keep back straight

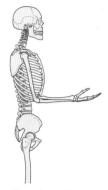 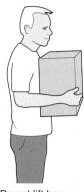

• Do not lift heavy weights – get someone to help you   • Place large heavy boxes on the floor – do not lift onto high shelves

Figure 1.3 Lifting technique

- Feet apart on either side of the load for a balanced stable base.
- Good posture; maintain natural curves.
- Tuck chin in, keep a straight back, lower and bend the knees.
- Take a firm grip.
- Keep the arms into the sides; hold the load close to the body. If you hold it away from the body, this increases the leverage and risk of injury.
- Lift smoothly; do not jerk or twist the body as you lift. Move the feet and place the load in position.
- Do not twist the trunk when placing the load down.

In the workplace

Back strains and injuries can also occur as a result of incorrect posture and stance when performing massage. Ensure that you adopt the correct stance. Keep the back straight and bend the knees. Do not twist the body as you work and avoid stretching over the client.

Fire precautions

Regulatory Reform (Fire Safety) Order 2005

This requires you, as an employer, to ensure that safety measures are in place to prevent and deal with the outbreak of fire in the workplace. You must assess the fire risks, keep a written record of these risks and inform all employees of the findings. The following precautions and measures must be in place:

Be aware

This order replaces The Fire Precautions (Workplace) Regulations 1997.

- A detailed fire risk assessment (see page 14).
- Smoke alarms or other fire detection equipment must be fitted, checked regularly and maintained in good working order.
- Fire-fighting equipment must be in good working order and suitable for the type of fire.
- Fire-fighting equipment must be clearly visible and easily accessible.
- Fire doors should be fitted if the risk of fire is assessed as high.
- A means of escape must be provided and marked Fire Exit.

- Doors should be left unlocked and kept free of obstruction for quick escape.
- All employees must be kept informed and trained in fire procedures.
- Notices for fire procedures and evacuation should be clear and prominently displayed.

Fire risk assessment

- Identify possible dangers and risks: possible sources of ignition; sources of fuel; sources of oxygen.
- Identify who is at risk: know how many people are on the premises at all times; be aware of people who may be particularly at risk, e.g. those who have poor mobility or impaired vision.
- Minimise risk from fire as far as possible: remove fire hazards; establish fire precautions.
- Plan: establish evacuation procedures and prepare an emergency plan.
- Train: ensure all staff know procedures and discuss them at staff meetings.
- Record: Using a risk-assessment form (see Table 1.2, page 16), keep a note of the findings, procedures and actions taken. Keep in an easily accessible place.
- Review: have regular updates and checks.

All members of staff should ensure that they receive training in fire drill and fire evacuation procedures.

Fire evacuation procedures must be practised regularly.

All staff should know:

- how to recognise the fire or smoke alarm
- who to report to and how to raise the alarm
- how to contact the emergency services or inform the person who is responsible for doing this
- the exact position of the fire-fighting equipment and how to use it should the fire be small and easy to control
- the colour coding on the fire extinguishers and what type of fire they are suitable for (read the instructions on each one and, if you are unsure of any detail, ask the supervisor or the person responsible)
- where the exit doors and exit routes are and in what order the workplace is to be evacuated (depending on location of fire)
- what and how checks are to be made on the numbers of staff and clients or others to ensure that everyone is safe
- how to contain the fire and limit the damage by closing any doors other than exit doors, closing windows, switching off electrical equipment and using a fire blanket to smother the

fire. *Note: These actions must only be taken if it is safe to do so and would not put yourself or anyone else at risk.*

KNOW YOUR FIRE EXTINGUISHER COLOUR CODE

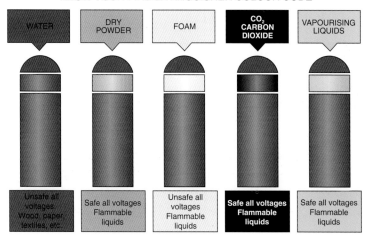

Figure 1.4 Types of fire extinguisher

Fire is a hazard in any place of work and it is very important that you familiarise yourself with the fire procedures and evacuation drill in the workplace. If a fire occurs you will need to act very quickly; it is therefore very important to know exactly what to do to ensure your own safety and the safety of others. Knowing exactly what procedure to follow beforehand will enable you to act promptly.

In the workplace
Obtain a copy of the Regulatory Reform (Fire Safety) Order (2005), which details the responsibilities of employers and staff.

Activity ✳ ✳ ✳
Identify anything that may be a fire hazard in your workplace and take every precaution to avoid risk to yourself and others. It is also useful to do this in the home.

Activity ✳ ✳ ✳
Draw a plan of the position of all the fire-fighting equipment in your workplace. Label each piece, state its colour coding and the type of fire it is suitable for.

Risk assessment

You may be required to carry out a risk assessment in your workplace to ensure that everything possible is in place to prevent anyone being harmed or contracting illness.

Consider the following:

- safe maintenance, care and use of equipment
- the safe use, handling and storage of hazardous substances
- safe and hygienic working practices
- personal hygiene and hygiene in the workplace

Best practice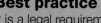
It is a legal requirement to keep a written record of the risk assessment if there are five or more employees but it is good practice to do so even if there are fewer employees.

What is the hazard?	Indicate the people at risk	Describe the possible risk	Assessment of the level of risk: High Med Low	What controls do you have in place?	What further actions need to be taken?	By whom	By when (agree specific date)	Review date (agree specific date)	Comments
Organisation:					**Recorded by: Date:**				
Positioning infra-red lamp directly over client	Client and therapist	Lamp falling on client and causing burns	Medium	Manufacturer's instructions available in central file. Training in appropriate use of equipment. Checking equipment for loose angle poise joints and dents to reflectors.	Regular staff meeting agenda item regarding all aspects of health and safety and electrical equipment.				
		Bulb exploding and causing burns or other injury	Low	Clear procedures for reporting faulty equipment.	Regular staff training and updates on use of equipment.				

Table 1.2 Sample risk assessment form

- adequate procedures for dealing with emergencies such as fire, electric shock
- appropriate temperature, ventilation, noise levels, etc.

Procedure

- Identify possible hazards that pose a risk of harm to anyone on the premises.
- Identify who is at risk: clients, staff, visitors, etc.
- Identify what the risk is; i.e. what might happen as a result of the hazard.
- Assess the level of risk; low, medium or high.
- Check the controls and procedures already in place.
- Plan for any changes or updates to those controls and procedures.
- Identify a person responsible for further actions.
- Train: ensure all staff know procedures and discuss them at staff meetings.
- Record using risk assessment forms and keep in an easily accessible place.
- Review: have regular updates and checks.

Local authority requirements

The Local Government (Miscellaneous Provisions) Act (1982)

Local Authorities issue licences and register businesses offering massage treatments. They also issue regulations with which, by law, you must comply. Before setting up a business you must contact your Local Authority to ensure that you comply with the exact requirements. When you meet all the requirements you will be issued with a **Certificate of Registration**. These bye-laws are mainly concerned with issues of hygiene and safety as explained in this text. Environmental Health officers have the right under this law to inspect your business and can issue fines or withdraw your registration if you are not complying with the regulations.

Hygiene

Hygiene deals with the precautions and procedures necessary for maintaining health and preventing the spread of disease. In the workplace, the highest priority must be given to preventing infection, cross-infection and infestation. You carry a heavy responsibility for protecting yourself, other staff and the clients from the risk of contamination by micro-organisms that cause disease.

Be aware
Local Authorities will vary in their requirements. Check with your own LA for details of legislation.

Learning point
An **infection** or infectious disease is caused by micro-organisms invading the body. The symptoms and severity of the illness will depend on the type of invading micro-organism and the part of the body that is affected.
An **infestation** is the invasion of the body by animal parasites such as lice, fleas etc; they may live in or on the body. Some parasites merely cause itchy irritation, while others cause serious illness.

Micro-organisms or microbes

There are many different types of micro-organism present in the environment. The main groups which may be present in your workplace include:

- bacteria
- viruses
- fungi, yeasts.

Bacteria

Bacteria are single-cell organisms varying in size from 0.2μm to 2.0μm in diameter. They are found everywhere in the environment but can only be seen through an optical microscope. Many bacteria are harmless and may be useful to humans. These are called **non-pathogenic bacteria**. Some are used in the production of food such as cheese and yoghurt. Others help to dispose of unwanted organic material, such as the breakdown of sewage, rendering it harmless. Some bacteria in the human intestine help to synthesise vitamins K and B_2. Bacteria are the simplest of living organisms, composed of a single cell with cytoplasm, surrounded by a protective cell membrane but devoid of organelles.

Some bacteria have whip-like projections on the surface of the cell, called flagella: these enable the bacteria to move around. Bacteria may be aerobic (requiring oxygen to sustain life,) or they may be anaerobic (able to survive without oxygen).

The aerobic variety is found invading surface tissues of the skin and mucous membranes of the respiratory tract. The anaerobic variety is found in the bowel or deep wounds. Some bacteria develop into spores; these can lie dormant for long periods of time and become active when conditions are suitable. Spores develop a hard, thick outer shell that protects the contents and makes them very difficult to destroy. They are more resistant to heat and disinfectants: higher temperatures and strong chemical disinfectants are required to kill spores.

Bacteria cause disease by producing toxins or poisons that are harmful to body cells. They grow and multiply if the conditions are right.

Types of bacterium

Bacteria are classified according to their shape:

- **Cocci:** these spherical-shaped bacteria may form clusters known as staphylococci, or chains known as streptococci, or pairs known as diplococci. They can cause a wide variety of conditions, such as boils, carbuncles, impetigo, sore throat, meningitis, pneumonia.
- **Bacilli:** these rod-shaped bacteria cause serious illness, such as diphtheria, tuberculosis, and typhoid fever.

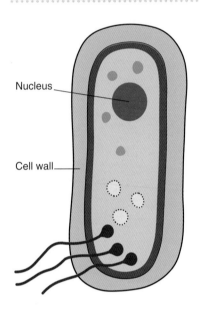

Nucleus

Cell wall

Figure 1.5 A bacterium

- **Spirochetes:** these spiral- or curved-shaped bacteria include spirillium and vibros and cause venereal disease, such as syphilis, and serious disease such as cholera.

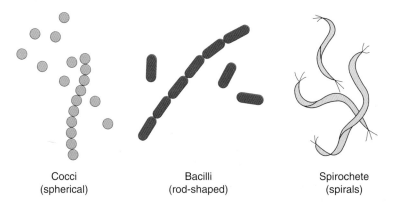

Cocci
(spherical)

Bacilli
(rod-shaped)

Spirochete
(spirals)

Figure 1.6 Three types of bacterium: cocci, bacilli and spirochete

The body protects itself against bacterial infection by producing:

- antitoxins, which neutralise the toxins produced by the bacteria
- large numbers of white cells, macrophages and granulocytes, which circulate in the blood and which engulf and destroy bacteria
- antibodies, which attack and destroy the bacteria.

The discovery of penicillin and development of other antibiotics and antibacterials mean that bacterial infections can usually be brought under control. Antibiotics must be used in adequate doses for at least five days (depending on the condition and the medication used). Some antibiotics kill the bacteria directly, while others prevent multiplication of the bacteria.

Viruses

Viruses are the smallest known infective particles: smaller than bacteria, they can only be seen through an electron microscope. They are between 0.1μm and 0.2μm in size, and vary in shape from spheres, cubes or rods.

They consist of a core of nucleic acid, ribonucleic acid (RNA) or deoxyribonucleic acid (DNA), enclosed in a protein shell or capsid. Viruses cannot metabolise, nor can they reproduce: they are parasitic, living inside a host cell. Once inside a host cell, a virus causes the host cell to make copies of the virus. Eventually, the host cell is destroyed and hundreds of new viruses are released that attack other cells. After the virus enters the host cell there is a period of incubation when the host cells show no sign of disease. Many cycles of viral spread occur and more and more host cells are affected. Eventually, typical signs and symptoms of the disease occur. By the time the symptoms appear, the viruses are so numerous that antiviral drugs have limited effect. The body protects itself against viral infection by producing specific antibodies. These will also provide future immunity to some

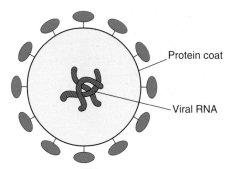

Protein coat

Viral RNA

Figure 1.7 A virus

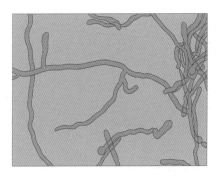

Figure 1.8 Fungi

diseases. Immunity can be produced artificially to combat some viral infections.

Body cells also produce interferons, which interfere with the multiplication of viruses. Antiviral drugs are now available, some of which prevent the multiplication of viruses, while others alter the DNA within the cell, preventing the virus from using it. In this way the spread of infection is halted.

The Hepatitis B virus and the Human Immunodeficiency Virus (HIV), which causes AIDS, are the two most serious viral infections that could be transmitted between clients and staff in the workplace. Both are carried in the blood: even minute amounts of blood or organic material, which may not be visible to the naked eye, can carry the viruses. The particular danger to you and your clients is contact with blood or tissue fluid through cuts or abrasions in the skin or anything that pierces the skin. The correct hygiene procedures must be adhered to prevent any possibility of infection (see page 25).

Fungi

Fungi are larger than bacteria: they may be **unicellular**, as in yeasts, or **multicellular**, as in moulds. The cells contain nuclei and other cell components but do not contain chlorophyll. They obtain their food by secreting enzymes through the cell walls: this digests any organic matter, which is then absorbed as liquid food. Fungi may be **saprophyte**s, which obtain food from dead organic matter, or they may be **parasites**, which live off plants, animals or humans, feeding off skin and mucous membranes and producing diseases. They reproduce by forming spores. The unicellular fungi and spores are not visible to the naked eye but the filamentous fungi-forming mycelia are visible (e.g. moulds and mildews).

Diseases caused by fungi

- **Ringworm**: this may affect different parts of the body and is named according to the part affected:
  - **Ringworm** of the foot is **tinea pedis** (athlete's foot).
  - **Ringworm** of the body is **tinea corporis**.
  - **Ringworm** of the head is **tinea capitis**.
  - **Ringworm** of the nail is **tinea unguium**.
- **Thrush**, which is caused by the fungus **Candida albicans**.
- More serious internal fungal infections of the lungs and heart, which can be fatal.

How the body deals with micro-organisms

Micro-organisms entering the body do not always produce disease, as the immune system is stimulated to protect the body. However, if the invading organisms are in large enough numbers to overcome the immune system then disease and illness will occur. Disease will also occur if the body has little immunity to the invading microbes or if the immune system has itself been damaged by disease, as in AIDS. If the body's defences are overcome then the microbes will cause damage to or destruction of the cells. Some microbes release toxins that destroy the cells, while others multiply and directly destroy them. The various micro-organisms produce a wide variety of diseases, each one showing particular symptoms.

When the immune system fails to contain a disease, drugs are necessary to treat the infections:

- Antibacterial or antibiotic drugs are used to treat bacterial infections.
- Antiviral drugs to treat viral infections.
- Antifungal drugs to treat fungal and yeast infections. Some anti-fungal drugs are applied onto the areas, while others are taken by mouth. They destroy the fungal cell wall and the cell dies.

Immunity

This is the ability of the body to resist or overcome infection and invasion by micro-organisms. The lymphatic system protects and defends the body against disease.

Natural active immunity

This is obtained when a person comes into contact with a particular microbe and produces antibodies to repel and control it. The antibodies produced to fight that infection remain in the body to control any future infection. Many infectious diseases occur only once in a lifetime, as immunity is lifelong, while others may recur, as immunity may last for only a few years.

Natural passive immunity

This involves the transfer of antibodies from an immunised donor to a recipient. Immunity may be passed from mother to baby via placenta or mother's milk.

Artificial active immunity

Artificial immunity can be provided by the use of vaccines. These are prepared from altered or diluted forms of the organism. Once they are introduced into the body they stimulate the immune system in the same way as an infection but are not strong enough to cause the disease.

Artificial passive immunity

This is another type of immunisation that relies on transferring antibodies from someone who has recovered from that particular disease. The transfer is made via a serum containing the antibodies.

> **Learning point**
> An antibody is a protein that recognises and neutralises foreign substances called antigens.

Invasion of the body

Micro-organisms enter the body via many routes:

- through broken or damaged skin
- through orifices such as the nose, mouth, anus, vagina, urethra
- through eyes and ears
- into hair follicles
- into the bloodstream by way of bites from blood-sucking insects such as mosquitoes and lice.

Some micro-organisms produce immediate symptoms. Others can lie dormant for a long time and attack when the body's immune system is low.

Transmission

Micro-organisms can be transmitted in many ways:

- By droplet infection: an infected person coughing and sneezing or spitting will expel organisms into the air where they may be inhaled by others.
- By handling contaminated articles such as clothing, towels and equipment, when micro-organisms may be transmitted to the handler.
- Dirty surfaces or dusty atmospheres will contain micro-organisms, which may be inhaled or may enter via the eyes or ears.
- Organisms present in faeces and urine may be transferred to others if the hands are not thoroughly washed after use of the toilet.
- Food may become contaminated by handling with unwashed hands and flies carrying contamination from excreta and rubbish. Water may become contaminated and then organisms will be transmitted through eating and drinking these foods.
- Organisms may be spread through contact with animals.
- Through direct contact with others, hand contact or touching.
- Organisms may be spread through an intermediary host, such as fleas and blood-sucking insects.
- Contaminated blood, if transmitted to another person, can cause serious and sometimes fatal illness. Organisms can be transmitted through blood transfusion, infected needles or at any time when the blood of the carrier (infected person) enters the body of the recipient. Hepatitis B and the human immunodeficiency virus (HIV), which causes AIDS, are transmitted in this way. These are very serious, life-threatening illnesses and great care must be taken to avoid any blood contact at any time. Any blood spillages should be dealt with by wearing gloves and using an appropriate solution. (See page 4 for disposal of contaminated materials soiled with body fluid.)

Conditions required for the growth of micro-organisms

These include:

- a food supply
- a water supply or moisture
- warmth: pathogenic bacteria favour a body temperature of 37°C (low temperatures found in the refrigerator or freezer will prevent growth of bacteria but will not destroy them)
- dark conditions (strong ultraviolet light (UVL) will kill bacteria)
- oxygen – required by some bacteria for aerobic respiration but others are anaerobic and survive without oxygen
- slightly alkaline conditions (The acidity of the skin – acid mantle composed of sebum and sweat – helps to protect against growth of bacteria.)

Ways in which the body resists infection

These include the following:

- Unbroken skin forms a physical barrier.
- Mucous membranes, mucus, hairs and cilia help to trap and filter microbes.
- Saliva washes microbes from teeth and mouths.
- Tears wash microbes from the eyes.
- Urine washes microbes from the urethra.
- Faeces remove microbes from the bowel.
- The acidic pH of the skin limits growth of bacteria.
- Sebum produces an oily film that protects the skin.
- Gastric juices destroy bacteria in the stomach.
- Various antibodies are produced by the body in response to infection.
- Macrophages and granulocytes ingest and destroy micro-organisms by a process of phagocytosis.

Animal parasites

Parasites are living organisms that live in or on another living organism and derive their food supply from that host. The parasites you are most likely to encounter in the workplace are called **ectoparasites**. These live outside the host, e.g. lice, fleas.

The presence of any parasite on the body is known as an **infestation**.

Ectoparasites

Head lice (Pediculus capitis)

The head louse is an insect found on the human scalp. It obtains its nourishment by piercing the skin and sucking blood.

Be aware

Endoparasites live inside the host, e.g. tapeworms or threadworms, roundworms and flukes.

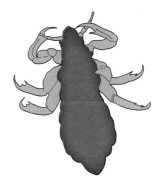

Figure 1.9 Head louse

The adult female is slightly larger than the male, about 2–3mm long and 1mm wide. The female lays white, shiny, oval-shaped eggs called nits, which are cemented to the hair close to the scalp. They take approximately one week to mature and can reproduce in another week. The life cycle of a louse lasts 4–5 weeks, during which time the female will lay around 300 eggs. They cause intense itching, and secondary infections may result due to scratching. Lice and nits may be killed by special shampoos or lotions containing insecticide and combing out with a fine tooth comb.

Body lice (Pediculus corporis)

These are similar to but larger than head lice. They obtain nutrients by sucking blood and laying eggs in underclothing. The crab louse is smaller and is found in pubic and underarm hair. Treatment is by insecticidal shampoo. Fabrics that have been in contact (clothing, towels, etc.) must be washed in insecticidal soap and boil-washed.

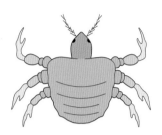

Figure 1.10 Body louse

Itch mites (Sarcoptes scabies)

This is a tiny animal that burrows into the skin, producing a condition called scabies. It has 8 legs and is around 0.3mm long and 0.2mm wide. The fertilised female burrows into the skin forming dark lines about 1cm long. She lays around 60 eggs in the burrows, which hatch in 4–8 days. The burrows are seen between the fingers, on the front of the wrists and forearms and may be on male genitalia. They cause intense irritation, vesicles, papules and pustules. They are easily passed from person to person. Medical opinion should be sought and any clothing, towels etc. that have come into contact with the infected client must be burned.

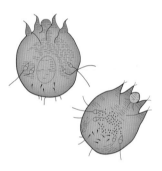

Figure 1.11 Itch mite

Fleas

The flea is an insect with three pairs of legs that enable it to jump long distances from host to host. It obtains nourishment by biting and sucking the blood of the host. The bites cause red spots that are usually found in groups. They are intensely itchy. Fleas lay eggs in dust, carpets or furniture. They can be eliminated by spraying with insecticides, washing clothing and bedding and thorough cleaning of soft furnishings. The flea is responsible for carrying plague infections.

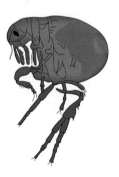

Figure 1.12 A flea

Methods of controlling micro-organisms

The process of controlling micro-organisms in the workplace is your responsibility and it must be taken seriously. Correct hygiene procedures must be adopted as a matter of routine. Any instruments and equipment used must always be cleaned after use, then sterilised or disinfected, according to requirements.

Several terms are used to refer to hygiene methods and procedures. Their meaning must be clearly understood so that the appropriate methods are selected. The terms and their definitions are as follows.

Antibiotic: an organic chemical substance that, in dilute solution, can destroy or inhibit growth of bacteria and some other micro-organisms. Antibiotics are used to treat infectious diseases in humans, animals and plants.

Antiseptic: a chemical agent that destroys or inhibits growth of micro-organisms on living tissues, thus limiting or preventing the harmful results of infection (usually used on wounds, sores or skin cleansing).

Aseptic methods: procedures adopted for creating conditions for avoiding infection.

Bactericide: a chemical agent that, under defined conditions, is capable of killing bacteria but not necessarily the spores.

Bacteriostat/fungistat: chemical agents that, under defined conditions, are capable of inhibiting the multiplication of bacteria/fungi.

Biocide, fungicide, virucide, sporicide: these terms imply the destruction of bacteria, fungi, viruses and spores. Biocides are effective on all harmful organisms.

Disinfectant: chemical agent that destroys micro-organisms but not spores (usually used on implements, surfaces, drains, etc).

Sanitation: the establishment of conditions favourable to health and preventing the spread of disease.

Sepsis/septic: infected by bacteria: usually associated with pus formation.

Sterilisation: the total destruction or removal of all living micro-organisms and their spores.

Procedures to prevent cross-infection in the workplace

While it is impossible to create a perfectly sterile environment in the workplace, every effort must be made to limit the growth and to destroy micro-organisms by practising high standards of hygiene. Procedures must be in place and adhered to, in order to protect yourself and others from cross-infection. This is a legal requirement.

- Hands *must* be washed frequently, before touching every client and after treatment, after handling equipment and after using the toilet. An antibacterial product should be used. Hands should be dried with a disposable towel or hot air dryer.

- Nails must be kept short and clean to prevent harbouring micro-organisms under the nails.

- Hands and nails must be examined for any cuts, abrasions or infections. If small, the damage may be covered with a waterproof plaster.
- Therapists or clients with any infection or infestation should not give or receive treatment until the conditions have been medically treated and cured.
- Feet should be cleaned before treatment with an appropriate solution or wipes.
- Clean towels and linen must be provided for every client, therefore a plentiful supply of good-quality towels should be available for covering the couch and for client use. Disposable paper sheets can also be used and should be disposed of after each client.
- Commodities should be chosen with care. Creams, lotions, oils etc. should preferably be contained in dispensers, or failing this, in tubes or narrow-necked bottles, which have a smaller surface to be contaminated than wide-necked jars.
- A new, clean spatula must be used to remove medium from containers to avoid contaminating the product. Lift the required amount of product in one scoop if possible and place it on a dish ready for use. Do not return unused product to the jar: dispose of it. Wash and disinfect the dish after use.
- If bleeding occurs for any reason, even the smallest amount must be dealt with immediately. Do not touch the blood: wear gloves. Clean the skin with a sterile dressing and cover with a waterproof dressing. If there is blood on any surface, such as the couch or floor, use a hypochlorite solution to disinfect, diluted according to the MSDS (the material safety data sheet).
- The workplace should always be clean, neat and tidy. All surfaces and equipment should be wiped down frequently during the day using a hypochlorite solution diluted according to the MSDS, and again at the end of the day.
- Bins with lids and plastic liners should be easily reachable. All waste should be immediately disposed of. Wet waste should first be wrapped in paper. The waste bins should be emptied and disinfected every night and clean liners inserted.
- Any equipment used must be free of debris before being cleaned according to manufacturer's instructions.
- Toilet and hand-washing facilities should be easily accessible. These should be well ventilated and disinfected at least once a day.
- A cloakroom should be available for leaving outdoor clothes and changing into uniform. This reduces the risk of carrying micro-organisms from the outside into the workplace.

Questions

1. Which of the following is the main legislation covering health and safety in the workplace?

   a. The Local Government (Miscellaneous Provisions) Act 1982.

   b. Health and Safety at Work Act 1974.

   c. Health and Safety Executive.

   d. The Workplace (Health, Safety and Welfare) Regulations 1992.

2. If materials are contaminated by body fluids how should you dispose of them?

   a. Place in a black refuse sack for the recycling advisors to collect.

   b. Place in a sturdy box and add to the general waste.

   c. Place in a yellow refuse sack for the registered waste carrier to collect.

   d. Place in a blue polythene bag and take it to the doctor's surgery or pharmacist.

3. A product that has a hazardous warning symbol with a black cross on it shows the substance is:

   a. an irritant

   b. toxic

   c. corrosive

   d. an oxidising agent.

4. The Health and Safety Executive is the:

   a. person responsible for carrying out a risk assessment

   b. person responsible for health and safety in the workplace

   c. local authority under the (Miscellaneous Provisions) Act 1982

   d. body of people appointed to enforce health and safety law.

5. What is risk assessment?

   a. A requirement for employers to assess only the most likely serious dangers to employees.

   b. Mathematical formulae used to assess danger in the workplace.

   c. A legal requirement for an employer to assess the dangers of harming employees and clients.

   d. A review to assess workplace policies and procedures.

6. An improvement notice can be:

   a. imposed on an employer by the Health and Safety Executive requiring the employer to improve a specified system of work

   b. given to an employee by a Health and Safety representative from a trade union

   c. given as a warning to an employee following a disciplinary hearing by their manager

   d. imposed on an employer who does not follow employment laws when recruiting staff.

7. Which of the following causes tinea pedis?

   a. Fungus.

   b. Bacterium.

   c. Parasite.

   d. Virus.

8. Which of the following is a virus transmitted through body tissue?

   a. Meningitis.

   b. HIV.

   c. Tinea corporis.

   d. Thrush.

9. Artificial active immunity means:

   a. transferring antibodies from a person who has had the disease

   b. producing own antibodies

   c. passing of antibodies from mother to baby via the placenta

   d. preparing vaccines from diluted forms of the organism.

10. When lifting a heavy box you should:

    a. keep the legs straight and bend your back

    b. bend the knees and keep your arms out to the side

    c. place feet on either side of the load and bend your knees

    d. hold the load away from your body and tuck your chin in.

2 Body systems and the physiological and psychological effects of massage

Learning point
Anatomy is the study of the structure of the body.
Physiology is the study of how the body functions.

Organisational levels

Massage is applied directly to the body and produces effects on the body tissues. An understanding of the structure of the body and how it functions is therefore essential to plan effective treatments and explain them to the client.

The following section will provide you with basic information relating to the structure and function of each of the body systems and will explain the effects of massage on each one. The body is made up of billions of cells containing chemical elements that carry out all the functions that are essential for maintaining life. These cells group together to form tissues, which further group together to form the body organs; many organs join together to form the systems of the body. We can study these organisational levels in greater detail.

The organisational levels are shown in Figure 2.1.

Chemicals

↓

Cells

↓

Tissues

↓

Body Organs

↓

Body Systems

Figure 2.1 Organisational levels

Chemicals

At the very basic level, these are the **chemical** substances within the cell. Reactions in which these chemicals combine or break down underlie all the processes essential for life.

Cells

These are the basic structural and functional units of the body. The cells carry out all the activities that maintain life. The body is made up of billions of cells. They all have a similar structure, but are modified to suit their function, e.g. blood cells differ from fat cells.

Tissues

Groups of similar cells form the **tissues** of the body. All the cells of one tissue will be identical, but will be different for different tissues, e.g. epithelial tissue covers the body and skeletal muscle tissue produces movement.

Body organs

Different tissues group together to form the **organs** of the body. Each organ will perform a specific function, e.g. the heart pumps blood around the body.

Body systems

Many different organs link together to form the **systems** of the body. They work together to carry out an essential function, e.g. the digestive system deals with food.

Cells

The structure of a typical cell is as follows.

The cell membrane or plasma membrane

This is the outer layer or boundary of the cell. It gives shape to the cell and protects it, separating things inside the cell (intracellular) from those outside the cell (extracellular). It regulates the passage of substances in and out of the cell.

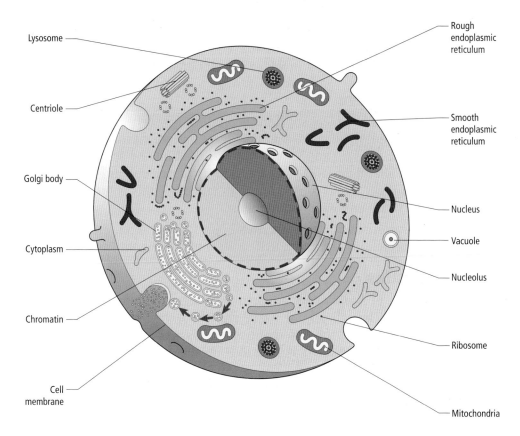

Figure 2.2 Structure of a cell

The cytoplasm

This is a soft jelly-like substance where the functions of the cell are carried out. It contains various structures called organelles (mini-organs), each of which has a specific function. Also in the cytoplasm are various chemical substances called inclusions.

The organelles

These mini-organs each have a characteristic shape and role to perform. The type and number of organelles in different kinds of cell vary depending upon the activities of the cell, e.g. muscle cells have large numbers of mitochondria, because they have a high-level energy output. The organelles are:

- the nucleus – the largest of the organelles. It controls the activities of the cell and contains the body's genetic material, deoxyribonucleic acid (DNA)
- the nucleolus, which is located within the nucleus and consists of ribonucleic acid (RNA), deoxyribonucleic acid (DNA) and protein. Its function is to manufacture protein
- mitochondria, which generate adenosine triphosphate (ATP/energy) – there are large numbers in muscle cells
- ribosomes, which synthesise protein
- lysosomes, which digest and deal with waste
- the Golgi apparatus or Golgi body, which is concerned with the production of membrane and protein lipids and lipoproteins
- endoplasmic reticulum – a series of channels for transporting substances within the cell
- the centrosome – involved in cell division.

The inclusions

These are chemical substances produced by cells. They may not be present in all cells, e.g. melanin is a pigment found in certain cells of the skin and hair: it protects the body by screening out ultraviolet light, and gives the skin its brown colour on exposure to sunlight. Lipid (fat) is found in fat cells – this is broken down to provide energy when required.

Characteristics of cells are metabolism, respiration, growth, reproduction, excretion, irritability and movement.

Tissues

Groups of similar cells are organised together to form the body tissues. The cells of one tissue will all be the same, but they will be different for the different tissues. Tissues are classified into four types: epithelial, connective, muscular and nervous.

Type of Tissue	Description	Where found: examples	Function: examples	Diagram
Simple squamous epithelium	Made up of a single layer of flat cells	This lines the heart, blood and lymphatic vessels and the air sacs of the lungs	It enables the exchange of gases, nutrients, and waste products	Figure 2.3
Simple cuboidal epithelium	Made up of a single layer of cube-shaped cells	This lines the kidney tubules; covers the ovaries	It allows the secretion of substances (e.g. tears and saliva) and the absorption of water in the kidneys	Figure 2.4
Simple columnar epithelium	Made up of a single layer of columnar-shaped cells	This lines the gastrointestinal tract from the stomach to the anus	Secretion and absorption as part of the digestive process	Figure 2.5

Table 2.1 Epithelial tissue: simple epithelium

Type of Tissue	Description	Where found: examples	Function: examples	Diagram
Simple ciliated columnar epithelium	Made up of a single layer of column-shaped cells with fine hair-like projections	This lines the upper respiratory tract and the Fallopian tubes	It enables the movement of mucus. It transports the zygote through the Fallopian tubes to the uterus	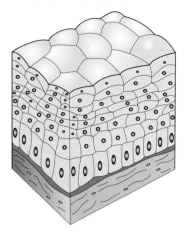 Figure 2.6

Table 2.1 *Continued*

Figure 2.7 Stratified squamous epithelium

Stratified epithelium is categorised according to the shape of the cells on the surface layers. They are:

- **stratified squamous epithelium**, which consists of layers of flat cells on the surface and cuboidal to columnar in the deeper layers. The keratinised cells protect the skin from injury and bacterial invasion. The non-keratinised cells line the mouth, tongue, oesophagus and vagina.
- **stratified cuboidal epithelium**, which is made up of layers of cuboidal cells that line the sweat glands and pharynx. Its function is to protect.
- **stratified columnar epithelium**, which consists of layers of columnar cells that line part of the male urethra and some excretory ducts. Its main function is to protect.
- **transitional epithelium**, which is a type of stratified epithelium that consists of rounded cells, which line the bladder, and parts of the ureters and urethra. Its function is to allow the tissues to expand.

Learning point

Stratified squamous epithelium cells can be further divided into **keratinised** and **non-keratinised** cells. Keratinised cells have dried out to form the protein keratin, e.g. the outer layer of the epidermis. Non-keratinised cells line moist surfaces, e.g. mouth, tongue, oesophagus and vagina.

Type	Function
Areolar	Connecting skin to tissues and muscles, lying around muscle bundles and binding muscles together
Adipose	Stores fat under skin and around organs
Dense fibrous	Gives tensile strength – ligaments and tendons
Yellow elastic	Gives elasticity to skin and walls of arteries

Table 2.2 Connective tissue

Type	Function	
Reticular	Found in lymphatic tissue	
Cartilage	**Fibro-cartilage** – intervertebral discs; act as shock absorbers	
	Elastic cartilage – outer ear; maintains shape	
	Hyaline cartilage – covers the ends of bones at joints	
Bone	**Compact** – outer layer of bones	
	Cancellous – inner mass of bones	
Blood	Fluid connective tissue contains erythrocytes, leucocytes and thrombocytes. Transports substances around the body and regulates body temperature	
Muscular tissue	**Skeletal** Produces body movement, maintains posture and produces heat	
	Cardiac Heart muscle maintains pumping action	
	Smooth Walls of blood vessels and intestines – peristalsis	
Nervous tissue	**Neurons** Pick up stimuli and conduct impulses to other neurons, muscle fibres or glands	
	Neuroglia Supporting substance that protects neurons	

Table 2.2 *Continued*

> **Learning point**
> Some columnar and ciliated columnar cells contain goblet cells that secrete mucus.

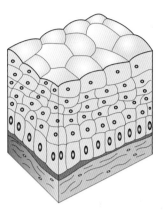

Figure 2.8 Transitional epithelium

Membranes

There are four membranes that cover or line body parts:

1. **cutaneous**: skin
2. **mucous**: lines body tracts that open to exterior – respiratory and gastro-intestinal
3. **serous**: lines body cavities, thorax and surrounds lungs
4. **synovial**: lines joints up to the cartilage.

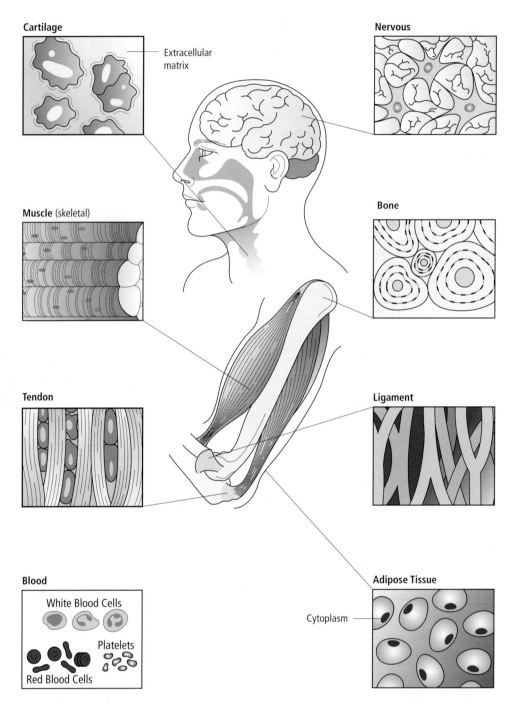

Figure 2.9 Types of connective tissue

Body organs

Many tissues will be organised to form the organs of the body. Each organ has a specific function or functions to perform, e.g. the stomach digests food, lungs exchange gases, the heart pumps blood, kidneys form urine and filter fluids, and ovaries produce and release ova. Organs form parts of the systems of the body.

Body systems

Each body system consists of many organs that link together to perform a common function. All the systems are interrelated and function together to maintain life. There are 11 body systems.

System	Structure	Function
Integumentary	The skin and all its structures – nails, hair, sweat and sebaceous glands	Protects, regulates temperature, eliminates waste, makes vitamin D, receives stimuli
Skeletal	The bones, joints and cartilages	Supports, protects, aids movement, stores fat and minerals, protects cells that produce blood cells
Muscular	Usually refers to skeletal muscle but includes cardiac and smooth	Produces movement, maintains posture and produces heat. Cardiac muscle pumps blood around the body. Smooth muscle is responsible for involuntary movements involved in processes such as digestion.
Cardiovascular	Heart, blood vessels and blood	Transports substances around body, helps regulate body temperature and prevents blood loss by blood clotting
Lymphatic	Lymphatic vessels, nodes, ducts, lymph, spleen, tonsils and thymus gland	Returns proteins and plasma to blood. Carries fat from intestine to blood. Filters body fluid, forms white blood cells, fights infection and protects against disease
Respiratory	Pharynx, larynx, trachea, bronchi and lungs	Supplies oxygen and removes carbon dioxide
Digestive	Gastro-intestinal tract, salivary glands, gall bladder, liver and pancreas	Physical and chemical breakdown of food. Absorption of nutrients and elimination of waste
Nervous	Brain, spinal cord, nerves and sense organs	Communication system for the body; processing, storing and responding to information
Urinary	Kidneys, ureters, bladder and urethra	Regulates chemical composition of blood. Helps to balance the acid/alkali content in the body and eliminates urine
Endocrine	All the hormone-producing ductless glands	Hormones regulate a wide variety of body activities, e.g. growth, and maintain body balance (homeostasis)
Reproductive	All organs of reproduction – ovaries, testes, etc	Involved in reproduction and production of sex hormones

Table 2.3 Classification of body systems

The integumentary system

This system includes the skin, hair, nails, sweat and sebaceous glands and various sensory receptors that convey sensations to the spinal cord and brain.

Skin

The skin forms a tough, waterproof protective covering over the entire surface of the body. It is continuous with the membranes lining the orifices. It covers a surface area of approximately two square metres, and varies in thickness from 0.05 mm to 3 mm, being thickest on the soles of the feet and palms of the hands and thinnest on the lips, eyelids, inner surfaces of the limbs and on the abdomen. The skin includes hair, nails, glands and various sensory receptors.

Skin colour

Skin colour varies from person to person and depends on ethnic origin. Skin colour is determined by the pigment melanin, the quantity of blood flowing through the blood vessels, and the amount of the pigment carotene present. The number of melanocytes is approximately the same in all human skin, but colour varies because of the amount and type of melanin produced.

Skin disorders associated with pigmentation include:

Naevus: this is an abnormality in the pigmentation of the skin

- Spider naevus: this presents as a central dilated blood vessel with small ones radiating from it like a spider. Frequently found on the face.

- Strawberry mark: this is an area of pink to red skin. Often present at birth.

- Port wine stain: this may be quite a large area of dark red to purple skin and is often present at birth. It is usually found on the face but can appear anywhere on the body. It does not usually fade.

Freckles (ephelides): small, brown-pigmented areas of skin that become darker when exposed to sunlight.

Macule: this is a mark or discoloured patch that lies flat on the skin.

Chloasma: this is a light-brown pigmentation of the cheeks, nose and forehead. Usually occurs during pregnancy and disappears after the birth.

Vitiligo: this is a total loss of pigmentation of the skin. It starts as small white patches, which can join up to form quite large areas of white skin.

Papilloma (moles): these are small growths on the skin that vary in size and colour. They may be pale to dark brown and may lie flat to the surface or be raised above the surface attached by a

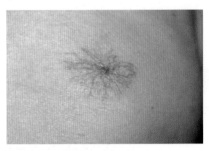

Figure 2.10 Spider naevus

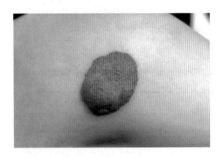

Figure 2.11 Strawberry mark

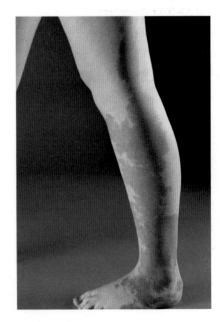

Figure 2.12 Port wine stain

short stalk. There is a danger of trapping these with the fingers when massaging.

Healthy skin is smooth, soft and flexible and has a good colour. A grey, ashen or yellow tinge may indicate health problems. (See Chapter 3 for more information on skin types.)

Skin structure

The skin is composed of two main layers with a subcutaneous fatty layer underneath. The two main layers are:

- the epidermis
- the dermis.

These layers may be further subdivided, as follows.

The epidermis has five layers:

- stratum corneum (horny layer - this is the superficial layer)
- stratum lucidum (clear layer)
- stratum granulosum (granular layer)
- stratum spinosum (prickle cell layer)
- stratum germinativum (basal cell layer – this is the deepest layer).

The dermis has **two** layers:

- the papillary layer
- the reticular layer.

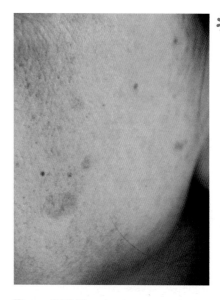

Figure 2.13 Macule

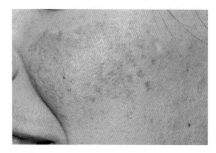

Figure 2.14 Chloasma

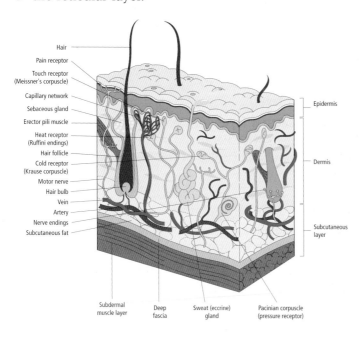

Figure 2.16 Structure of the skin

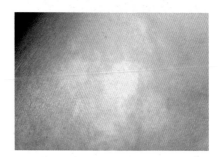

Figure 2.15 Vitiligo

Epidermis

The epidermis is composed of five layers of stratified squamous epithelium. The living cells of the two deepest layers contain nuclei. The dead cells of the upper three layers lose their nuclei and become filled with a protein called **keratin**. As the cells of the stratum basale multiply, they push upward, forming the next layer.

Stratum germinativum (basal cell layer)

This is the deepest layer of the epidermis. It is a single layer of cells on a basement membrane and lies directly on the papillary layer of the dermis. The capillary network of the dermis provides nutrients for these living cells.

The cells have a nucleus and multiply by mitosis (cell division).

Approximately one in ten of these basal cells are specialised cells called melanocytes. They produce the pigment melanin from the amino acid tyrosine. Melanin is produced to protect the cells against the damaging effect of ultraviolet radiation. It gives the skin its brown colour.

This layer also contains the nerve endings sensitive to touch (Merkel's discs).

Stratum spinosum (prickle cell layer)

This is composed of between eight and ten layers of living cells. Granules of melanin pass into this layer. The cells begin to lose their shape and have projections or spines, which join the cells together.

Stratum granulosum (granular layer)

This consists of three to five layers of flattened cells. Enzymes break down the nucleus and the cells die. Keratohyaline is laid down in the cytoplasm, giving the first stages of keratinisation.

Stratum lucidum (clear layer)

This is composed of several layers of clear, flat, dead cells that are translucent and filled with keratin. This layer is found only on the palms of the hands and soles of the feet, where it provides extra protection.

Stratum corneum (horny layer)

This is the superficial layer, composed of many rows of flat, dead, scaly cells filled with keratin, which are constantly shed and replaced (this shedding of cells is known as desquamation). Rubbing or friction of the skin will increase the rate of desquamation. Sebum secreted by the sebaceous glands helps to keep this layer soft and supple.

Dermis

The dermis lies under the epidermis and is composed of two layers: the upper papillary layer and the lower reticular layer.

> **Learning point**
>
> The protein keratin protects the skin from injury and invasion of micro-organisms and makes it waterproof.

> **Learning point**
>
> It takes approximately 28 days for the live cells in the basal layer to reach the horny layer as dead plaques of keratin.

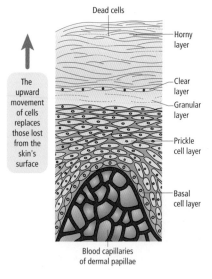

Figure 2.17 Layers of the epidermis

The surface of the papillary layer is ridged, forming an uneven surface. These finger-like projections increase the surface area and are called **dermal papillae**.

They produce the pattern known as fingerprints. The blood capillary loops of the dermis transport nutrients and oxygen to basal layer cells and remove waste products. Some elastin and collagen fibres are found in the matrix.

The reticular layer is composed of dense irregular connective tissue with more collagen and elastin fibres. This gives the skin strength, extensibility and elasticity.

The skin's ability to stretch and recoil is necessary during pregnancy and obesity. The ground substance or matrix retains water, helping the skin to remain firm and turgid.

Many structures are found in the dermis. They include blood vessels, lymphatic vessels, sebaceous glands, sweat glands, nerves and nerve endings, hair in hair follicles, erector pili muscles, fibres (white fibres and yellow elastic fibres), fibroblasts, mast cells, plasma cells and macrophages.

> **Learning point**
> A macrophage is a type of white blood cell that engulfs and digests debris and pathogens.

Blood vessels

The dermis is well supplied with blood vessels, partly to provide nutrients to the actively dividing cells of the epidermis (which has no direct supply), but also to enable the skin to play its part in the regulation of body temperature. Small vessels leave the dermal plexus at right angles and pass upwards to the skin's surface, ending in the dermal papillae. Nutrients and oxygen pass out into the tissue fluid and into the basal cells, and waste products pass out of the cells into tissue fluid through capillaries to the small veins.

The amount of blood flowing near the surface of the skin is controlled by nerve endings in the artery walls. If the body is becoming too hot, the small arteries dilate (get bigger). This causes flushing of the skin known as **erythema** and the body loses heat via the skin. If the body becomes too cool, the arteries constrict, preventing heat loss. Massage stimulates the nerve endings and by reflex action the blood vessels dilate, producing an erythema.

Lymphatic vessels

There is a network of fine lymphatic capillaries and vessels throughout the dermis. They are blind-end tubes with walls of greater permeability than blood capillaries – larger particles can enter these vessels and be drained away in the lymph. The broken-down products of infection by micro-organisms are also drained away in the lymph.

Sebaceous glands

These glands secrete an oily substance called **sebum**. (It consists mainly of waxes, fats and fatty acids, and dehydrocholesterol, which forms vitamin D in sunlight.)

The glands are found in all areas except the soles and palms and between the fingers and toes. They are numerous on the scalp, forehead, nose, chin, chest and between the shoulders.

The glands are sac-like and are usually attached to the side wall of hair follicles, into which the secretions enter via a duct, but some open directly onto the skin surface.

The glands are composed of epithelial cells that multiply, grow larger towards the centre and become filled with sebum. Eventually they burst, discharging sebum into the hair follicle.

The production of sebum is controlled by hormones (secreted by the endocrine glands). Hormonal imbalance increases the flow of sebum, often causing problems such as acne vulgaris, acne rosacea and seborrhoea.

The function of the sebum is to coat the skin and hair and keep the surface smooth and supple. It prevents loss of water from the skin.

It also has antiseptic and antifungal properties, protecting the skin from bacterial and fungal infections.

Sebum is gradually lost by washing and desquamation but is continually replaced. Massage stimulates the glands to produce more sebum.

Acid mantle

Together with the sweat secreted by sweat glands, sebum forms a coating on the skin known as the **acid mantle** because the secretions have a pH of between 5.5 and 5.6 (acidic). The acid mantle prevents the growth of bacteria. It is neutralised when the skin is washed with an alkaline product, but the acid mantle is restored after a few hours.

Sweat glands

There are two types of sweat gland:

- **eccrine glands** (sudoriferous): these consist of a coiled tube lying in the dermis with a straight duct opening in a pore on the skin surface. They are most numerous on the soles of feet and palms of hands.
- **apocrine glands** (odoriferous glands): these consist of coiled tubes larger than eccrine glands. They open into hair follicles, usually above the sebaceous glands. Sometimes they open directly onto the skin surface near a follicle. They are found in limited areas only, e.g. armpits and pubic areas. Development takes place at puberty. The secretion is somewhat viscous and sticky; when bacteria act on it, it results in unpleasant body odour (BO).

Sweat

Sweat is a clear liquid containing 98 per cent water, 2 per cent sodium chloride and other substances, including urea and lactic acid. Sweat takes heat from the skin during evaporation. It therefore helps to maintain constant body temperature. Massage produces heat and therefore stimulates the sweat glands to produce more sweat.

Nerves

The skin is richly supplied with sensory nerve endings, which relay information about the environment to the nervous system. Most of the nerve endings lie in the dermis, but a few that detect pain lie in the lower layers of the epidermis. There are various types of nerve ending, modified according to their function. They detect cold, heat, pain and pressure (Meissner's corpuscles – touch; Merkel's discs – pressure; Pacinian corpuscles – vibration and deep pressure). These warn the body of harmful changes so that it can protect itself. The few motor nerves control secretion of sweat and contraction of erector pili muscles. These nerve endings may be soothed by massage, but if the massage is too light they may be irritated and if it is too deep, pain is increased. These factors will increase tension and must be avoided.

Hair

Hairs are dead, horny structures composed of keratinised cells. They are found all over the body except on the soles and palms. They vary in length, texture and colour. Hairs are embedded in a depression called a hair follicle. The hair follicle consists of epithelial cells that form a tube passing obliquely into the dermis. It encases the hair bulb and hair root. The hair bulb is the expanded part of the hair that lies at the base of the follicle in the dermis. The hair root grows from the bulb and up through the follicle to the skin's surface. The hair shaft is the part that extends beyond the surface of the skin. Massage is more comfortable if it is performed in the direction of the hair growth, but this is not always possible.

Erector pili muscles

These are small involuntary muscles connected to the hair follicles. When they contract they pull the hair follicles straight. This happens during extreme fright or cold – the skin around the follicle becomes raised, forming 'goose bumps'.

Fibres

These consist of white collagen fibres and yellow elastic fibres.

White fibres are formed from non-elastic fibres of the protein collagen, lying in layers. They give the skin tensile strength and flexibility, and they bind structures together.

Yellow elastic fibres are formed from the protein elastin. They are scattered throughout the matrix. These highly elastic fibres are capable of stretch and recoil. They give the skin elasticity, enabling it to stretch and return to normal. This is important for pregnancy and obesity. If the skin is over-stretched, small tears occur in the dermis. These can be seen as white lines called 'stretch marks'. With ageing, the skin loses elasticity and becomes wrinkled. Care must be taken when massaging older clients not to further stretch the skin. All fibres are embedded in a jelly-like matrix. This is capable of absorbing water, giving firmness to the skin.

Cells

Fibroblasts produce the matrix and fibres.

Mast cells release **histamine** following injury or reaction to an allergen. Histamine initiates an inflammatory response, causing dilation of capillaries and increasing the permeability of cell walls. This process aids tissue repair.

Plasma cells produce antibodies.

Leucocytes destroy, and protect the body against, micro-organisms.

Macrophages clean up cellular debris.

Subcutaneous layer

This lies between the reticular layer and the underlying structures. It is a type of connective tissue and contains adipose and areolar tissue and nerve endings that are sensitive to pressure (Pacinian corpuscles). Adipose tissue helps protect the body from injury, acts as an insulating layer to prevent heat loss and stores excess fat, so that it is ready to convert into energy when required.

Functions of the skin

Sensitivity

The skin contains many sensory receptors, which register changes in the external environment. These receptors are sensitive to touch, pressure, pain, heat and cold. From the nerve endings in the skin, impulses are transmitted to the brain where an appropriate response is initiated.

Heat regulation

The skin is one of the main organs for body temperature control. Normal body temperature is 37°C (98.4°F). Heat regulation is achieved by:

- evaporation of sweat: body heat is used for the evaporation of sweat – this lowers body temperature.
- dilation and constriction of blood capillaries in the skin: if the body becomes too hot, the surface capillaries dilate and more

blood flows to the surface, giving off heat. When this happens the skin becomes pink or red; this reddening of the skin is known as erythema. If the body becomes too cold the blood vessels constrict and less blood flows to the surface, so less heat is lost and body temperature is maintained.

- insulating properties of adipose tissue: the fatty tissue in the dermis and subcutaneous layer acts as an insulating layer that helps to retain body heat.

Absorption

The absorption of substances through the skin is limited. The keratin in the cells and the covering of sebum prevent the absorption of water, making the skin waterproof. However, the skin will allow certain substances to pass through so that drugs, hormones and other substances are sometimes administered through the skin.

Protection

This is a very important function. The skin forms an effective barrier, which protects the body from harm. The skin gives protection against:

- dirt and chemical attack: the keratin and flat dead cells in the superficial layers of the skin protect against dirt and chemical attack.
- invasion by micro-organisms: the mixture of sebum and sweat forms an acid mantle over the surface of the skin. The pH of the skin is around 5.5 or 5.6 and this slightly acidic environment discourages the growth of micro-organisms.
- minor injuries: through the sensory nerve endings in the skin the brain can quickly respond to painful stimuli, thus protecting the body from damage.
- UV radiation, the melanocytes (cells that produce melanin) in the stratum germinativum produce the pigment melanin, which protects the underlying tissues from the harmful effects of ultra-violet rays.

Excretion

The skin plays a minor role in the excretion of urea and other waste products through sweating.

Secretion and storage

The sebaceous glands secrete sebum, which, with sweat, forms the protective acid mantle. Sebum also lubricates the skin, keeping it soft and supple. The skin stores water and fat.

Formation of vitamin D

This is an important function of the skin. It forms vitamin D from the action of sunlight on the chemical 7-dehydrocholesterol in the skin.

Effects of massage on the skin

- Massage improves the condition of the skin because the increased blood supply increases the delivery of nutrients and oxygen and speeds up the removal of metabolic waste. Metabolism is increased, which stimulates the cells of the stratum basale and increases mitosis (cell division). More cells move upwards towards the surface, improving the condition of the skin as old cells are replaced.

- Massage aids desquamation (shedding of dead cells). Increased mitosis will increase the shedding of the flaky dead cells of the stratum corneum. Also, the friction of the hands on the skin will rub off these dead cells on the surface.

- The colour of the skin is improved. Massage produces dilation of surface capillaries: this results in hyperaemia and erythema, which improve the colour of sallow skin.

- Sebaceous glands are stimulated to produce and release more sebum. This lubricates the skin and keeps it soft and supple.

- The oil or cream used as a medium also lubricates and softens the skin.

- Sweat glands are stimulated to produce more sweat, which aids cleansing and elimination of waste.

Effects of massage on adipose tissue

Adipose tissue is a connective tissue composed mainly of specialised cells called adipocytes, which are adapted to store fat. It is found under the skin in the subcutaneous layer and around organs. Fat is the body's energy reserve. It is *stored* when energy intake is greater than energy output and *utilised* if energy intake is less than energy output. Therefore, the only way of losing fat is through sensible eating and increasing activity or exercise. However, massage is thought to help the dispersal of fat because the deeper movements stimulate blood flow to the area. This softens the area and may speed up removal via the circulating blood from that area, providing the client also reduces intake of food.

The effect of massage on cellulite (very hard consolidated fat) is dealt with in Chapter 6.

The skeletal system

The skeletal system is made up of bones, joints and cartilages. The human skeleton is made up of 206 bones. These are grouped into two main divisions: the **axial skeleton**, which forms the core or axis of the body, and the **appendicular skeleton**, which forms the girdles and limbs. It is important to identify skeletal bones, particularly those with bony points or prominences, which must be avoided when massaging.

Learning point
The study of the structure and function of bones is called osteology.

Remember
Bone is a connective tissue. It is also called osseous tissue.

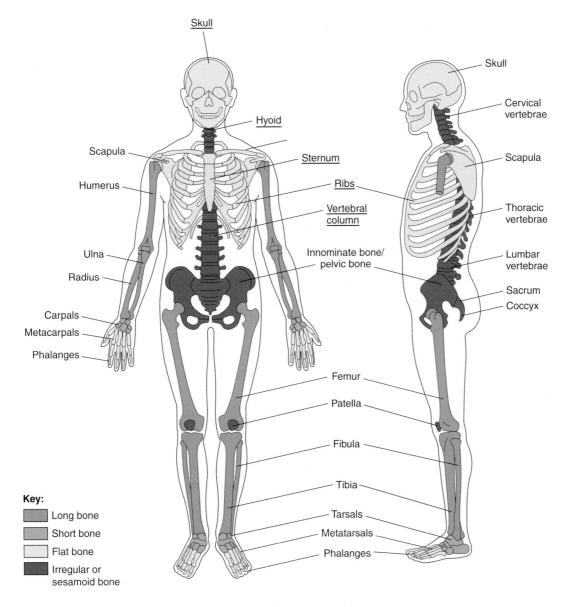

Figure 2.18 Anterior and side views of the skeleton

The axial skeleton

The bones of the axial skeleton include the:

- skull (the cranium and bones of the face)
- vertebral column (spine)
- sternum (breast bone)
- ribs
- hyoid bone (small bone in neck below mandible).

Appendicular skeleton

The bones of the appendicular skeleton include the following.

Upper limb:

- clavicle (collar bone)
- scapula (shoulder bone)

- humerus (upper arm bone)
- radius (forearm – lateral)
- ulna (forearm – medial)
- carpals (wrist)
- metacarpals (palm)
- phalanges (fingers).

Lower limb:

- innominate or pelvic bone (hip bone)
- femur (thigh bone)
- patella (knee cap)
- tibia (large bone of lower leg – medial)
- fibula (thin bone of lower leg – lateral)
- tarsals (ankle)
- metatarsals (foot)
- phalanges (toes).

Vertebral column

The vertebral column (also known as the spinal column) is composed of 33 vertebrae. Some are fused together, making 26 bones. The vertebrae are separated by intervertebral discs of fibro-cartilage, which act as shock absorbers. The bones and discs are bound together by strong ligaments.

The column is divided into five regions:

cervical: 7 vertebrae (neck), concave when viewed posteriorly

thoracic: 12 vertebrae (upper back), convex when viewed posteriorly

lumbar: 5 vertebrae (lower, small of back), concave when viewed posteriorly

sacral: 5 fused vertebrae (sacrum), convex when viewed posteriorly

coccygeal: 4 fused vertebrae (coccyx).

Functions of the skeleton

The functions of the skeleton are as follows:

Support – the bony framework gives shape to the body, supports the soft tissues and provides attachments for muscles.

Protection – the bony framework protects delicate internal organs from injury, e.g. the brain is protected by the skull; the heart and lungs are protected by the rib cage.

Movement – produced by a system of bones, joints and muscles. The bones act as levers, and muscles pull on the bones, resulting in movement at the joints.

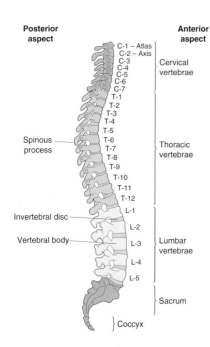

Figure 2.19 Vertebral column

Learning point
Ligaments attach bone to bone.

Storage of minerals – bones store many minerals, particularly calcium and phosphorus.

Storage of energy – fats or lipids stored in the yellow bone marrow provide energy when required.

Storage of tissue that forms blood cells – both red and white blood cells are produced by red bone marrow, which is found in the spongy bone of the pelvis, vertebrae, ribs, sternum and in the ends of the femur and humerus.

Joints

A joint is where two or more bones join or articulate. There are three main groups: fibrous, cartilaginous and synovial.

Types of joint

Fibrous

Immoveable joints, the bones fit tightly together and are held firmly by fibrous tissue. There is no joint cavity. Examples are the sutures of the skull.

Cartilaginous

Slightly moveable joints, the bones are connected by a disc or plate of fibro-cartilage. There is no joint cavity. Examples are the symphysis pubis (between the pubic bones) and the intervertebral joints (between the vertebral bodies).

Synovial

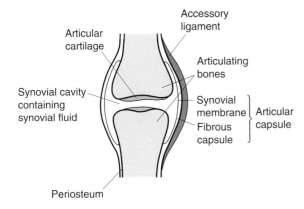

Figure 2.20 Synovial joint

Freely moveable joints, these are the most numerous in the body. There are six different types of synovial joint. They are classified according to their planes of movement, which depend on the shape of the articulating bones. All the freely moveable joints of the body are synovial joints and, although their shape and movements vary, they all have certain characteristics in common:

a) a **joint cavity** (space within the joint)

b) a **synovial membrane** lining the capsule of the joint up to the hyaline cartilage, which produces synovial fluid

c) **synovial fluid** or synovium – a viscous fluid that lubricates and nourishes the joint

d) **hyaline cartilage**, which covers the surfaces of the articulating bones. It is sometimes called articular cartilage. It reduces friction and allows smooth movement

e) a **capsule**, or articulating capsule, which surrounds the joints like a sleeve. It holds the bones together and encloses the cavity. The capsule is strengthened on the outside by ligaments, which help to stabilise and strengthen the joints. Ligaments may also be found inside a joint, holding bones together and increasing stability. Massage is used around joints to increase the circulation and to free ligaments that may have become bound down following injury.

Discs (menisci)

Some joints have pads of fibro-cartilage called discs. They are attached to the bones and give the joint a better 'fit'. They also cushion movement, e.g. cartilages of the knee.

Bursae

Any movement produces friction between the moving parts. In order to reduce friction, sac-like structures containing synovial fluid are found between tissues. These are called bursae and are usually found between tendons and bone.

Classification of the six synovial joints

Although synovial joints differ in shape and movement range,
they all have similar characteristics

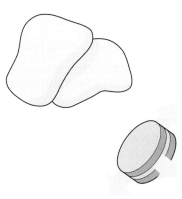

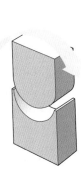

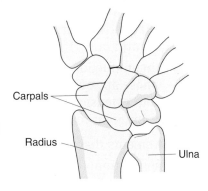

A gliding joint: found in the wrist between the carpal
bones. Two bones have a small range of gliding
movement limited by connecting ligaments

A hinge joint: found at the elbow and knee.
The range of movement is limited to one
plane, such as a door hinge

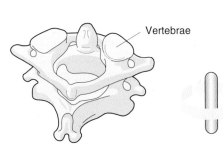

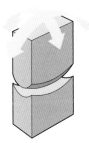

A pivot joint: found in the neck. Part of the
bone fits into another ring of bone as in atlas
and axis, allowing rotation of the head

A condyloid joint: found at the
wrist and ankle. Movement in two
planes, but not such a full range
as in the ball and socket joint

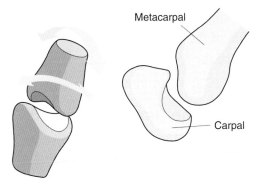

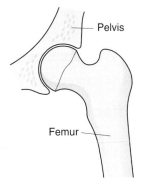

A saddle joint: found at the base of the thumb. This
joint allows the thumb to be moved in two directions
and circled around

A ball and socket joint: found in the shoulder and the
hip. Designed to allow a wide range of movement

Figure 2.21 Types of synovial joint
a) **gliding joint,** e.g. intercarpal or intertarsal joints
b) **hinge joint,** e.g. elbow or knee

c) **pivot joint,** e.g. atlas on axis or superior radio-ulnar joint

d) **ellipsoid joint** (condyloid), e.g. wrist or knuckle joints

e) **saddle joint,** e.g. base of the thumb

f) **ball-and-socket joint,** hip or shoulder joint.

Direction of joint movement

The following terms are used to describe the direction of joint movement:

- **flexion:** the bringing together of two surfaces (a bending movement), e.g. bending the elbow or knee
- **extension:** movement in the opposite direction to flexion (a straightening movement), e.g. straightening the elbow or knee
- **abduction:** movement away from the mid-line, e.g. taking the arm from the body
- **adduction:** movement towards the mid-line e.g. taking the arm back to the body
- **rotation:** movement around a long axis, which may be medial rotation, e.g. turning the arm in or lateral rotation, e.g. turning the arm out
- **circumduction:** a movement where the limb describes a cone whose apex lies in the joint: a combination of flexion, abduction, extension and adduction e.g. circling the shoulder joint or hip joint round and round.

Movements that occur between the radius and ulna:

- **supination:** turns the hand forwards or upwards
- **pronation:** turns the hand backwards or downwards.

Movements of the ankle joint:

- **dorsi-flexion:** pulling the foot upwards
- **plantar flexion:** pointing the foot downwards.

Movements of the foot occurring between the tarsal joints:

- **inversion:** turning the sole of the foot inwards
- **eversion:** turning the sole of the foot outwards.

See Chapter 7 for more information about joint movements.

Effects of massage on bone tissue and joints

- Bones are covered by a layer of connective tissue known as the 'periosteum'. Blood vessels from the periosteum penetrate the bone. Deep massage movements will stimulate blood flow to the periosteum and hence indirectly increase blood supply to the bone.
- Massage around joints will increase the circulation and nourish the structures surrounding the joint.

- Massage is effective in loosening adhesions in structures around joints. For example, frictions across a ligament help to loosen it from underlying structures.
- Massage and passive movements will help to maintain full range of movement.

The muscular system

There are three types of muscle tissue:

- **skeletal muscle** – forms the body flesh and produces body movement
- **cardiac muscle** – forms the walls of the heart and pumps blood around the body
- **smooth muscle** – found in the walls of the intestines (viscera), which contract to move food along in the digestive tract (peristalsis).

Skeletal muscle forms the body flesh. The function of skeletal muscle is to produce movement, maintain posture and produce body heat. Skeletal muscle tissue is totally under the control of the nervous system: impulses transmitted from the brain via motor nerves initiate contraction of muscle fibres. This muscle contraction pulls on bones and movement occurs at joints.

Structure of skeletal muscle

Skeletal muscle is composed of muscle fibres arranged in bundles called **fasciculi**. Many bundles of fibres make up the complete muscle. The fibres, bundles and muscles are surrounded and protected by connective tissue sheaths.

Skeletal muscle fibres are long, thin multi-nucleated cells. These fibres are made up of even smaller protein threads called myofibrils. These run the whole length of the fibre and are the elements that contract and relax. Each myofibril is composed of actin and myosin protein threads that slide into each other so that the myofibril shortens. When these myofibrils shorten, the whole muscle contracts.

- The connective tissue around each fibre is called the **endomysium**.
- The connective tissue around each bundle is called the **perimysium**.
- The connective tissue around the muscle is called the **epimysium**.

> **Learning point**
> The contraction of skeletal muscles help to increase venous return and lymphatic drainage back towards the heart.

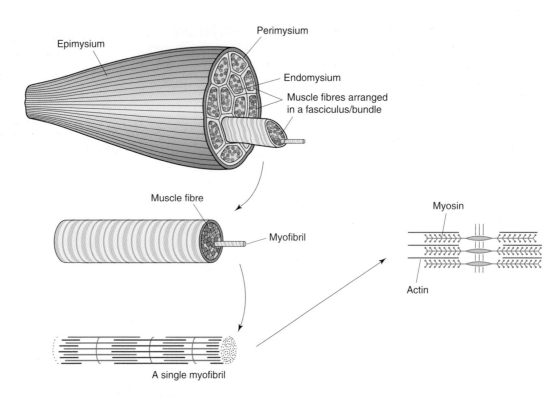

Figure 2.22 Construction of skeletal muscle

Learning point

Muscles form the flesh and help to give the body its shape.

Learning point

Proximal means a structure that is towards the root or origin, i.e. nearer the trunk. **Distal** means a structure that is further away from the root or origin, i.e. further away from the trunk.

If this connective tissue becomes tight or adheres to underlying structures, the muscle function is impaired. Petrissage movements and myofascial stretching techniques are very effective in freeing and stretching the tissue, allowing the muscle fibres to function normally.

Muscle fibres

Muscle fibres are long, thin, multi-nucleated cells. The fibres vary from 10 to 100 microns in diameter, and from a few millimetres to many centimetres in length. The long fibres extend the full length of the muscle while the short fibres end in connective tissue intersections within the muscle.

Muscle attachments

As previously explained, a muscle is composed of muscle fibres and connective tissue components – the endomysium, perimysium and epimysium. Certain muscles have connective tissue intersections dividing the muscle into several bellies, as seen in *rectus abdominis*.

These sheets of connective tissue blend at either end of the muscle and attach the muscle to underlying bones. Muscles are attached via tendons or via aponeuroses.

- **Tendons** are tough cord-like structures of connective tissue that attach muscles to bones.
- **Aponeuroses** are flat sheets of connective tissue that attach muscles along the length of bone.

A muscle has at least two points of attachment, known as the origin and insertion of the muscle.

- The **origin** is usually **proximal** and stationary or immoveable.
- The **insertion** is usually **distal** and moveable.

In the workplace

Following over-use or injury, tendons may become inflamed. Massage around the area can restore function. Transverse frictions are useful for freeing tendons held by adhesions.

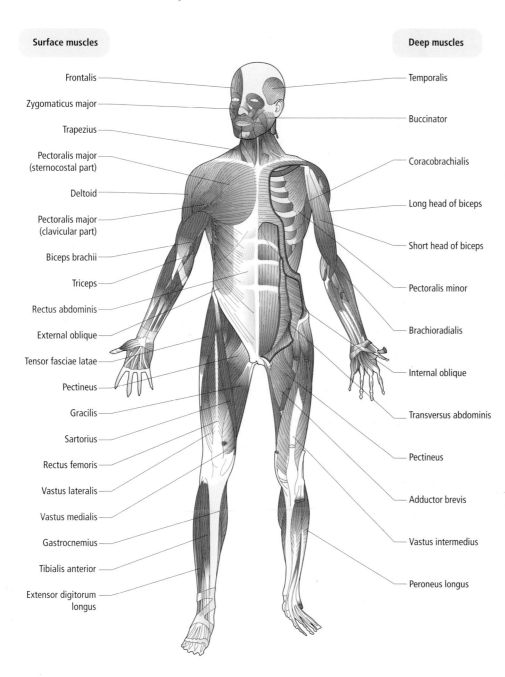

Surface muscles	Deep muscles
Frontalis	Temporalis
Zygomaticus major	Buccinator
Trapezius	
Pectoralis major (sternocostal part)	Coracobrachialis
Deltoid	Long head of biceps
Pectoralis major (clavicular part)	Short head of biceps
Biceps brachii	
Triceps	Pectoralis minor
Rectus abdominis	
External oblique	Brachioradialis
Tensor fasciae latae	
Pectineus	Internal oblique
Gracilis	
Sartorius	Transversus abdominis
Rectus femoris	
Vastus lateralis	Pectineus
Vastus medialis	Adductor brevis
Gastrocnemius	
Tibialis anterior	Vastus intermedius
Extensor digitorum longus	Peroneus longus

Figure 2.23 Muscles of the body – anterior

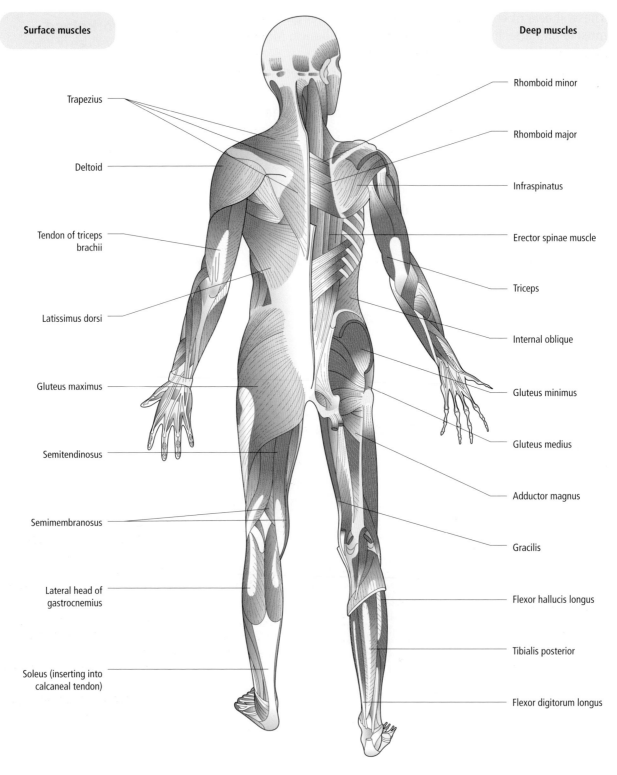

Surface muscles		Deep muscles

Trapezius

Deltoid

Tendon of triceps brachii

Latissimus dorsi

Gluteus maximus

Semitendinosus

Semimembranosus

Lateral head of gastrocnemius

Soleus (inserting into calcaneal tendon)

Rhomboid minor

Rhomboid major

Infraspinatus

Erector spinae muscle

Triceps

Internal oblique

Gluteus minimus

Gluteus medius

Adductor magnus

Gracilis

Flexor hallucis longus

Tibialis posterior

Flexor digitorum longus

Figure 2.24 Muscles of the body – posterior

Muscle shape

Muscle shape varies depending on the function of the muscle. The fleshy bulk of the muscle is known as the belly. The muscle fibres that form bundles lie parallel or obliquely to the line of pull of the muscle. Parallel fibres are found in strap-like and fusiform muscles. These long fibres allow for a wide range of movement. Oblique fibres are found in triangular and pennate muscles. These shorter fibres are found where muscle strength is required.

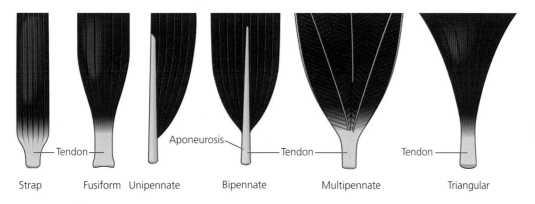

Tendon — Aponeurosis — Tendon — Tendon —

Strap   Fusiform Unipennate   Bipennate   Multipennate   Triangular

Figure 2.25 Muscle shapes

Blood supply to skeletal muscle

Supplies of oxygen and nutrients required by muscles to produce energy for muscle contraction are transported in the blood via the arteries supplying the muscle; the waste products are removed via the veins. The arteries branch to form smaller arteries and arterioles within the perimysium. They then further divide forming capillary networks within the endomysium, where they join venules that lead to veins. When muscles are relaxed, the capillary network delivers blood to the muscle fibres. When muscles contract, the pressure impedes the flow of blood through the capillary beds, which reduces the supply of oxygen and nutrients and limits removal of waste. During exercise, muscle fibres alternately contract and relax, and the capillaries deliver blood during the relaxation phase. However, repeated or sustained contractions, such as isometric work or exercising without sufficient rest periods, prevent blood flow to the muscle fibres, due to compression on blood vessels and capillaries. This results in **muscle fatigue**, due to lack of oxygen and nutrients and the accumulation of waste products such as lactic acid. The strength and speed of contraction becomes progressively weaker until the muscle finally fails to relax completely, resulting in muscle spasm and pain.

Muscle tone

Muscle tone is the state of partial contraction or tension found in muscles even when at rest. Only a small number of muscle fibres will be in a state of contraction. This is sufficient to produce tautness in the muscle but not to result in full contraction and movement. Different groups of fibres contract alternately, working a 'shift' system to prevent fatigue. Changes in muscle tone are

> **Learning point**
> Long effleurage strokes speed up venous return and the circulation to the muscle is increased. Accumulated waste is removed and pain and stiffness relieved. The squeezing movements of petrissage also increase the circulation. When tension in the muscle is relieved, pressure is decreased and circulation flows normally through the capillary beds.

adjusted according to the information received from sensory receptors within the muscles and their tendons. **Muscle spindles** transmit information on the degree of stretch within the muscle. **Tendon receptors** called Golgi organs transmit information on the amount of tension applied to the tendon by muscle contraction. Too much stretch and tension will result in reduction in muscle tone. Too little will result in increase in muscle tone. Muscle tone is essential for maintaining upright postures.

Effects of massage on muscle tissue

- Massage aids the relaxation of muscles, due to the warmth created, reflex response and removal of accumulated waste.

- Massage pushes the blood along in the veins. Deoxygenated blood and waste are removed and fresh oxygenated blood and nutrients are brought to the muscles. The metabolic rate is increased and the condition of the muscles will improve.

- Massage will reduce pain, stiffness and muscle fatigue produced by the accumulation of waste following anaerobic contraction. The removal of this metabolic waste, i.e. lactic acid and carbon dioxide, is speeded up and normal function is more quickly restored. This is particularly important following hard training, sport and athletic performance, for example, when massage will speed up the recovery of muscles, allowing the athlete to return to training more quickly. The increased nutrients and oxygen will also facilitate tissue repair and recovery.

- Massage warms muscles due to the increased blood flow, the friction of the hands moving over the area and the friction of the tissues as they move over each other. This reduces tension and aids relaxation of the muscles. Warm muscles contract more efficiently and are more extensile than cold muscles. Thus performance is enhanced and the likelihood of strains, sprains, micro-tears or other injury is reduced. Massage prior to exercise must be used in conjunction with (but not instead of) warm-up and stretch exercise.

- The elasticity of muscles is improved because manipulations such as kneading, wringing and picking up, stretch the fibres and separate the bundles. Any restricting fibrous adhesions are broken down and any tight fascia surrounding the bundles are stretched, allowing muscle fibres to function normally.

- Massage will break down adhesions and fibrositic nodules that may have developed within the muscle as a result of tension, poor posture or injury.

The cardiovascular system

The cardiovascular (blood circulatory) system is a closed circuit. It is composed of a pump called the heart, a network of interconnecting tubes called blood vessels, and the fluid flowing through the circuit known as blood. The parts that make up the system are:

- heart
- arteries and arterioles
- veins and venules
- capillaries
- blood.

The system is designed to carry blood to and from the organs and cells of the body. Blood carries oxygen, nutrients, hormones and enzymes to the cells, and takes away the waste products of metabolism from the cells.

Tissue fluid

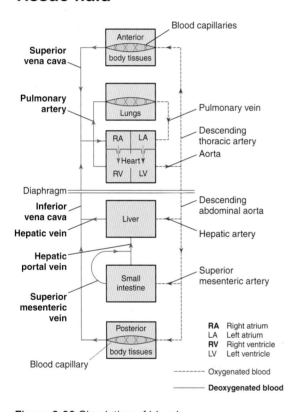

Figure 2.26 Circulation of blood

All body cells are bathed in interstitial fluid (tissue fluid). This fluid provides a medium for substances to move across from the blood to the cells and from the cells to the blood.

Oxygenated blood flows from the heart, through the arteries and arterioles, and into the capillaries.

The walls of the capillaries are very thin: consequently the oxygen and nutrients pass out through the walls into the tissue fluid and from there into the cells.

The waste products of metabolism pass out of the cells into the tissue fluid and into the capillaries in the same way. This deoxygenated blood is transported via the venules and veins back to the heart.

The heart then pumps it to the lungs to be reoxygenated.

Some fluid and larger particles of waste are removed from the tissues via the thinner-walled lymphatic vessels. These lie alongside blood vessels among the tissues.

The heart

The heart lies in the thoracic cavity between the lungs. It is somewhat cone-shaped, with the base above and the apex below. The walls of the heart are made up of three layers:

- **pericardium**: a tough outer coat of fibrous tissue
- **myocardium**: the middle coat of cardiac muscle
- **endocardium**: the inner lining of squamous epithelium.

The heart is divided into a right and left side by a muscular wall or septum. The left side of the heart deals with **oxygenated** blood. The right side deals with **deoxygenated** blood. Each side is further divided into two chambers separated by valves. The upper chambers are called **atria** (singular: atrium); the lower chambers are called **ventricles**.

Flow of blood through the heart

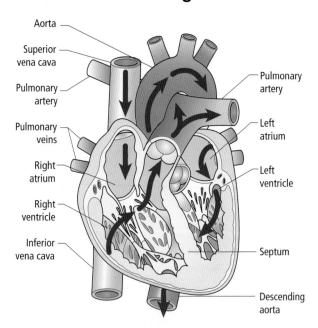

Figure 2.27 The heart

- The inferior and superior venae cavae (veins) collect deoxygenated blood from the body and empty it into the right atrium.
- This blood then passes through the tricuspid valve into the right ventricle.

- From the right ventricle it is pumped into the pulmonary artery (the only artery carrying deoxygenated blood) and carried to the lungs.
- Interchange of gases occurs in the lungs and the oxygenated blood is carried by the pulmonary vein (the only vein carrying oxygenated blood) back to the left atrium of the heart.
- This blood passes through the bicuspid valve into the left ventricle.
- From the left ventricle, blood is pumped into the aorta – the first artery of the general circulation. The aorta branches into numerous arteries, which carry oxygenated blood to all body parts.

Blood vessels

There are three main types of blood vessel: arteries, veins and capillaries.

Arteries transport oxygenated blood from the heart around the body to all tissues and organs. The main artery, the large **aorta**, leaves the left ventricle of the heart and divides to form other arteries, which further subdivide forming a network of arteries all over the body. Arteries finally divide into small thinly-walled vessels called arterioles, which enter the capillary networks among the tissues. Arteries transport blood carrying oxygen, nutrients, hormones etc around the body. Artery walls have three layers of tissues: a fibrous outer layer, a muscular middle layer and an inner lining of smooth epithelium. The middle muscular layer of arteries is thicker than the muscular layer of veins and their lumen is smaller. Blood is pumped through the arteries, around the body, by the contraction of the heart; with each contraction the blood is forced along. The rate at which the heart is beating can be felt as a pulse at arteries that lie near the surface, such as the radial artery at the wrist.

Veins transport deoxygenated blood back to the heart. The walls are similar in structure to those of arteries but the middle muscular layer is thinner. The inner layer of epithelial cells is folded to form valves. These valves prevent the backward flow of blood. The lumen of veins is larger than that of arteries.

Blood is pumped along the veins by the contraction and relaxation of muscles and by the expansion and contraction of the thorax and diaphragm during breathing. If muscles are not contracting, e.g. during long periods of standing and inactivity, gravity exerts a downward force. If the valves are weak, blood 'pools' in the veins. This pressure overloads the veins and the wall bulges outwards, causing the condition known as varicose veins. Regular leg massage speeds up the flow of blood through the veins. This prevents overloading of the veins, which helps prevent varicose veins.

During periods of prolonged inactivity, such as bed rest or sitting in cramped conditions for a long time, the flow of blood through the veins slows down and there is a risk of blood clots forming in the veins. A clot may attach to the vessel wall where it is called a **thrombus** or it may become detached and be carried in the bloodstream, where it is known as an **embolus**. The clot may end up blocking the blood supply to the lung with potentially fatal consequences. This is one of the greatest dangers of massage, making thrombosis an absolute contra-indication to massage (see page 129).

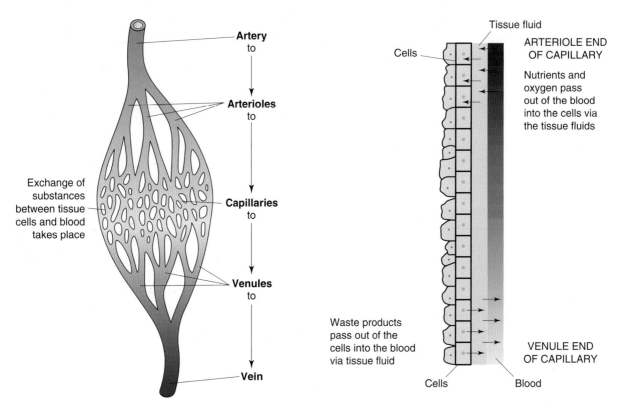

Figure 2.28 Blood flow from artery to vein

Figure 2.29 Transfer of substances between the blood and cells

Capillaries are thin-walled, tiny vessels that form networks among the tissue spaces. Arterioles enter capillary networks and venules leave. The primary function of capillaries is to allow the exchange of gases, nutrients and metabolic waste between the cells and the blood. Arterioles bring oxygen and nutrients to the capillaries. These pass through the thin vessel walls into the tissue fluid and then through the cell wall into the cell. Carbon dioxide and metabolites pass out of the cell and into the blood in the same way.

Venules leave the capillary networks and join to form larger veins that transport the deoxygenated blood and the waste products of metabolism (metabolites) back to the heart via the largest veins, namely the **inferior vena cava** and the **superior vena cava**. These two large veins empty into the right atrium of the heart.

When the metabolic needs of the tissues are low, parts of the capillary network can shut off, limiting blood flow. More blood is then available for those tissues with greater metabolic needs. Thus blood flow can be shunted in this way to areas that require a greater supply of oxygen and nutrients, e.g. exercising muscles.

Massage aids the dilation of these surface capillaries by reflex action, promoting blood flow. An accumulation of waste products in the tissues, or tension in muscle fibres, exerts pressure on the capillaries and restricts blood flow. Massage helps to relieve this pressure, as it speeds up the removal of waste products and promotes muscle relaxation. Thus the pressure is reduced and normal blood flow through the capillaries is restored. This helps the recovery of the muscles and restores normal function.

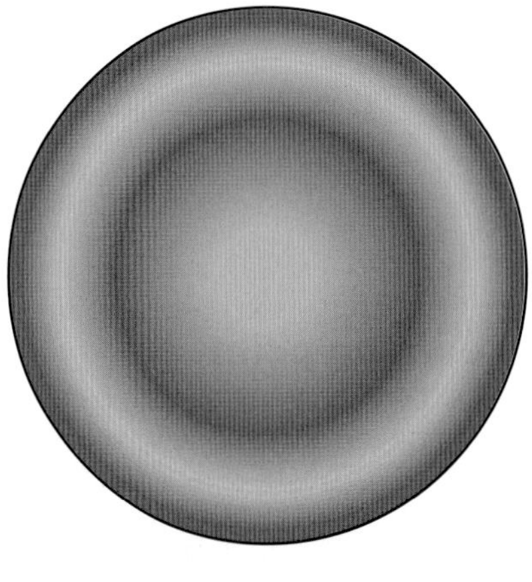

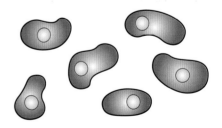

Figure 2.30 An erythrocyte

Blood

Blood is a viscous fluid (slightly sticky) that flows through the heart and blood vessels. It is composed of 55 per cent plasma and 45 per cent cells. (Plasma is a faintly yellow transparent fluid composed of 91 per cent water, 7 per cent proteins and 2 per cent other solutes.) Its temperature is around 38°C and its pH is around 7.4 (slightly alkaline). The total volume of blood in the human body is 5–6 litres in men and 4–5 litres in women.

Blood cells

There are three main types of blood cell:

- **erythrocytes**: red blood cells, which contain haemoglobin that transports oxygen and carbon dioxide
- **leucocytes**: white blood cells, which protect the body against invading micro-organisms; they play a part in the body's defence system and immune reaction
- **thrombocytes** or **platelets**: they play an important role in blood clotting.

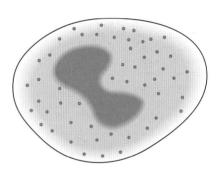

Figure 2.31 A leucocyte

Functions of the blood

Blood *transports*:

- oxygen from the lungs to body cells
- carbon dioxide from the cells to the lungs
- nutrients from the digestive tract to body cells
- metabolic waste products from cells to excretory organs
- hormones from endocrine glands to cells
- any drugs taken for medicinal purposes.

It *regulates*:

- the water content of cells
- body heat, maintaining normal body temperature
- pH by means of buffers.

Figure 2.32 A thrombocyte

It *protects*:

- against disease and infection, by the action of leucocytes, which destroy micro-organisms through phagocytic action and production of antibodies
- against blood loss, by the process of blood clotting.

Blood pressure

This is the force or pressure the blood exerts on the walls of the blood vessels. The blood pressure in arteries is higher than that in veins.

Normal average blood pressure rises to around 120 mmHg (millimetres of mercury) as the heart contracts (systolic pressure), and falls to around 80 mmHg as the heart relaxes (diastolic pressure). Blood pressure is measured using a **sphygmomanometer** and expressed as: BP = 120/80 mmHg

Pulse

The pulse rate is the same as the heart rate, being around 74 beats per minute. The pulse can be felt in arteries because of the expansion and recoil of their walls during each ventricular contraction of the heart. The pulse is strongest in the arteries closest to the heart. The pulse is usually taken at the radial artery at the wrist, but can also be taken at the carotid artery in the neck and the brachial artery in the arm, medial to the biceps muscle.

Effects of massage on blood circulation

- Massage is thought to increase the blood flow through the area being treated, i.e. it produces hyperaemia (increased blood supply) and erythema (reddening of the skin).
- It speeds up the flow of blood through the veins. Veins lie superficially (nearer the surface than arteries). As the hands move over the part in the direction of venous return, the blood is pushed along in the veins towards the heart. The deeper and faster the movements, the greater the flow. This venous blood carries away metabolic waste products more quickly. If these are allowed to accumulate in muscle tissue they produce pain and stiffness, and exert pressure, which further restricts the circulation. Therefore, massage will relieve pain and stiffness by flushing out metabolic waste and relieving pressure on the capillaries, which restores free flow of blood within the tissues.
- It increases the supply of fresh, oxygenated blood to the part. As the deoxygenated blood is moved along, the capillaries empty and fresh oxygenated blood flows into them more quickly. The nutrients and oxygen nourish the tissues and aid tissue recovery and repair.
- Massage dilates superficial arterioles and capillaries, which improves the exchange of substances in and out of cells via tissue fluid. This will improve the metabolic rate, which, in turn, will improve the condition of the tissues. This dilation of the superficial capillaries produces an erythema (redness of the skin).

Learning point

Blood pressure varies with sex, age and weight, and with activities, stress levels or anxiety. The condition of the heart and vessels also affects pressure.

- Warmth is produced in the area due to the increased blood flow and friction of the hands on the part.
- Massage is thought to reduce the viscosity of the blood, reducing its rate of coagulation.
- Relaxing slow massage may reduce high blood pressure.

The lymphatic system

The lymphatic system is closely associated with the cardiovascular system and connects with it. The lymphatic system removes tissue fluid and proteins from the tissue spaces and returns it to the blood via the subclavian veins. This fluid in the lymphatic vessels is called **lymph**. The system also transports fats from the small intestine to the blood, and it plays an important role in protecting the body against infection.

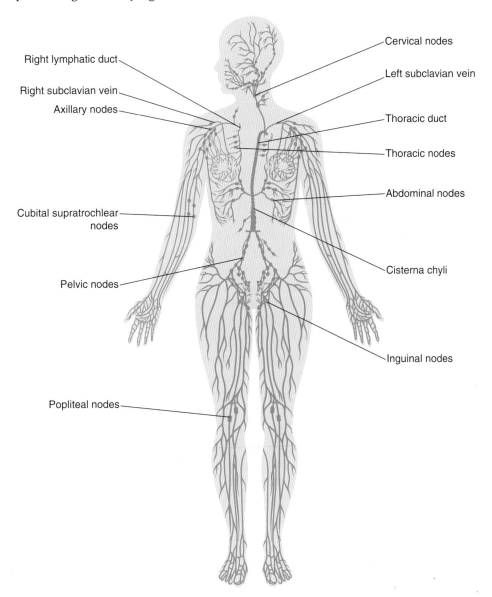

Figure 2.33 The lymphatic nodes of the body

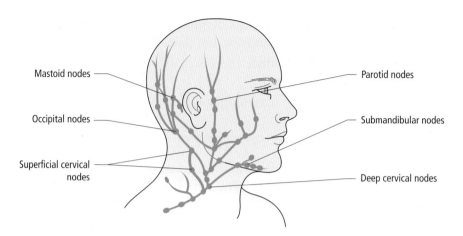

Figure 2.34 Lymphatic nodes of the head and neck

The parts of the lymphatic system are:

- **lymphatic capillaries, vessels and trunks:** these are tubes that carry the fluid
- **lymphatic nodes:** arranged in groups throughout the body
- **lymphatic organs:** such as the spleen, thymus gland and tonsils
- **lymphatic ducts:** there are two ducts, the right lymphatic duct and the thoracic duct, which empty into the right and left subclavian veins
- **lymph:** the fluid flowing through the vessels.

Lymphatic capillaries begin as blind-end tubes, which form a network among the tissue spaces. Their walls are very thin and allow fluid, larger proteins and particles to pass through. Because these larger particles and proteins are unable to pass through blood vessel walls, they are returned to the blood via the lymphatic system. These minute lymphatic capillaries then join together to form larger lymphatic vessels. Lymphatic vessels are very similar to veins in structure, but have thinner walls and a greater number of valves to prevent backward flow.

All lymphatic vessels drain into lymphatic nodes. These are strategically placed in groups along the path of the vessels. Many afferent vessels enter a node, but only one or two efferent vessels leave. Lymphatic nodes are small, bean-shaped structures up to 2 cm in length. Here the lymph is filtered, foreign substances are trapped and destroyed, and lymphocytes are produced that combat infection and disease. The efferent vessels leaving the nodes join to form lymphatic trunks. These empty into two main ducts:

- **the thoracic duct**, which receives lymph from the left arm, left side of the head and chest and all the body below the ribs, then empties into the left subclavian vein
- **the right lymphatic duct**, which receives lymph from the right upper quarter of the body, i.e. the right arm, right side of head and chest, then empties into the right subclavian vein.

In this way, the lymph is transported from the tissue spaces back to the blood. Any malfunction or blockage of the lymphatic system will result in swelling of the tissues known as **oedema**.

The speed at which lymph flows through the system depends on many factors, for example the contraction and relaxation of muscles help its return, as do negative pressure and movement of the chest during respiration. Exercise is therefore very important in aiding the flow of lymph. Areas of stasis and oedema can be improved by moving the joints and exercising the muscles of the swollen area. The volume of lymph passing into the capillaries and vessels depends on the pressure inside and outside the vessels.

Massage is very effective at speeding up the flow of lymph in the lymphatic vessels and thereby increasing the drainage of tissue fluid. Long effleurage strokes exert pressure and push the lymph along in the vessels towards the nearest set of lymphatic nodes (remember always move towards the nearest set of lymphatic nodes). The pressure (petrissage) manipulations squeeze the tissues. This pressure increases the amount of tissue fluid passing into the vessels to be drained away.

Functions of the lymphatic system

The lymphatic system:

- drains tissue fluid from the spaces between cells.
- transports this tissue fluid and proteins to subclavian veins and so returns it back into the blood.
- transports fats from the small intestine to the blood.
- produces lymphocytes, which protect and defend the body against infection and disease.
- filters and removes broken-down foreign substances and waste from the nodes.

Effects of massage on the lymphatic system

- The flow of lymph in the lymphatic vessels is speeded up. As the hands move along in the direction of lymph drainage to the nearest group of lymphatic nodes, the speed of lymph flow is increased. Massage strokes should always be directed towards the nearest set of lymphatic nodes.
- Pressure on the tissues will facilitate the transfer of fluid across vessel walls. Fluid from the tissues will pass into the lymphatic vessels and will drain away more quickly: this will prevent or reduce oedema (swelling of the tissues).
- Larger particles of waste that are able to pass through the lymphatic vessel walls are removed more quickly.

The pressure and squeezing movements of petrissage are the most effective in reducing oedema, followed by effleurage. This effect is assisted if the part is elevated while being massaged, as gravity will assist drainage. Treatment of oedema using massage is described in Chapter 6.

The respiratory system

This system is responsible for the exchange of oxygen and carbon dioxide between the external environment and the internal environment of the body. It is closely linked with the cardiovascular system, as the exchange of gases takes place between the alveoli of the lungs and the blood in the pulmonary capillaries.

The system is composed of the:

- nose and nasal passages
- pharynx
- larynx
- trachea
- bronchi and bronchioles
- lungs, which are composed of alveoli.

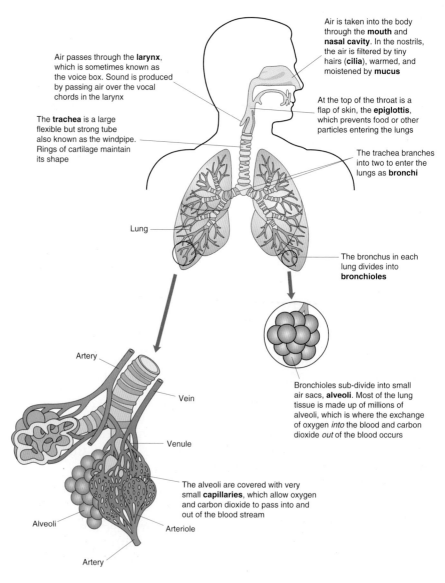

Air passes through the **larynx**, which is sometimes known as the voice box. Sound is produced by passing air over the vocal chords in the larynx

The **trachea** is a large flexible but strong tube also known as the windpipe. Rings of cartilage maintain its shape

Air is taken into the body through the **mouth** and **nasal cavity**. In the nostrils, the air is filtered by tiny hairs (**cilia**), warmed, and moistened by **mucus**

At the top of the throat is a flap of skin, the **epiglottis**, which prevents food or other particles entering the lungs

The trachea branches into two to enter the lungs as **bronchi**

Lung

The bronchus in each lung divides into **bronchioles**

Bronchioles sub-divide into small air sacs, **alveoli**. Most of the lung tissue is made up of millions of alveoli, which is where the exchange of oxygen *into* the blood and carbon dioxide *out* of the blood occurs

Artery

Vein

Venule

The alveoli are covered with very small **capillaries**, which allow oxygen and carbon dioxide to pass into and out of the blood stream

Alveoli

Arteriole

Artery

Figure 2.35 The respiratory system

The nose

The nose serves as the first section of the passageway for air going into the lungs. It is also the organ of smell, as the olfactory receptors are located in the nose. The inner lining of the nose is a ciliated mucous membrane with a rich supply of blood vessels. It has two functions:

- to filter the air as it enters the system – the tiny hairs trap organisms and dust particles, preventing their entry into the lungs
- to moisten and warm the air as it passes through.

The pharynx

Both the respiratory and digestive tracts share the pharynx, as both air and food pass through this passageway. The tonsils are located here.

The larynx

This is the voice box, which lies between the pharynx and the trachea. It is composed of cartilages and smooth muscle tissue. The larynx plays a part in respiration, speech and swallowing. Air passes through the larynx to the trachea: the passage of air over the vocal chords causes them to vibrate, producing sound. Between the base of the tongue and the upper opening of the larynx lies the **epiglottis**. This covers the larynx during the swallowing of food, protecting and shutting off the airway to prevent food entering.

The trachea

This is a tube about 11 centimetres long and 2.5 centimetres in diameter, which extends from the larynx to the bronchi. It is composed of smooth muscle with C-shaped bands of cartilage at regular intervals along its length. These cartilaginous bands prevent the walls of the trachea from collapsing inwards. The function of the trachea is to maintain a permanently open pathway to the lungs. Any obstruction of this vital airway, even for a few minutes, will result in asphyxia (suffocation) and death.

The bronchi

The trachea eventually divides into two primary bronchi:

- the right bronchus leads into the right lung
- the left bronchus leads into the left lung.

In structure, each bronchus is similar to the trachea, being composed of smooth muscle with C-shaped rings of cartilage at intervals along its length. As the bronchi enter the lungs they further subdivide into smaller secondary bronchi and then into even smaller bronchioles. The bronchioles further divide into minute tubes called alveolar ducts, which terminate in sponge-like sacs called alveoli.

The lungs

The left and right lungs are cone-shaped organs that extend from their base on the diaphragm below, to their apex above the clavicles. They lie within the thoracic cavity protected by the ribs and the sternum. The left lung is composed of two lobes and the right lung is composed of three lobes. They are covered by the visceral pleura containing serous fluid, which reduces friction and facilitates movement of the lungs during breathing. The lungs are composed of the tubes of the bronchial tree and the numerous sponge-like alveoli. The alveoli are surrounded by dense capillary networks.

The function of the lungs is to provide a large surface area where the inspired air can come into close contact with the blood, thus facilitating the rapid exchange of gases. This exchange takes place across the alveoli pulmonary capillary interface. Oxygen from inspired air diffuses through the walls of the alveoli, through the walls of the surrounding capillary networks, into the blood to be transported around the body to the tissue cells. Carbon dioxide from tissue cells is carried via the blood to the lungs. Here it diffuses through the capillary walls then through the walls of the alveoli to be expired out of the lungs.

> **Learning point**
> Diffusion is the movement of molecules across a permeable membrane.

Ventilation

Ventilation is the movement of air in and out of the lungs. Ventilation is brought about by the contraction of the skeletal muscles, which expands the thorax. The muscles involved are the diaphragm and the intercostal muscles that lie between the ribs. Ventilation is composed of *two* phases: **inspiration**, taking air into the lungs and **expiration**, expelling air out of the lungs.

During inspiration:

- The external intercostal muscles contract, swinging the ribs outwards and upwards.
- The sternum is pushed forward.
- The diaphragm contracts.
- This increases the volume of the thoracic cavity, causing the pressure within to drop below atmospheric pressure, sucking air into the lungs.

During expiration:

- The external intercostal muscles relax, allowing ribs to return to normal.
- The sternum drops back.
- The diaphragm relaxes.
- This decreases the volume of the thoracic cavity, causing the pressure to be higher in the lungs than atmospheric pressure, forcing air out of the lungs.

> **Learning point**
> When the diaphragm is relaxed, it is dome-shaped. When it contracts, it flattens. Hiccoughs are the result of involuntary spasms of the diaphragm, rapidly sucking air into the lungs.

Effects of massage on the respiratory system

The air passages are lined with a mucous membrane that continuously secretes a small quantity of mucus. This moistens the tubes and traps any organisms and particles in the inspired air. Any irritation of this membrane will result in an increase in the production of mucus. This mucus may thicken and become difficult to remove through coughing. Shaking and vibration manipulations performed over the chest can help to loosen these secretions so that they can be coughed up more easily. Deep breathing exercises will also help to move the mucus. See also Chapter 6.

The digestive system

The digestive system is concerned with the intake, breakdown and absorption of food substances. Carbohydrates, fats (lipids) and proteins are broken down into small molecules that can pass through the walls of the digestive tract into the bloodstream and then into body cells. Here they are used for energy, growth and repair of tissues.

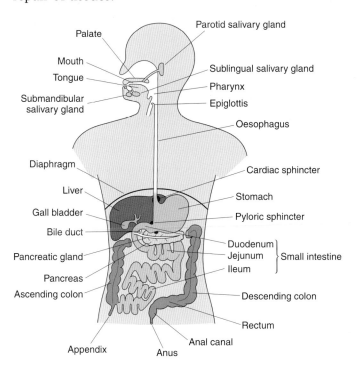

Figure 2.36 The digestive system

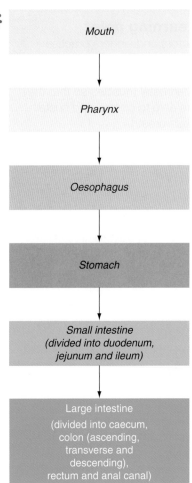

Figure 2.37 Route of the gastro-intestinal tract

The digestive system can be divided into two main parts: the gastro-intestinal tract and the accessory structures.

The **gastro-intestinal tract** or alimentary canal is a tube approximately 7m in length. It starts at the mouth and ends at the anus. The parts of the gastro-intestinal tract are shown in Figure 2.37.

Accessory structures and organs connect with the tract and play an important role in the digestive process. They are the

- teeth
- tongue
- salivary glands
- gall bladder
- pancreas
- liver.

Substances move along the tract by a series of muscle contractions known as **peristalsis**. Massage stimulates peristalsis and also aids the movement through the tract.

The digestive processes

The activities of the digestive system can be divided into four processes:

- **Ingestion**: taking food into the body.
- **Digestion**: the breaking down of food, which involves two processes:
  - *mechanical* breakdown by chewing and movements of the tract that churns the food
  - *chemical* breakdown by enzymes secreted into the tract at various stages, e.g. saliva from salivary glands in the mouth; gastric juices in the stomach; pancreatic juice from the pancreas; bile from the gall bladder; intestinal juice in the small intestine.
- **Absorption**: the process by which digested food passes out of the tract into blood vessels and lymphatic capillaries and into cells.
- **Elimination**: the passage of waste substances out of the body.

Digestion involves all the processes that break down and convert the food we eat into substances that can be absorbed and used by the body.

Food is broken down *mechanically* into minute particles and *chemically* into smaller molecules that are more easily absorbed. These changes begin as soon as food is taken into the mouth and continue through the gastro-intestinal tract until the processes of ingestion, digestion, absorption and elimination have been completed. The movement of food through the digestive system is by **peristalsis**: this is a wave-like contraction of the circular muscles in the wall of the intestines.

The mouth

Food is taken into the mouth (ingestion), where the process of digestion begins. When the food is chewed (mastication), the teeth mechanically break down food into small particles.

The salivary glands produce saliva, which pours into the mouth. This contains the enzyme **amylase** (ptyalin), which begins the *chemical conversion* of starch into simple sugars. The food is moistened by the saliva and rolled by the tongue into a round ball called a **bolus**.

This is swallowed and passes through the pharynx into the oesophagus. It moves down the oesophagus by the wave-like contraction and relaxation of the muscles. This is known as **peristalsis**.

The stomach

This is a J-shaped sac that provides a reservoir for food and continues its breakdown. There are sphincter muscles at the entrance and exit of the stomach that open and close to control the food coming in and passing out: the **cardiac sphincter** at the entrance and the **pyloric sphincter** at the exit. Food can be held in the stomach for up to five hours while it is being digested.

The churning action of the stomach *mechanically* breaks the food down. The stomach produces gastric juices that break food down *chemically*.

The gastric juices include:

- **pepsin**, which begins the chemical breakdown of protein to amino acids
- **hydrochloric acid**, which aids digestion and destroys any ingested bacteria.

This mixture of partially digested food in the stomach is known as **chyme**. Very little **absorption** of food takes place in the stomach apart from water, alcohol and some drugs such as aspirin.

The small intestine

The small intestine is composed of three parts: the **duodenum**, the **jejunum** and the **ileum**.

After the contents of the stomach are thoroughly churned, the chyme passes into the first part of the small intestine called the duodenum. In the duodenum, **bile** formed in the liver (and stored in the gall bladder) enters the tract to begin emulsifying (breaking down) fats into fatty acids.

Pancreatic juice from the pancreas also enters here, containing enzymes that further break down starches, proteins and fats. These enzymes are:

- **amylase**, which breaks down starch
- **trypsin**, which breaks down proteins
- **lipase**, which emulsifies fats.

The juices from the mucous membrane lining the wall of the small intestine, containing **lactose, maltose** and **sucrose,** further break down sugars into **glucose**. The walls of the small intestine are lined with finger-like projections called **villi** that greatly increase the surface area, for **absorption** to take place. Each **villus** (singular) contains a network of blood and lymphatic capillaries. The digested, broken-down food products pass through the walls of the villi into the blood capillaries and hence into the bloodstream. Some fatty acids are absorbed into the lymphatic system and then returned in the lymph into the blood circulation via the thoracic duct.

The products that are not absorbed move on to the large intestine as waste.

The large intestine

This is divided into three parts: the **ascending colon,** which passes upwards on the right side of the abdomen; the **transverse colon,** which runs horizontally across the top of the abdomen and the **descending colon,** which passes downwards on the left side of the abdomen. This ends in the rectum and anus.

The colon reabsorbs water from the waste material as it passes through. Healthy bacteria in the colon also help to synthesise vitamins B and K. The colon forms the waste into faeces, which are stored in the rectum until they are **eliminated** through the anus.

Effects of massage on the digestive system

- Abdominal massage stimulates peristalsis and the movement of digested food through the colon.
- Massage may be helpful to relieve constipation and flatulence.

The nervous system

The nervous system is the communication and control system of the body. It works with the endocrine system to maintain homeostasis (body balance). The nervous system will sense changes inside and outside the body, interpret them and initiate appropriate action. The nervous system is made up of:

- the **central nervous system,** comprising the brain and spinal cord
- the **peripheral nervous system,** comprising 12 pairs of cranial nerves arising from the brain and 31 pairs of spinal nerves arising from the spinal cord
- the **autonomic system**.

The peripheral nerves carry impulses inwards from sensory receptors in sense organs to the brain. They also carry impulses from the brain to muscles and glands.

> **Remember**
> The ascending colon is on the right side of the person whose colon it is, not on the right as you look at their body. It can be confusing when you are used to looking at diagrams showing a supine body.

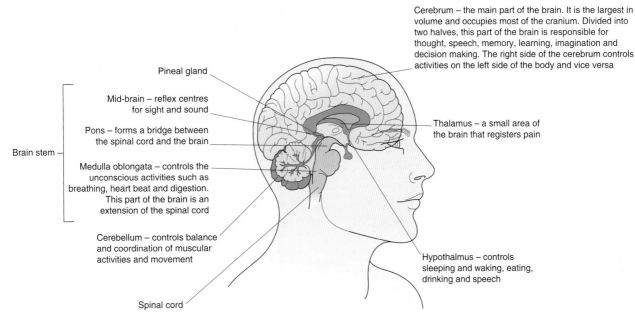

Cerebrum – the main part of the brain. It is the largest in volume and occupies most of the cranium. Divided into two halves, this part of the brain is responsible for thought, speech, memory, learning, imagination and decision making. The right side of the cerebrum controls activities on the left side of the body and vice versa

Pineal gland

Mid-brain – reflex centres for sight and sound

Pons – forms a bridge between the spinal cord and the brain

Brain stem

Medulla oblongata – controls the unconscious activities such as breathing, heart beat and digestion. This part of the brain is an extension of the spinal cord

Cerebellum – controls balance and coordination of muscular activities and movement

Spinal cord

Thalamus – a small area of the brain that registers pain

Hypothalmus – controls sleeping and waking, eating, drinking and speech

Figure 2.38 Principal parts of the brain

Nervous tissue is composed of functional units called **neurons**, which conduct impulses, and the supporting tissue called **neuroglia**.

There are three types of neuron:

- **sensory** neurons, which transmit stimuli *from* sensory organs *to* the spinal cord and brain. They convey sensations of pain, pressure, temperature, taste, sight, etc.

- **motor** neurons, which transmit stimuli *from* the brain and spinal cord *to* muscles and glands. They initiate the contraction of muscles and the action of glands.

- **interneurons**, which form connections *between* neurons. They convey impulses from one neuron to another.

Structure of a neuron

All neurons have a similar structure: they have a **cell body**, one long nerve fibre called an **axon** and several short nerve fibres called **dendrites**.

Axons carry impulses *away* from the cell body; dendrites carry impulses *towards* the cell body.

The nerve impulse

When receptors or sense organs are stimulated, an impulse is initiated that is transmitted along the sensory nerve towards the spinal cord and brain.

The brain then decides upon the corrective action and initiates impulses that are transmitted along the motor nerves to appropriate muscles or glands. Impulses are transmitted in axons and

Learning point

An easy way to remember this is that <u>a</u>xons and <u>a</u>way both start with A; den<u>t</u>ri<u>t</u>es and <u>t</u>owards both have **T** sounds in them.

dendrites in one direction only, as shown in Figure 2.39. More than one neuron will be involved in the transmission of a nerve impulse and the point at which the impulse passes from one neuron to another is called a synapse.

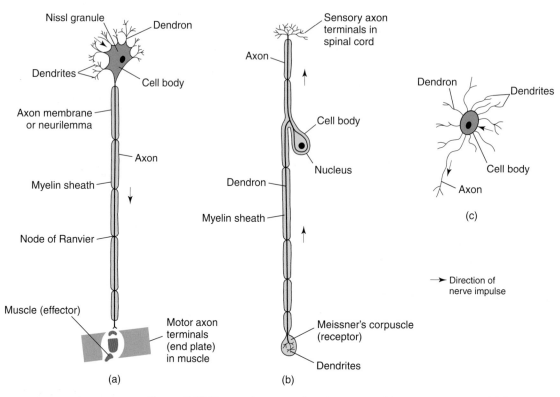

Figure 2.39 Types of neuron: a) motor neuron, b) sensory neuron, c) interneuron

Synapses

A synapse is known as a nerve-to-nerve junction. It is the point where two neurons connect. The neurons do not make direct contact: there is a gap between them called a **synaptic cleft**. The nerve impulse must be transmitted across this gap. Chemicals called neurotransmitters conduct the impulses across the gap. These chemicals may facilitate the passage of the impulse or they may inhibit the passage of the impulse:

- acetylcholine (Ach) facilitates the passage of an impulse.
- gamma-aminobutyric acid (GABA) inhibits the passage of an impulse.

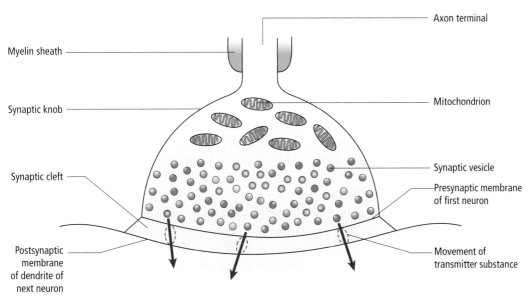

Myelin sheath

Synaptic knob

Synaptic cleft

Postsynaptic
membrane
of dendrite of
next neuron

Axon terminal

Mitochondrion

Synaptic vesicle

Presynaptic membrane
of first neuron

Movement of
transmitter substance

Figure 2.40 The conduction of a nerve impulse across a synapse

Nerve-to-muscle junction

The point at which a nerve connects with its muscle fibre is known as the **neuro-muscular junction**, which is very similar to a synapse. The impulse is transmitted across the gap from the axon end of the nerve to the **motor end plate** on the muscle fibre, by the chemical transmitter acetylcholine.

Receptors

The nervous system has millions of receptors, which are the distal ends of the dendrites of the sensory nerves. These receptors detect changes in the external and internal environment. All sensations are felt through the stimulation of these receptors. In response to these stimuli, nerve impulses are initiated and transmitted along the nerve to the spinal cord and brain, where they are interpreted and the appropriate responses selected.

The main groups of receptors are:

- **exteroceptors**. There are many types, which tend to lie on the surface of the body: they detect changes in the external environment. They are found in skin, mucous membranes, and register cold, heat, touch, pressure, pain etc. Highly specialised ones are found in the eye and ear for sight and sound. Those in the skin include **Meissner's corpuscles**, which sense light touch, **Merkel's discs** sense touch and stretch, and **Pacinian corpuscles** sense deep pressure.

- **interoceptors** or **visceroceptors**. These lie internally and detect changes in the internal environment. They are found in the internal organs such as the intestine, stomach, liver, kidneys etc and in the walls of blood vessels. These register changes in the internal organs.

> ### Learning point
> If the receptors register cold, these stimuli are conducted to the brain, where they are interpreted and the brain sends impulses to stimulate muscles to contract rapidly: this produces body heat, which we know as shivering.

- **proprioceptors.** These are located in muscles, tendons and joints and register the degree of stretch or tension in a muscle, while others provide information of joint position and the spatial location of body parts.

Reflexes

There are many types of physiological reflex resulting in responses, such as coughing, sneezing, blinking: these are involuntary actions (not under conscious control).

Reflex action

A reflex action is a rapid involuntary response to a stimulus. When a rapid response to a particular stimulus is required the impulses do not always ascend to the brain, they simply enter the spinal cord, where an automatic response is initiated.

A reflex arc

This is the pathway taken by an impulse, from the sensory receptors in the skin, along the sensory nerve into the spinal cord, via an interneuron and along the motor nerve to the muscles, which contract in response.

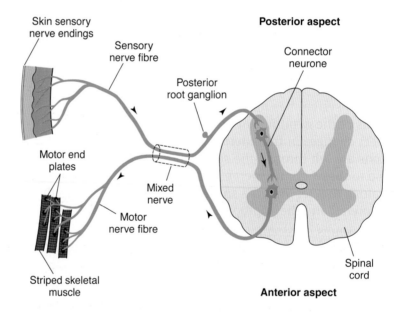

Figure 2.41 A simple three-neuron reflex arc

Example: If a hot object is touched, the sensory nerve endings in the skin register something hot and the flexor muscles of the arm will contract to withdraw the hand.

Pain

Palpation or massage of the tissues may produce pain. The pain may be in the exact location of the problem and may be due to increased tension in the underlying tissues, or it may be referred from another area. Problems affecting internal organs may refer tension and pain to an area of skin and subcutaneous tissue where the sensory fibres share the same spinal segment as the nerve supply of the affected organ. Specific neuromuscular techniques over that area will produce an automatic reflex response in the affected organ. Tension points or nodules that become chronic can develop into trigger points. These may lie deep within a muscle but may refer pain to another area called the target zone, which shares the same nerve pathway.

The autonomic system

The autonomic system consists of two parts: the **sympathetic** and the **parasympathetic** parts, which exercise involuntary control of smooth muscle, cardiac muscle, and glands. The sympathetic system has similar effects on the body as those produced by the hormones adrenaline and noradrenaline: they bring about physiological changes that help the body to cope quickly under conditions of stress, the fight and flight reaction. Stimulation of the sympathetic system tends to speed up processes while stimulation of the parasympathetic system tends to slow things down. The systems work together to maintain a stable internal environment.

Sympathetic	Parasympathetic
Stimulation of this system includes the following changes	**Stimulation of this system balances the effect of the sympathetic system**
The heart rate and strength of contraction increases	Slows the heart rate and decreases the strength of contraction
The coronary arteries dilate, increasing the blood supply to the heart	Constricts coronary arteries, decreasing the blood supply to the heart
Stimulates the release of adrenaline and noradrenaline from the Adrenal medulla	No effect
The blood supply to the organs of digestion decreases thus providing more blood for skeletal muscle contraction	Increases blood supply to the digestive system and stimulates peristalsis
The rate of respiration, oxygen consumption and carbon dioxide output increases	Reduces the rate of respiration and oxygen consumption
Increase in the rate of conversion of glycogen in the liver, making more glucose available for energy	Increases the secretion of bile
Increase in the quantity of sweat excreted, with increased heat loss	No effect
The pupils dilate giving a wide-eyed look	Constricts the pupils

Table 2.4 Effects of sympathetic and parasympathetic nervous systems

During massage, the sensory receptors in the skin convey impulses of touch and pressure to the central nervous system. If pressure is too light it can be irritating, if it is too deep or uneven it may be irritating or painful. Muscles then respond with increased tension. Slow, rhythmical, deep massage has a soothing effect on the nerve endings, promoting relaxation.

Effects of massage on the nervous system

- Slow, rhythmical massage produces a soothing, sedative effect on sensory nerve endings, promoting general relaxation.
- Vigorous brisk massage will have a stimulating effect, producing feelings of vigour and glow. Light hacking on either side of the vertebral column is particularly effective.
- If massage technique is poor or too heavy, the pain sensors in the skin will be stimulated. Painful manipulations will increase tension, which is counter-productive, and care must be taken to avoid this. Similarly, if movements are too light, i.e. barely touching the skin or tickling, this will have an irritating effect that will also increase tension and must be avoided.

The urinary system

The urinary system is *one* of the excretory systems of the body.

The body takes in food, liquid and air, all of which are necessary for the metabolic activities of cells that sustain life. These metabolic processes release waste substances that must be eliminated from the body.

Excretory organs

- The excretory organs of the body are the kidneys, skin, lungs and large intestine.
- The kidneys form urine, which passes to the bladder and is excreted through urination.
- The skin eliminates water and mineral salts through perspiration.
- The large intestine eliminates waste from digested food through defecation.
- The lungs eliminate carbon dioxide and water vapour through exhalation.

The urinary system is made up of:

- two **kidneys**, which filter the blood and form urine
- two **ureters**: two tubes that carry urine from the kidneys to the bladder
- the **bladder**: a hollow sac where urine is stored until it is excreted
- the **urethra**: a tube that carries the urine from the bladder out of the body.

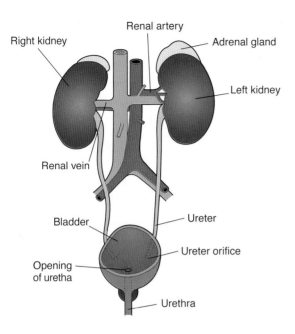

Figure 2.42 The urinary system (top of bladder removed to show openings)

The kidneys

The kidneys are bean-shaped organs, approximately 10cm in length. They are situated on the posterior wall of the abdominal cavity and lie on either side of the spine at the level between the twelfth thoracic and the third lumbar vertebrae. Their medial surface is concave and have an indentation or notch called the **hilum**. They are covered and held in place by fibrous connective tissue and protected by adipose tissue (fat), which insulates and protects the kidneys.

Blood is brought to the kidneys via the renal artery and taken away via the renal vein. These vessels enter the kidney at the hilum, together with the nerves and lymphatic vessels. One ureter leaves each kidney at the hilum and leads into the bladder.

The kidneys are composed of three distinct layers:

- a tough fibrous outer layer or **capsule** that encases and protects the kidney
- the **cortex**, which lies in the middle, and is dark red in colour
- the **medulla**, which is the inner layer, and is reddish brown in colour.

Each kidney is made up of over a million functional units called **nephrons**, where the kidney processes of **filtration** and **selective reabsorption** occur.

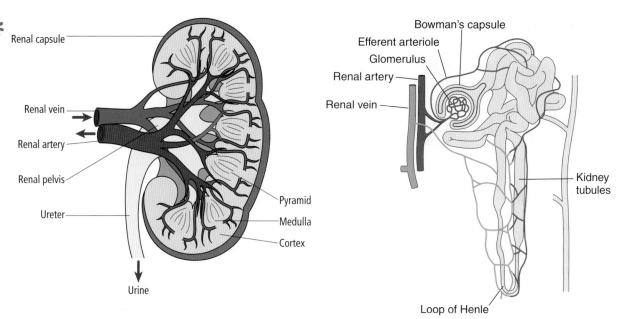

Figure 2.43 Structure of a kidney

Figure 2.44 The nephron

Blood entering the kidney via the renal artery passes into fine capillary networks, which surround the tubules of the nephrons. The first phase of kidney function is the **filtration** of substances from the capillary blood into the kidney. These substances pass from the blood in the glomerulus into the Bowman's capsule of the kidney: they include water, mineral salts, glucose, toxins, uric acid and urea. These pass through the tubules to be eliminated but some substances are reabsorbed if the body needs them.

The substances to be eliminated from the body form urine and include the waste products of protein metabolism, i.e. urea, uric acid, ammonia; toxins; certain mineral salts and some water. These substances pass along the tubules into the ureters and bladder to be eliminated.

Other substances, needed by the body, are reabsorbed into the bloodstream. These substances pass from the kidney tubules back into the capillary blood: this is known as **selective reabsorption**. Most of the water, all of the glucose, some sodium ions and vitamin C are reabsorbed into the blood. Hormones regulate the reabsorption of water and sodium depending on body requirements.

Through these functions of filtration and reabsorption, the kidneys adjust the balance of water, sodium ions and other substances leaving the body, with those entering the body. In this way the kidneys regulate the composition and volume of blood and maintain a stable internal environment for the tissues, known as **homeostasis**.

Functions of the kidneys

The functions of the kidneys are as follows:

- formation of urine
- elimination of toxic waste substances that are harmful to the body
- regulation of water balance in the body
- regulation of sodium level and other electrolytes
- maintenance of normal pH level of the blood
- influence blood pressure.

These functions maintain homeostasis and are vital for sustaining life: kidney failure will result in death if not rectified.

Kidney dialysis

This is a treatment for maintaining life if the kidneys fail to function. The patient is connected to a machine that circulates their blood through special tubing, which is immersed in dialysing fluid that contains prescribed substances necessary for treatment. Any unwanted or harmful substances are removed from the blood and its constituents are balanced. The procedure must be carried out at regular intervals to sustain life.

The ureters

The right and left ureters are two tubes extending from the kidneys to the bladder. The upper end opens out into a funnel called the renal pelvis, where the urine is collected. The ureter leaves the hilum of the kidney, and its lower end enters the posterior surface of the bladder. There is a small valve at this entrance to the bladder that shuts to prevent the backward flow of urine when the bladder is full.

The walls of the ureters are composed of three coats:

- an *inner lining* of mucous membrane,
- a *middle coat* made of two layers of smooth muscle,
- an *outer fibrous* coat.

Urine is collected from the kidney and moved along the ureters by peristalsis (wave-like contractions of the muscle wall) to the bladder.

The bladder

The bladder is a muscular sac that acts as a reservoir for the urine. Its walls are composed of three layers of smooth muscle lined with a mucous membrane. The bladder is capable of distension, which occurs as the bladder fills. **Stretch receptors** in the bladder wall stimulate an awareness that the bladder needs to be emptied and also initiate a reflex contraction of the bladder. At the same time there is a reflex relaxation of the internal sphincter followed by relaxation of the external sphincter, and

> **Learning point**
> A kidney transplant will offer the chance of near normal life to those fortunate enough to receive one. Unfortunately, there are not enough kidneys available to meet the demand. Many people choose to carry donor cards, offering their organs in the event of their death.

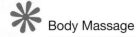
the bladder empties. The passage of urine through the urethra, known as **micturition**, occurs when the two sphincters controlling the opening relax.

It is possible to control the passage of urine out of the urethra by voluntary contraction of the external sphincter. The ability to exercise this control will diminish if there is nerve damage, or the sphincter muscle is weak: voluntary control is lost and urine leaks out of the urethra. The leakage is worse if abdominal pressure is increased, as in coughing or laughing. This involuntary passage of urine is known as urinary incontinence. Many women suffer from this condition especially after childbirth when the pelvic floor muscles are stretched, or with ageing when the muscles lose tone. This condition can be helped and these women should be encouraged to seek medical advice.

Effects of massage on the urinary system

Massage movements, and in particular abdominal massage, will improve the circulation to the kidney and may slightly increase the output of urine and hence the elimination of toxins.

Precautions

Heavy percussion manipulations should not be performed over the area of the kidneys, as there is a risk of damage.

When massaging the abdomen, too heavy a pressure over the bladder area can be uncomfortable.

Pain in the lower thoracic and lumbar region radiating around to the abdomen on one side may indicate a kidney problem. If you are unsure of the cause of pain in this loin region, seek medical advice.

Make sure that the client empties the bladder before treatment, as it is impossible to relax if the bladder is full.

The endocrine system

The endocrine system is made up of separate glands located in different parts of the body. Each gland makes chemical substances called hormones, which regulate and influence body processes such as growth, development, metabolism, reproduction and responses to stress.

The endocrine system and the nervous system control and co-ordinate body functions and maintain the body's internal balanced state (**homeostasis**).

Endocrine glands are known as ductless glands because the hormones they secrete pour directly into the bloodstream (unlike exocrine glands, which pass their secretions into ducts, e.g. sebaceous glands).

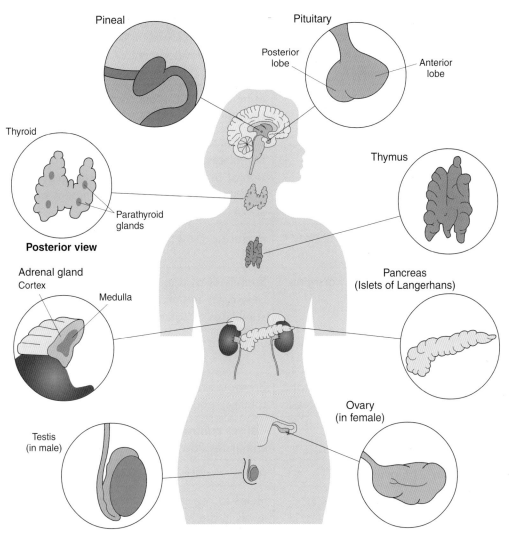

Figure 2.45 The endocrine system

Hormones are known as 'chemical messengers'. They are released from the gland and carried by the bloodstream to their target organs. One gland may produce a number of different hormones that influence and control the activities of many organs. The responses in the target organ are usually slow and continue over a long period of time. Some endocrine glands control the function of other endocrine glands.

The **pituitary gland** controls the function of other glands and because of this it is known as the **'master gland'**.

Gland	Location	Hormone	Function
Pituitary (anterior)	Cranium under the brain	ACTH (Adrenocorticotropin)	Promotes development of the adrenal cortex; helps in conditions of stress
		Thyroid-stimulating hormone (TSH) or thyrotropin	Stimulates the thyroid to produce thyroxine
		Follicle-stimulating hormone (FSH)	Stimulates growth and oestrogen production of ovarian follicles; stimulates growth of testes; promotes the development of sperm
		Growth hormone (GH)	Promotes growth of all body tissues
		Luteinising hormone (LH)	Stimulates ovaries and the production of oestrogen and progesterone in females; stimulates testosterone in males
		Prolactin (lactogenic hormone)	Stimulates secretion of milk by the breasts
Pituitary (posterior)	Base of the brain	Antidiuretic hormone (ADH) or Vasopressin	Promotes reabsorption of water in kidney tubules; reduces volume of urine
		Oxytocin	Causes contraction of pregnant uterus; stimulates flow of milk from breasts;
Adrenal cortex	Above the upper end of the kidney	Cortisol	Aids in metabolism; active to reduce stress
		Aldosterone	Helps to regulate sodium and potassium levels in the blood
		Sex hormones	Contribute to the secondary sexual characteristics in males and females
Adrenal medulla	Above the upper end of each kidney	Adrenaline, Noradrenaline	Stimulates smooth and cardiac muscle; increases BMR, blood pressure and heart rate; prepares for 'fight and flight'
Pancreas (Islets of Langerhans)	Below the stomach	Insulin	Helps the transport of glucose into cells; decreases blood sugar levels
		Glucagon	Increases blood sugar levels
Parathyroid	In the throat in front of the trachea	Parathormone (PTH) or Parathyroid hormone	Increases calcium level in blood
Thyroid	In the throat in front of the trachea	Thyroxine	Regulates metabolic rate, growth and development of tissues
		Calcitonin	Decreases calcium level in blood

Table 2.5 Classification of endocrine glands

Gland	Location	Hormone	Function
Ovaries (Ovarian)	Each side of the uterus	Oestrogen	Stimulates the growth of sexual organs, e.g. uterus, breasts, etc
Corpus luteum	In the ovaries	Progesterone	Stimulates the development of the breasts; helps in maintaining pregnancy
Testes	In the scrotum	Testosterone	Stimulates development of sexual organs; hair growth on the body and face; maturation of sperm cells
Thymus	Behind the sternum	Thymosin	Stimulates the production of antibodies by lymphocytes
Pineal	In the brain	Melatonin	Stimulated by darkness; affects body rhythms

Table 2.5 *Continued*

Under normal conditions the amount of hormone produced and secreted by the glands is carefully regulated by the nervous system. Under- or over-production of a hormone can result in a number of endocrine disorders.

Effects of massage on the endocrine system

- The increase in blood circulation helps in the transport of hormones to target organs.
- Massage helps to reduce secretion of the hormone adrenaline, the body's 'fight or flight' response to stress.
- It helps to reduce secretion of cortisol, the hormone responsible for the body's long-term stress response. High levels of this hormone can have a negative effect on the body e.g. higher blood pressure and low immunity.
- A relaxing massage can stimulate the parasympathetic nervous system by slowing down the heart rate, increasing peristalsis and relaxing tense muscles.

The reproductive system

The reproductive system is the only body system that has a different structure, as well as some differences in function, in men and in women. It is also the only system that does not function continually from birth. Instead, it is activated at puberty and, in women, it changes again at menopause, when its reproductive function ceases. Its principal function is the creation of new life, but there are other associated functions, such as the production of the hormones that determine male and female characteristics. Unlike the other body systems, it is not a necessity for the maintenance of life of an individual, but it is necessary to ensure the survival of the species.

Reproduction involves the gonads (sex glands) of the male and female, and takes place when an ovum (egg) from the woman is fertilised by a sperm cell from the man. This generally takes place through sexual intercourse, although some fertility treatments involve artificial fertilisation in laboratories.

The male reproductive system

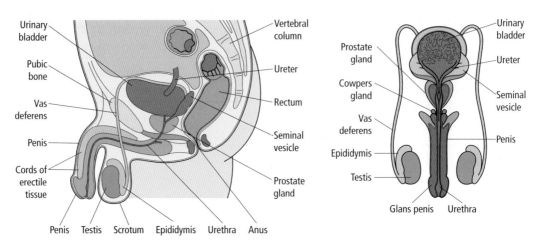

Figure 2.46 The male reproductive system

The parts of the reproductive system in men are:

- the testes, where sperm cells are produced
- the epididymis, where sperm is stored until it has matured
- the vas deferens, a tube through which sperm travels to the urethra
- the urethra, a tube which releases sperm (in the form of semen), as well as excreting urine
- the penis, the external sex organ through which semen is ejaculated and urine excreted.

The testes

The testes are a pair of oval-shaped glands; the male gonads. They hang outside the body in the scrotum or scrotal sac, a bag of skin, which helps to keep the temperature of the testes below body temperature. The production of sperm cells is hampered by overheating. The testes also produce male sex hormones called **androgens**. The most important of these is **testosterone**. Testosterone is responsible for the secondary sexual characteristics of the male, which develop at puberty. These characteristics include the growth and development of the male sex organs, growth of body and facial hair, the deepening of the voice and the broadening of the shoulders. Testosterone also affects sex drive (libido) and is linked to aggression.

Learning point
Androgens are also produced by women. In women they are produced in the adrenal cortex, not the gonads, and in smaller quantities than in men.

The epididymis

The **epididymus** is composed of tightly coiled tubes leading from each of the testes, where the sperm cells are produced. Sperm cells are stored here and nurtured to maturity. Mature sperm cells are propelled from the epididymis through peristalsis.

The vas deferens

The **vas deferens** is a long tube from the epididymis to the urethra, along which the sperm cells travel through peristalsis.

The seminal vesicles

The seminal vesicles are a pair of glands located behind the bladder, where semen is added to the sperm cells during ejaculation. **Semen** is an alkaline fluid, which helps to neutralise the acidity of the vagina. It contains nutrients to help the sperm generate energy, and prostaglandins which stimulate the vaginal walls to contract and aid the journey of the sperm.

The urethra

The urethra transports both semen and urine out of the body. A sphincter muscle at the base of the bladder prevents ejaculation of semen and excretion of urine from happening simultaneously.

The penis

The penis is composed of erectile tissue and many blood vessels. Sexual stimulation causes the blood vessels to dilate and fill with blood, which results in the penis becoming erect.

The female reproductive system

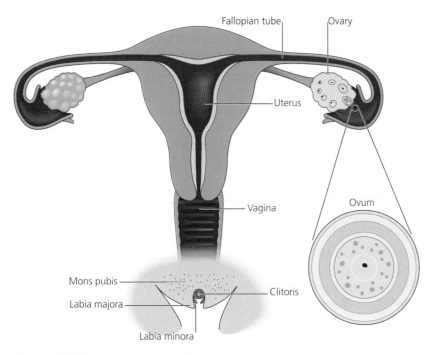

Figure 2.47 The female reproductive system

The parts of the reproductive system in women can be divided into internal and external.

The internal parts are:

- the **ovaries** (where ova (eggs) are produced)
- the **Fallopian tubes** (along which ova are carried to the uterus – fertilisation occurs in the Fallopian tubes)
- the **uterus** (a hollow, muscular organ in which the foetus will develop and grow)
- the **vagina** (a passageway from the uterus to the vulva, connecting the internal sex organs with the external sex organs).

The external parts, or genitalia, are known as the vulva and consist of:

- the **mons pubis** (fatty tissue covered by skin and coarse hair which protects the **pubis symphysis**)
- the **labia** (majora and minora) or outer and inner lips (fleshy folds that lie at the entrance to the vagina)
- the **clitoris** (a sensitive, conical organ composed of erectile tissue and nerve endings: like the penis, it responds to sexual stimulation and can become erect)
- the **hymen** (a thin membrane protecting the entrance to the vagina)
- the **vestibule** (the area between the labia minora, which contains the vaginal opening, the opening of the urethra and several mucus-producing glands which lubricate the vulva).

The ovaries

The **ovaries** are the female gonads: a pair of almond-shaped glands, located either side of the uterus towards the top of the pelvic cavity. They contain ovarian follicles, in which the ova develop. The ovarian follicle releases one ripened ovum each month from puberty until the menopause.

The ovaries also produce the female sex hormones oestrogen and progesterone. Oestrogen is responsible for the development of the female secondary sexual characteristics. These include the development of breasts, growth of body hair, widening of the hips and redistribution of adipose tissue over the abdomen. Progesterone, together with oestrogen, regulates the changes that occur to the uterus during a woman's menstrual cycle and leading up to and during pregnancy.

The Fallopian tubes

The **Fallopian tubes** carry the ovum from the ovary to the uterus by peristalsis. Fertilisation takes place in the Fallopian tube, when a single sperm cell penetrates the ovum to form a zygote. The zygote then travels down the Fallopian tube to the uterus.

Learning point

Girls are born with all the ovarian follicles they will produce in their lifetime already in their ovaries. By the time of puberty (which usually occurs between the ages of 12 and 14) girls will have many thousands of follicles. However, only about 400–500 of these will produce ova for fertilisation.

Learning point

Fertilisation can only occur within 24 hours of ovulation.

The uterus

The **uterus** is situated behind the bladder and in front of the rectum. It is composed of:

- an outer membrane
- a middle layer of muscle fibres
- an inner mucus membrane.

The muscles produce the strong contractions during labour, pushing the baby out along the vagina. The mucus membrane thickens each month in readiness for receiving a fertilised ovum; if fertilisation does not occur, the surface of the mucus membrane is shed. This is known as **menstruation**.

The uterus joins the vagina at the **cervix** – an area of fibrous muscle, which forms the narrow opening between the two. The cervix is capable of dilating to around 10cm during labour to allow the baby to pass through.

The vagina

The **vagina** is a muscular tube, which enables the passage of blood during menstruation, semen during sexual intercourse and the foetus during labour. It contains erectile tissue, which responds to sexual stimulation, causing the area to become engorged with blood. The muscles respond to prostaglandin in semen and contract rhythmically, aiding the transport of semen to the uterus. The walls of the vagina are able to expand to accommodate the foetus during childbirth.

Accessory reproductive organs

The breasts or **mammary glands** are referred to as accessory reproductive organs. They do not develop until puberty, when the release of oestrogen stimulates the secondary sexual characteristics. Their function is to provide milk for the baby, but they are not capable of producing milk (a process known as lactation) until the end of pregnancy. The breasts are composed of lobes, separated by adipose tissue. The lobes form into lobules, which contain milk-secreting cells. They are supported by ligaments, called Cooper's ligaments.

Processes of the female reproductive system

Menstruation

Menstruation takes place from puberty to menopause, approximately every 28 days. It is regulated by hormones that are produced in the pituitary gland: follicle-stimulating hormone (**FSH**) and luteinizing hormone (**LH**). The duration and frequency of menstruation varies from woman to woman, but usually lasts up to five days, when the lining of the womb breaks down and is shed. FSH is released to stimulate the development of the ovum. The lining of the womb starts to build up. Around the fourteenth day an ovum is released, ready to be fertilised. Hormones secreted cause the lining of the womb to thicken in readiness for a fertilised ovum. If the ovum is not fertilised it starts to degenerate and the resulting lack of oestrogen and progesterone causes the thickened lining of the womb to break down, when it will be expelled as menstrual flow. During menstruation many women suffer from fluid retention, mood swings and stomach cramps.

Pregnancy

Pregnancy begins with fertilisation and ends with birth. Typically, pregnancy lasts for 38 weeks. A baby's due date is calculated as 40 weeks from the last menstruation. A woman is fertile from puberty until the menopause. Some women experience back pain, nausea and tiredness during pregnancy.

Menopause

Menopause marks the end of a woman's ability to reproduce. It usually occurs between the ages of 45 and 55, but some women may have a much earlier or later menopause. Menstruation becomes less frequent and eventually stops completely; oestrogen and progesterone production reduces; the uterus shrinks and the ovaries thicken and harden so that no more ova are produced. The vagina loses elasticity and becomes drier. The lack of oestrogen affects the density of the bones, which can become thin and brittle, resulting in osteoporosis. Other physical symptoms may include hot flushes, loss of libido, sweating, hair loss, headaches, insomnia, weight gain, anxiety and mood swings.

Learning point

Ageing also has an effect on the male reproductive system. The production of testosterone reduces, which can lead to a loss of libido, the testes atrophy and soften and sperm production decreases. Male fertility, however, does not necessarily stop completely.

Effects of massage on the reproductive system

- The increase in blood circulation and lymphatic drainage can help to reduce fluid retention.
- During pregnancy a back massage can help to reduce pain in the lower back by bringing oxygen and nutrients to the muscles and removing waste products.
- Regular massage treatments for clients experiencing pre-menstrual tension, painful periods and menopausal symptoms will help to balance hormone levels in the body.

Psychological effects of massage

The psychological effects of massage must also be considered.

- It creates feelings of well-being and health.
- It promotes feelings of vigour and increases energy.
- It increases postural awareness.
- It promotes feelings of being cared for and cosseted, which in turn promote relaxation, contentment and satisfaction.
- It reduces mental stress, which also enhances feelings of contentment and relaxation.

Questions

CELLS AND TISSUES

1. Which of the following describes the levels of structural organisation of the body from the simplest to the most complex level?
   a. Tissue, cell, chemical, system, organ.
   b. Chemical, cell, tissue, organ, system.
   c. Cell, chemical, organ, system, tissue.
   d. System, organ, chemical, tissue, cell.

2. The outer boundary of the cell is the:
   a. intracellular
   b. cytoplasm
   c. extracellular
   d. plasma membrane.

3. The role of mitochondria in the cells is to:
   a. deal with waste products
   b. transport substances
   c. generate energy
   d. synthesise lipids.

4. The Golgi apparatus:
   a. contains the body's genetic material
   b. detoxifies chemicals
   c. moves molecules in and out of the nucleus
   d. produces proteins and lipids.

5. Simple squamous epithelium lines the:
   a. blood vessels
   b. stomach
   c. respiratory tract
   d. mouth.

6. The tissue that lines the bladder is:
   a. simple cubodial
   b. compound transitional
   c. simple columnar ciliated
   d. stratified squamous.

7. Which of the following covers the ends of bones at joints?
   a. Hyaline cartilage.
   b. Adipose tissue.
   c. Cancellous bone.
   d. Reticular tissue.

8. Skeletal muscle tissue:
   a. maintains the pumping action of the heart
   b. aids peristalsis
   c. produces heat
   d. lines the walls of the intestines.

9. The function of neuroglia is to:
   a. protect neurones
   b. clear neural pathways
   c. conduct impulses
   d. pick up stimuli.

10. The membrane that lines body tracts and opens directly to the exterior is:
    a. synovial
    b. mucous
    c. cutaneous
    d. serous.

INTEGUMENTARY SYSTEM

1. The strata of the skin from the deepest to most superficial are:
   a. lucidum, corneum, spinosum, granulosum, basale
   b. corneum, granulosum, spinosum, basale, lucidum
   c. spinosum, basale, granulosum, lucidum, corneum
   d. basale, spinosum, granulosum, lucidum, corneum.

2. Another term for 'cell division' is:
   a. papillae
   b. mitosis
   c. nucleus
   d. ribosomes.

3. Which layer of the skin is only found on the soles of the feet and the palms of the hands?
   a. Stratum lucidum.
   b. Stratum spinosum.

c. Stratum corneum.

    d. Stratum granulosum.

4. The acid mantle consists of:

    a. sweat and keratin.

    b. sebum and sweat.

    c. keratin and melanin.

    d. melanin and sebum.

5. The production of sebum is controlled by:

    a. blood flow

    b. neurones

    c. erector pili muscles

    d. hormones.

6. Histamine is produced by:

    a. mast cells

    b. plasma cells

    c. fibroblasts

    d. leucocytes.

7. Apocrine glands are found:

    a. on the scalp

    b. in the nostrils

    c. in the armpit

    d. on the face.

8. Vasoconstriction helps the body to:

    a. absorb substances

    b. regulate heat

    c. protect against infection

    d. produce sebum.

9. Adipocytes are found in the:

    a. subcutaneous layer

    b. papillary layer

    c. reticular layer

    d. stratum basale layer.

10. The chemical dehydrocholesterol in the skin helps to form:

    a. Vitamin A

    b. Vitamin B

    c. Vitamin D

    d. Vitamin E.

SKELETAL SYSTEM

1. The bones that form the axial skeleton include:

    a. humerus, skull, scapula

    b. ribs, hyoid, vertebral column

    c. sternum, clavicle, pelvic girdle

    d. skull, ribs, scapula.

2. The sutures of the skull are:

    a. cartilaginous joints

    b. gliding joints

    c. fibrous joints

    d. synovial joints.

3. How many sacral and coccygeal vertebrae are there in the spinal cord?

    a. 6.

    b. 7.

    c. 8.

    d. 9.

4. The mineral stored in bones is:

    a. phosphorus

    b. magnesium

    c. potassium

    d. sodium.

5. A function of yellow bone marrow is to:

    a. maintain levels of calcium

    b. strengthen bone tissue

    c. store lipids

    d. secrete salts to protect bones.

6. Red bone marrow produces:

    a. synovial fluid

    b. fats

    c. calcium

    d. blood cells.

7. The outer covering of bone is called:

    a. hyaline cartilage

    b. periosteum

    c. synovial membrane

    d. collagen.

8. An example of a hinge joint is the:

   a. knee joint

   b. wrist joint

   c. radio-ulnar joint

   d. intercarpal joint.

9. The atlas on axis joint is a:

   a. gliding joint

   b. ellipsoid joint

   c. saddle joint

   d. pivot joint.

10. The metatarsals are:

   a. long bones

   b. flat bones

   c. irregular bones

   d. short bones.

MUSCULAR SYSTEM

1. Skeletal muscle tissue is controlled by the:

   a. cardiovascular system

   b. skeletal system

   c. nervous system

   d. endocrine system.

2. Smooth muscle:

   a. causes peristalsis

   b. produces body heat

   c. maintains the posture

   d. pumps blood around the body.

3. The proteins actin and myosin in skeletal muscle are found in the:

   a. fasciculi

   b. myofibrils

   c. perimysium

   d. endomysium.

4. The function of tendons is to:

   a. increase the tone of muscles

   b. maintain the strength of bones

   c. protect organs

   d. attach muscles to bones.

5. The latissimus dorsi muscle is situated on the:

   a. arm

   b. back

   c. chest

   d. leg.

6. The adductor muscles of the leg include:

   a. longus, sartorius, gracilis

   b. magnus, rectus femoris, peroneus longus

   c. pectineus, biceps femoris, longus

   d. brevis, magnus, pectineus.

7. Muscle fatigue is due to:

   a. increase in potassium

   b. lack of oxygen

   c. increase in magnesium

   d. lack of carbon dioxide.

8. Another term for 'flaccid' muscle is:

   a. hypertonic

   b. spastic

   c. hypotonic

   d. receptor.

9. Adhesions in muscles are caused by:

   a. poor posture

   b. diet

   c. smoking

   d. mental stimulation.

10. Metabolic waste consists of:

   a. carbon dioxide and oxygen

   b. calcium and oxygen

   c. lactic acid and carbon dioxide

   d. oxygen and lactic acid.

CARDIOVASCULAR SYSTEM

1. Waste products pass out of cells and into the:

   a. capillaries

   b. tissue fluid

   c. venules

   d. arterioles.

2. The pericardium layer of the heart is composed of:
   a. fibrous tissue
   b. squamous epithelium
   c. reticular tissue
   d. cardiac muscle.

3. The inferior and superior venae cavae collect deoxygenated blood from the body and empty it into the:
   a. left ventricle
   b. right ventricle
   c. left atrium
   d. right atrium.

4. One of the main differences between arteries and veins is that:
   a. the walls of veins are composed of three layers of tissue
   b. the flow of blood in veins is faster
   c. arteries have a smaller lumen
   d. arteries have valves to stop the backflow of blood.

5. Blood is composed of:
   a. 30 per cent cells and 70 per cent plasma
   b. 40 per cent cells and 60 per cent plasma
   c. 50 per cent plasma and 50 per cent cells
   d. 55 per cent plasma and 45 per cent cells.

6. The blood cells involved in immunity are:
   a. thrombocytes
   b. leucocytes
   c. platelets
   d. erythrocytes.

7. A person's pulse rate is usually taken at the artery in the wrist known as the:
   a. pulmonary artery
   b. brachial artery
   c. radial artery
   d. carotid artery.

8. A clot that travels around the body via the bloodstream is called:
   a. an embolus
   b. an erythrocyte

c. a thrombus
d. a thrombocyte.

9. Blood pressure is defined as the:
   a. amount of blood flowing through the heart
   b. force exerted by blood on the walls of the blood vessels
   c. increase in heart rate due to specific hormones
   d. number of times the heart beats in one minute.

10. Erythrocytes contain:
    a. hormones
    b. carbon dioxide
    c. haemoglobin
    d. metabolic waste.

LYMPHATIC SYSTEM

1. The lymphatic system is closely associated with the:
   a. nervous system
   b. cardiovascular system
   c. urinary system
   d. endocrine system.

2. Lymph capillaries are different to blood capillaries because they:
   a. receive fluid but do not allow fluid to exit
   b. filter foreign substances and waste
   c. empty their content into venules
   d. carry carbon dioxide and waste.

3. Which of the following describes, in the correct sequence, the movement of lymph through the lymphatic system?
   a. Capillary, duct, node, vessel, trunk.
   b. Capillary, duct, trunk, vessel, node.
   c. Capillary, trunk, node, vessel, duct.
   d. Capillary, vessel, node, trunk, duct.

4. The function of a lymph node is to:
   a. speed up the flow of lymph
   b. prevent swelling in the tissues
   c. filter lymph
   d. produce leucocytes.

5. Which of the following is a lymphatic organ?

   a. Thymus gland.

   b. Pancreas.

   c. Pineal gland.

   d. Liver.

6. The thoracic duct receives lymph from the:

   a. left and right leg, left and right arm, left side of the chest

   b. right arm, right side of head and chest, left side of the trunk

   c. right side of the trunk above the ribs, right side of the head and right leg

   d. left arm, left side of the head and chest and all areas below the ribs.

7. The flow of lymph through the body is assisted by the:

   a. kidneys

   b. contraction and relaxation of skeletal muscles

   c. hormones

   d. protein haemoglobin found in red blood cells.

8. Which of the following veins receives lymph and returns it to the blood circulation?

   a. Subclavian.

   b. Femoral.

   c. Pulmonary.

   d. Axillary.

9. What does the lymphatic system transport from the small intestine to the blood?

   a. Proteins.

   b. Vitamins.

   c. Fats.

   d. Carbohydrates.

10. The posterior auricular lymph nodes are found:

   a. at the base of the skull

   b. behind the knee

   c. below the chin

   d. behind the ear.

RESPIRATORY SYSTEM

1. The larynx helps with:

   a. digestion and respiration

   b. swallowing and producing sound

   c. speech and digestion

   d. swallowing and gaseous exchange.

2. The air is warmed and moistened in the nostrils by:

   a. cilia

   b. oxygen

   c. mucus

   d. blood.

3. The epiglottis:

   a. helps to produce mucus

   b. lubricates the voice box

   c. assists food to pass through the larynx

   d. protects the opening of the larynx.

4. The tonsils are located in the:

   a. pharynx

   b. trachea

   c. larynx

   d. bronchi.

5. The trachea lies between the:

   a. nose and pharynx

   b. larynx and pharynx

   c. nose and larynx

   d. larynx and bronchi.

6. The serous membrane that covers the lungs is:

   a. pericardium

   b. pleural

   c. cutaneous

   d. peritoneum.

7. Gaseous exchange takes place in the:

   a. trachea

   b. larynx

   c. alveoli

   d. bronchioles.

8. During inspiration, the:
   a. external intercostal muscles relax and the diaphragm relaxes
   b. internal intercostal muscles contract and forces the diaphragm upwards
   c. external intercostal muscles contract and the diaphragm contracts
   d. intercostal muscles relax and forces the diaphragm upwards.

9. The most appropriate massage movements that help loosen excess mucus over the chest area are:
   a. petrissage and vibrations
   b. effleurage and petrissage
   c. tapotement and effleurage
   d. shaking and vibrations.

10. The larynx and trachea are composed of:
    a. smooth muscle tissue and cartilage
    b. skeletal muscle tissue and cartilage
    c. smooth muscle tissue and serous membrane
    d. skeletal muscle and serous membrane.

DIGESTIVE SYSTEM

1. The accessory structures of the digestive system include:
   a. pancreas, salivary glands, teeth
   b. caecum, tongue, gall bladder
   c. liver, gall bladder, oesophagus,
   d. teeth, pharynx, salivary glands.

2. Salivary amylase in the mouth begins the chemical breakdown of:
   a. fats
   b. vitamins
   c. starch
   d. proteins.

3. Hydrochloric acid secreted in the stomach helps to:
   a. lubricate the sphincter muscles
   b. create a part alkali and acid environment
   c. dilute the food into a liquid substance
   d. destroy microbes that have been ingested.

4. The function of the oesophagus is to transport the food to the:
   a. pharynx
   b. stomach
   c. duodenum
   d. ileum.

5. The two vitamins formed in the large intestine are:
   a. A and D
   b. B and D
   c. B and K
   d. E and K.

6. The semi-fluid content of the stomach is called:
   a. bolus
   b. sucrose
   c. peristalsis
   d. chyme.

7. Which of the following greatly increases the total surface area of the small intestine?
   a. Peristalsis.
   b. Gastric pits.
   c. Villi.
   d. Mucus.

8. Which of the following forms part of the large intestine?
   a. Duodenum.
   b. Caecum.
   c. Ileum.
   d. Jejunum.

9. The substance that enters the duodenum to continue to breakdown proteins is:
   a. lipase
   b. trypsin
   c. pepsin
   d. amylase.

10. Bile is formed in the:
    a. liver
    b. duodenum
    c. gall bladder
    d. stomach.

NERVOUS SYSTEM

1. The cerebellum controls:
   a. balance and coordination of movement
   b. memory and decision making
   c. eating and sleeping
   d. breathing and heart beat.

2. Motor neurones transmit stimuli:
   a. from sensory organs to the brain
   b. to the brain from muscles and glands
   c. to sensory organs from the brain
   d. from the brain to muscles and glands.

3. Which of the following systems works closely with the nervous system to maintain homeostasis?
   a. Cardiovascular system.
   b. Integumentary system.
   c. Endocrine system.
   d. Muscular system.

4. The central nervous system consists of:
   a. cranial nerves and spinal nerves
   b. brain and spinal cord
   c. spinal nerves and brain
   d. cranial nerves and brain.

5. What is the function of a synapse?
   a. Transmits nerve impulses away from the cell body.
   b. Forms a junction between two neurones.
   c. Protects and insulates neurones.
   d. Initiates nerve impulses.

6. Pacinian corpuscles sense:
   a. deep pressure
   b. heat
   c. taste
   d. touch.

7. Which of the following is an effect of the parasympathetic nervous system?
   a. Increases carbon dioxide output.
   b. Stimulates the spleen.
   c. Increases peristalsis.
   d. Stimulates contraction of skeletal muscle.

8. Proprioceptors are located in the:
   a. glands
   b. muscles
   c. bone
   d. skin.

9. How many pairs of cranial nerves arise from the brain?
   a. 6.
   b. 9.
   c. 12.
   d. 18.

10. The spinal nerves form the main part of the:
    a. parasympathetic nervous system
    b. central nervous system
    c. sympathetic nervous system
    d. peripheral nervous system.

URINARY SYSTEM

1. Which of the following are excretory organs of the body?
   a. Lymph and kidneys.
   b. Large intestine and lungs.
   c. Skin and small intestine.
   d. Spleen and liver.

2. The kidneys:
   a. transport urine to the bladder
   b. act as a reservoir for urine
   c. form urine
   d. store vitamin A.

3. The kidneys are protected by:
   a. adipose tissue
   b. simple squamous epithelium
   c. hyaline cartilage
   d. serous membrane.

4. The kidneys are located either side of the spine between the:
   a. 9th thoracic and 3rd lumbar vertebrae
   b. 10th thoracic and 1st lumbar vertebrae
   c. 10th thoracic and 5th lumbar vertebrae
   d. 12th thoracic and 3rd lumbar vertebrae.

5. The functional unit of the kidney is called:

a. hilum

b. glomerulus

c. Bowman's capsule

d. nephron.

6. The kidneys help to:

a. regulate water balance in the body

b. store glycogen

c. destroy worn out red blood cells

d. promote the growth of T-cells.

7. Urine leaves the kidneys at the:

a. loop of Henle

b. hilium

c. cortex

d. medulla.

8. The term 'homeostasis' means to:

a. maintain a stable internal environment for cells and tissues

b. reabsorb substances needed by the body

c. eliminate mineral salts through perspiration

d. store essential amino acids until they are needed by the body.

9. The blood supply to the kidney is by the:

a. splenic artery

b. common iliac artery

c. renal artery

d. hepatic artery.

10. The walls of the bladder are lined with:

a. yellow elastic tissue

b. smooth muscle

c. elastic cartilage

d. skeletal muscle.

ENDOCRINE SYSTEM

1. Which of the following glands is referred to as the 'master gland'?

a. Hypothalamus.

b. Adrenals.

c. Pituitary.

d. Thyroid.

2. The gland that controls body rhythms is the:

a. parathyroid

b. adrenal cortex

c. pineal

d. pituitary.

3. Follicle-stimulating hormone stimulates the:

a. secretion of milk from the breasts

b. production of oestrogen and progesterone

c. contraction of the uterus during labour

d. production of sperm.

4. Which of the following hormones helps the body to cope with stress?

a. Thyroxine.

b. Cortisol.

c. Melatonin.

d. Aldosterone.

5. Calcium levels are regulated by:

a. thyroxine and aldosterone

b. thymosin and adrenaline

c. parathyrin and calcitonin

d. glucagon and thyroxine.

6. The hormone that helps maintain pregnancy is:

a. progesterone

b. luteinising hormone

c. oestrogen

d. oxytocin.

7. The two hormones secreted by the posterior pituitary gland are:

a. growth hormone and thyroid-stimulating hormone

b. follicle-stimulating hormone and oxytocin

c. prolactin and luteinising hormone

d. antidiuretic hormone and oxytocin.

8. The action of thymosin is to:

  a. increase blood pressure

  b. stimulate the production of antibodies

  c. inhibit the secretion of the luteinising hormone

  d. promote growth of body tissues.

9. The hormone that regulates metabolic rate is:

  a. glucagon

  b. thyrotropin

  c. thyroxine

  d. parathyrin.

10. Aldosterone helps to:

  a. regulate sodium and potassium levels

  b. promote the development of sperm

  c. reduce the volume of urine

  d. raise blood pressure.

REPRODUCTIVE SYSTEM

1. Fertilisation takes place in the:

  a. Fallopian tubes

  b. uterus

  c. vagina

  d. ovaries.

2. Which of the following describes a fertilised egg?

  a. ovarian follicle

  b. embryo

  c. zygote

  d. ova.

3. The hormone that stimulates the development of the egg is:

  a. luteinizing hormone

  b. follicle-stimulating hormone

  c. progesterone

  d. oestrogen.

4. The cervix joins the:

  a. vulva and mons pubis

  b. ovary and Fallopian tube

  c. uterus and vagina

  d. Fallopian tube and uterus.

5. The hymen membrane protects the entrance to the:

  a. clitoris

  b. labia majora

  c. pubis symphysis

  d. vagina.

6. Semen:

  a. aids the multiplication of sperm cells

  b. neutralises the acidity of the vagina

  c. causes blood vessels to dilate in the penis

  d. helps to lower the temperature of the testes.

7. The vas deferens joins the:

  a. epididymis and urethra

  b. penis and urethra

  c. seminal vesicles and epididymis

  d. urethra and bladder.

8. Which structure stores sperm cells?

  a. Seminal vesicles.

  b. Testes.

  c. Epididymis.

  d. Vas deferens.

9. Sperm cells are produced in the:

  a. seminal vesicles

  b. urethra

  c. scrotum

  d. testes.

10. Which of the following stimulates the vaginal walls to contract to help propel sperm?

  a. testosterone

  b. prostaglandins

  c. bacteria

  d. oestrogen.

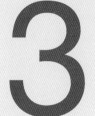

3 Professional conduct, consultation and preparation

After you have studied this chapter you will be able to:

1. list the factors that contribute to professional behaviour
2. explain the importance of safety and hygiene
3. prepare the working area, yourself and your client
4. explain the importance and purpose of detailed consultation and record keeping
5. carry out a detailed consultation
6. describe the contra-indications to massage.

Professional conduct and ethics

Professional conduct and ethics refers to the standards, moral principles and conduct of behaviour of an individual or professional group. You must undergo a reputable course of training to enable you to acquire the understanding and skills necessary to carry out safe and effective treatment. In addition, you must consider your standard of behaviour in relation to colleagues, clients and the general public.

A high standard of professional conduct will gain the confidence of clients and establish an excellent reputation, which is the basis for success. Abide by the following codes of practice:

- Look professional: be clean, neat and tidy.

- Be punctual, keep to appointment times and do not cancel appointments at the last minute.

- Be discreet and refrain from gossip. Remember that clients often confide personal problems during consultation. These facts and all personal details must be treated with the utmost confidentiality. Do not repeat information or gossip to colleagues or others.

- Be loyal to your employer, colleagues and clients. Create a friendly, but not over-familiar, working relationship with everyone you meet at work.

- Be honest and reliable: this will gain the trust of others and establish a high reputation. Do not make false claims for treatments: explain the benefits clearly and accurately.

- Speak correctly and politely to everyone. Do not use improper language. Consider the manner in which you answer or speak on the telephone. Be competent, helpful and pleasant.

In the workplace

There are various professional associations that you can join that offer members direct benefits, such as professional insurance deal, training opportunities, networking and access to websites. They also have indirect benefits, such as giving clients and employers confidence in you. Members of these associations agree to abide by a code of conduct, to observe bye-laws and follow disciplinary procedures in order to ensure the safety and well-being of their clients.

In the workplace

Always be aware of who can overhear your conversations, for example during breaks or standing at reception. You must present a professional image at *all* times. Clients want to feel that their privacy will be respected or they will take their custom elsewhere.

- Be polite and courteous at all times. There may be difficult clients to deal with: learn to handle tricky situations with tact and diplomacy.

- Know and abide by legal requirements and local authority byelaws, rules and regulations.

- Keep up to date with new theories, techniques and treatments. Attend courses and keep in touch with other professionals in your field.

- Always practise the highest standards of personal hygiene and hygiene in the workplace.

- Do your utmost to deliver the most effective treatment suited to the needs of the client.

- Organise yourself and your working practices to ensure a smooth-running, efficient service for the benefit of all concerned.

> **Best practice**
> Continuing Professional Development (CPD). For many of the professional associations CPD is a requirement for membership. However, even if you are not a member of a professional body, it is vital to maintaining the highest possible standards of knowledge and skill. This will improve your practice and enhance your earning power. (Chapter 9 has more on CPD).

Client consultation

Initial consultation

The consultation is a very important part of the treatment: sufficient time must be allowed so that it is not rushed. This is the time to gather and exchange information.

The initial consultation will be the longest and provide detailed information, which must be accurately noted on a consultation record. This must be filed in a safe and accessible place and used each time the client attends for treatment.

The client should be seated comfortably for the consultation. Position yourself alongside or opposite them. The environment should feel warm and private.

Detailed consultation is important for the following reasons:

- to introduce yourself and get to know the client
- to establish a rapport with the client and put them at ease
- to develop mutual trust and gain the client's confidence
- to gain information on the client's past and present state of mental and physical health
- to identify any contra-indications
- to gain insight into the client's lifestyle, responsibilities, work environment, leisure activities and any other relevant circumstances
- to identify the client's needs and expectations of the treatment
- to establish the most appropriate form of treatment and to discuss and agree this with the client

> **In the workplace**
> Each organisation will have its own method of recording and storing client information and the treatment plan. There are several names for these documents, e.g. 'record card', 'treatment record', 'client information'. In this book, the term 'consultation record' is used. On this you will record personal details, the treatment plan, the treatment evaluation and subsequent treatments.

> **Learning point**
> Before subsequent treatments, a brief consultation is usually sufficient to establish the effects and outcomes of the previous treatments and whether any changes are to be made or further action is to be taken.

- to explain the treatment fully to the client, including the procedure, expected effects, timing and frequency
- to agree a treatment plan, the timing and cost with the client so that they fully understand the financial commitment, and obtain a signature to confirm
- to answer queries and questions related to the treatment and to allay doubts and fears.

The information gathered will help you to formulate the best treatment plan to meet the needs of the client. The short- and long-term objectives should be discussed and agreed.

Examples of treatment objectives include:

- a relaxing massage to relieve stress and tension
- a stimulating massage to promote alertness
- an uplifting massage to reinforce positive feelings
- a targeted massage to stimulate and soften areas of cellulite
- engendering a feeling of wellbeing, taking time to focus on self.

You should also give the client information about the cost of any recommended products.

Essential information

The following personal, medical and lifestyle factors should be recorded on the consultation record, together with figure analysis. The information gathered will provide a baseline from which the appropriate treatment can be planned, the effectiveness of the treatment can be judged and any necessary changes or adjustments made.

The Data Protection Act 1998

A business that stores details about their staff and clients whether manually or on a computer may have to register with the Data Protection Register.

The Act protects peoples' personal details from being freely available to others. The Data Protection Register will issue a business with a code of practice. The main points are:

- Keep staff and clients' records safe and secure.
- Record personal information that is relevant.
- Do not release information to third parties unless you have the written consent of the individual.
- If an individual requests access to their information, you must provide it.

Observation, assessment and analysis

When you have gathered the essential information from the client, you then need to complete the consultation record. This is done through observation, assessment and analysis of the client.

In the workplace

Many businesses offer an incentive for a course of treatment, such as free products or the offer of free sessions at the end of the course.

Be aware !

In today's climate of personal injury claims being commonplace, you are potentially in a vulnerable position. Consultation records are evidence of your good practice, should such a claim be brought against you.

Be aware !

All the information given must be recorded and treated in confidence.

Be aware !

Treating minors. You must refer to your workplace policies to check whether there are any age restrictions for treatments. Some regulations allow the treatment of minors if a parent or guardian is present.

Personal Details

Name: (include title, Mr, Mrs, Miss, Ms or other) _____

Some clients may want to be addressed more formally than others. Also, when contacting clients by post or email you will know how to address them.

Address: (include postcode) _____

_____

To ensure letters arrive promptly.

Date of birth: _____

Under 20 ☐   21–30 ☐   31– 40 ☐   41–50 ☐

51–60 ☐   61–70 ☐   71 + ☐

Some clients do not want to acknowledge their age but will feel comfortable ticking a category.

Telephone: day_____   evening_____

Fax _____

Email _____

These are quick and efficient methods of contacting the client especially if you have to cancel or rearrange an appointment at short notice.

Client objectives _____

_____

_____

_____

Important to find out short and long-term objectives. Are they realistic and will the proposed treatment meet the client's needs?

Medical Details

Doctor's name _____

Address _____

_____

Tel no. _____

Should you need to liaise with the doctor about a contra-indication or give a progress report on treatment.

Past medical history

Surgical operations _____

Pregnancies _____

Serious illnesses _____

These details will enable you to establish the client's state of health; the likelihood of any contra-indications as a result of past illnesses; whether particular care must be taken over certain areas and whether medical referral is necessary. If the client suffers from a condition that is contra-indicated, then massage must not be given.

Present medical history

Medication _____

General health _____

These details will indicate whether massage will be helpful to this client and will influence the type of massage to be given.

Lifestyle

Occupation _____

Free time _____

Ability to relax _____

This information will help you judge what sort of massage will be most beneficial.

Diet _____

Exercise _____

Type and number of drinks per day _____

Alcohol consumption _____

Smoker/non-smoker _____

This information will impact on the homecare advice you give the client.

Emotional and mental factors

Stress levels (on a scale of 1–10 with
1 = no stress, 10 = very stressed) _____

Sleep pattern _____

Energy levels _____

Work/life balance _____

_____

_____

This helps you decide what sort of massage and what advice to give the client.

Massage Analysis

Contra-indications _____

Any allergies _____

Has client received massage in the past? _____

How long ago? _____

No. of sessions _____

Did client benefit from massage? _____

Reasons for requesting massage _____

Check if client has any contra-indications that may prevent, restrict or indicate certain precautions are needed. It is important to find out if the client has experienced any previous reaction to products or has any known allergies which may impact on your choice of medium. If the client has not experienced massage before then s/he may be apprehensive. Previous experience of massage will affect expectations and dictate preferences.

Assessment

Posture _____

> Assess if there are any postural conditions e.g. kyphosis, lordosis or scoliosis, where some muscles will be tight and shortened and others will be stretched and weakened. Think about the types of massage movements that would be beneficial.

Height _____

Weight _____

> These will help you work out the client's Body Mass Index (BMI) – a measure of body fat based on weight and height. If the client is overweight you will need to discuss their current lifestyle and diet and recommend alternatives.

Skin type (face) _____

> You will need to consider the type of media to use when carrying out the facial massage. If the client is wearing skin make-up, recommend the client removes it, as it is more beneficial for you to spend the treatment time on the massage and not removing make-up.

Skin (body) _____

Stretch marks _____

> Note dry, dehydrated and rough areas of skin – think about the retail products you could recommend at the end of treatment. Look for conditions such as eczema, psoriasis, bruises, thread and varicose veins and think how you are going to adapt your massage routine.

Areas of hard/soft fat/cellulite _____

> Consider how you can adapt the routine to address these areas.

General muscle tone _____

Fluid retention _____

> Well-toned clients often prefer a deeper massage than clients with poor muscle tone. If the client is stressed the upper fibres of the trapezius will probably be tight.

Other factors that may affect massage _____

> Ensure you find out through questioning the cause of the oedema. If in doubt advise the client to seek medical advice.

Treatment Plan _____

_____

> From the information you have gathered you will be able to prepare a plan of how you are going to adapt the treatment to suit the client's needs. This will detail the areas of the body to be included or excluded with reasons why, timing, depth of pressure, rhythm and how you will adapt the movements to achieve the outcome. You will also need to consider how often the client should attend and for how long.

Aftercare and homecare advice given

_____

_____

Any adverse reactions the client experienced

_____

_____

> This information should be recorded after each treatment to ensure good continuity of care and appropriate adaptation of future treatments. It is useful if another therapist has to take over future treatments for any reason.

The type of medium chosen and why

_____

Support used for client comfort.

_____

> You must ensure the client reads and signs the consultation record as this confirms their understanding and agreement with the details recorded and also gives their consent to treatment.

Client signature: _____

Therapist signature: _____

> By signing this document you are agreeing to keep the client's information confidential.

Date: _____

Figure 3.1 Sample consultation record

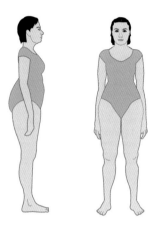

Figure 3.2 Endomorph body

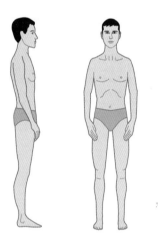

Figure 3.3 Ectomorph body

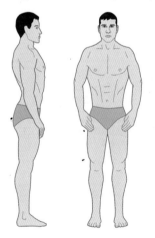

Figure 3.4 Mesomorph body

The information you need to note from the assessment includes:

- body type
- posture
- weight
- height
- measurements
- distribution and types of fat
- muscle tone
- fluid retention
- skin type and condition
- contra-indications.

Body types

Endomorph

People who have this body type are short, stocky, curvaceous and plump, often pear-shaped with small hands and feet. For this group, weight/fat gain is easy but weight loss is difficult.

Ectomorph

People of this type are long-limbed, slim and slightly muscular. They do not easily gain weight.

Mesomorph

People of this type are muscular and stocky with well-developed shoulders and slim, boyish hips giving an inverted triangle shape. They gain weight/fat slowly but increase muscle strength easily.

Individuals are predominantly of one type but may have aspects of another.

Posture

If there are postural problems then some muscles will be short-ened and tight, while others will be stretched and weakened. These factors will influence the types of massage manipulation used over certain muscles. Tight, shortened muscles will benefit from those manipulations that have a stretching effect, such as the petrissage movements, while the stretched muscles will ben-efit from the more stimulating percussion movements.

Clients with poor posture will also benefit from exercises to correct posture: these can be given after treatment or as part of home advice.

Posture is used to describe the alignment of the body, in other words how the body is held. Very few people have perfect pos-ture because it is influenced by both physical and psychological factors throughout life.

When the client comes into the salon, observe how they walk, stand and hold themselves: this alone will give some information regarding posture. Are the movements evenly balanced or is there tilting, stooping or unevenness in the way they move? When the client has undressed, a more accurate assessment can be made.

Assessment of posture

Ask the client to adopt a normal stance and assess the posture from the front, side and back. A plumb line may be used to check body alignment from the side. It should pass through the lobe of the ear, the point of the shoulder, the greater trochanter at the hip joint, behind the patella and in front of the ankle joint.

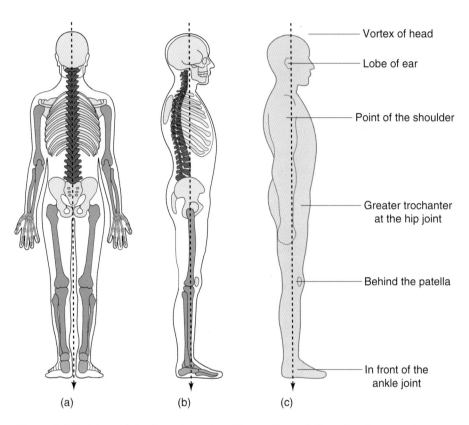

Vortex of head

Lobe of ear

Point of the shoulder

Greater trochanter at the hip joint

Behind the patella

In front of the ankle joint

(a)   (b)   (c)

Figure 3.5 Points that the line of gravity will pass through if posture is correct

From the front

Head position:

● Are the ear lobes level? If they are not, there is a muscle imbalance. The sterno-cleido-mastoid and the upper fibres of the trapezius are tight on the lower side, while those on the other side will be stretched.

Shoulders:

● Are they level, or is one higher than the other, indicating muscle imbalance? The upper fibres of the trapezius and levator scapulae are tight on the raised side.

● A difference in level may also indicate **scoliosis**, so check for that as well. This is a lateral curvature of the spine, which may be a long 'C' curve or an 'S' curve. The muscles that

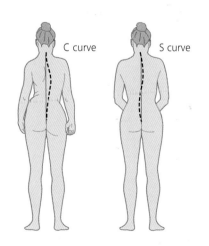

C curve   S curve

Figure 3.6 Scoliosis

will require strengthening will be those on the outside of the curve. The muscles that require stretching will be those on the inside of the curve. (A slight difference is considered normal.)

- Are both shoulders held high? This indicates tension in the muscles on both sides. The right and left upper fibres of the trapezius and the levator scapulae are tight.
- Are the shoulders drawn forward, rounded? This indicates muscle imbalance. The pectoral muscles are tight, but the middle fibres of the trapezius and rhomboids are stretched.
- Are there hollows above the clavicles? This indicates muscle tension, which may be due to respiratory problems such as asthma.

Breasts:

- Are the breasts held high or sagging? If there is breast sag and round shoulders, correction of the posture may help to lift the breasts.

Waist:

- Are the waist angles on the right and left level? If one is lower than the other, there may be spinal deformity or a difference in leg length.

Anterior superior iliac spines:

- Are they level? If not, there may be spinal deformity or a difference in leg length.
- Are they dropped forward? This indicates a **lordosis**. This is an exaggerated curve of the lumbar spine where the pelvis is tilted forwards.

  The weak stretched muscles that require strengthening are:
  - the abdominals – rectus abdominus, internal oblique and external oblique
  - the hip extensors – gluteus maximus and the hamstrings.

  The tight muscles that require stretching are:
  - the trunk extensors – erector spinae and quadratus lumborum
  - the hip flexors – ilio-psoas.

Are they dropped backwards? This indicates a **flat back** or sway back. This is a condition where there is little or no lumbar curve and the pelvis is tilted backwards. It may be accompanied by kyphosis of the thoracic spine.

- The weak, stretched muscles that require strengthening are the back extensors – erector spinae (in some cases the abdominals and gluteus maximus are weak).
- The tight muscles that require stretching are the hamstrings on the posterior thigh.

Patellae:

- Do they point forwards? If not, there may be 'knock knees' (genu valgum) or 'bow legs' (genu varum).

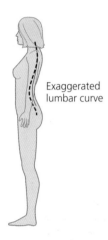

Exaggerated lumbar curve

Figure 3.7 Lordosis

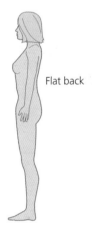

Flat back

Figure 3.8 Flat back

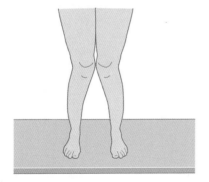

Figure 3.9 Knock knees

Toes:

- Do they point forwards? If they point outwards, there may be flattening of the medial arch and flat feet.
- If they point inwards or outwards, the weight distribution over the foot will be wrong, causing foot problems.
- Look for bunions, where the big toe deviates towards and sometimes lies across the other toes and there is swelling at the metatarso-phalangeal joint.
- Look for 'hammer toes', where the inter-phalangeal joints are deformed.

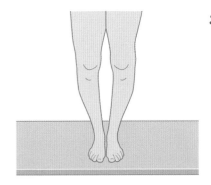

Figure 3.10 Bow legs

From the side

Use a plumb line.

Head position:

- Is the neck or cervical curve exaggerated and the chin forward? This means that the neck extensors, the upper fibres of the trapezius at the back of the neck, are tight and the neck flexors are weak.

Thoracic curve:

- Is there **kyphosis**? This is an exaggerated curve of the thoracic region.
- The weak, stretched muscles that require strengthening are: the middle fibres of trapezius, the rhomboids and the middle part of erector spinae.

  The tight muscles that require stretching are: pectoralis major and the neck extensors.

Abdomen:

- Is the abdomen protruding or sagging forwards, indicating weakness of the abdominal muscles? The pelvis may be tilted forward. This is known as visceroptosis, as the weak abdominals allow the viscera to sag forward.

Lumbar curve:

- Is there **lordosis**, i.e. an exaggerated lumbar curve with the spine curved inwards? (See 'From the front'.)
- If the lumbar region is flat, which is much less common, the erector spinae and quadratus lumborum will be weak.

Buttocks:

- Are the buttocks well toned with strong muscles, or are the gluteal muscles weak and sagging?

Knees:

- Are the knees hyper-extended?

From the back

Head:

- Are the ear lobes level, or is the head tilted, indicating muscle imbalance? (See 'From the front'.)

> **Remember**
> This should fall through the lobe of the ear, the point of the shoulder and the hip joint, behind the patella and just in front of the lateral malleolus.

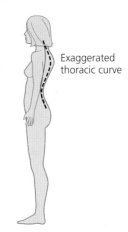

Exaggerated thoracic curve

Figure 3.11 Kyphosis

Shoulders:

- Are they level? (see 'From the front'.)
- Are there winged scapulae, i.e. the inferior angle and medial border of the scapulae lift away from the chest wall? This indicates a weakness of the serratus anterior and the lower fibres of the trapezius.

Spine:

- Is there **scoliosis**, i.e. a lateral deviation of the spine? This may be an 'S' or 'C' curve to the right or left. If you are unsure, pull a finger down the spinous process: the red line should be straight, and will show up any deviation. A scoliosis may be structural (present from birth), or it may be postural, and will straighten out when the body is flexed forward (see Figure 3.6).

Buttocks:

- Are the buttock folds level? If they are not, **scoliosis**, lateral pelvic tilt or different leg length may be present.

Heels:

- Are these square and firmly planted on the ground? If not, the weight distribution will be uneven.

Correction of the posture

Where required, the correction of the posture should be discussed with the client, and the following process should be explained. This exercise should then form part of the home care advice given to the client, perhaps suggesting they practise in front of a mirror.

Correction of the posture should begin at the feet. Each position should be maintained as the subsequent one is practised.

Feet

Stand with the feet 10 to 15 centimetres apart, with the toes pointing forward. The weight should be evenly distributed between the balls of the feet and the heels.

Practise the following:

- Raise the toes off the ground, feel the weight evenly distributed between the balls of the feet and the heels. Then lower the toes.
- Sway the body forward, feeling more weight on the balls of the feet.
- Sway the body backwards, feeling more weight on the heels.
- Position the body so that the weight is evenly distributed between the balls of the feet and the heels. Lift the medial arch slightly, but do not curl the toes.

Knees

- Press the knees backwards hard, ease the knees by bending them slightly, then find the mid-point and pull the kneecaps upwards by tightening the quadriceps muscle.

- If the knees are hyper-extended, ease them slightly and pull the kneecaps upwards as explained above.
- If the knees are bowed or knock-kneed, tighten the kneecaps, rotate the thighs outwards and tighten the buttocks to bring the kneecaps to point forward. Check the feet again after performing these movements.

Pelvis

- Tilt the pelvis forwards and then backwards; pull it forwards again tightly, tucking the tail under, and hold this balance. Pull the abdomen in and breathe out as the pelvis is pulled forward, then hold this position while breathing normally.

Thorax

- Pull the thorax upward from the waist as you breathe in, drawing the shoulders backwards and downwards. Hold this position while breathing normally. Do not thrust the chest forwards.

Neck and head

- Elongate the neck and pull the chin backwards. Feel as though someone is pulling the hair upwards at the crown.

Check the feet, knees, pelvis and thorax again, hold this position and then relax. Practise this correction several times a day and during various activities. Correct the posture during inhalation and hold the balance during exhalation.

If the new posture is maintained while walking around, it will eventually become habitual.

Weight and height

Weight measurement is needed to calculate the client's BMI, a measurement of the proportion of body fat. If a client wishes to lose weight, and this is appropriate, their weight can be monitored at each visit as an aid to motivation. In this case the client should be weighed at the same time of day, where possible, and in the same amount of clothing (ideally, underwear only). If the client prefers to remain dressed, you can allow about 1kg (2lbs) for outer clothing. Note the weight on the consultation record. It can then be measured against the healthy weight range (or BMI) tables for the client's height.

To measure height accurately, the client should be barefoot and the measuring scale should be fixed to the wall. The client should stand with the heels together and the back as straight as possible. The head should be level, with eyes looking straight ahead and shoulders should touch the wall.

Be aware

People generally weigh more towards the end of the day. Pre-menstrual water retention can also add weight temporarily.

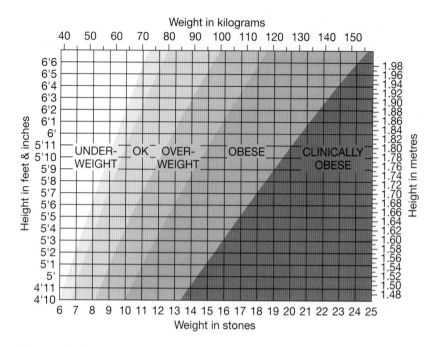

Figure 3.12 BMI chart

Taking measurements

Where a treatment is part of a client's weight loss goal, body measurements can be a useful guide to progress. Sometimes, even when the weight has not changed, the body shape may have improved with the toning of muscle, so measurements will reflect this and help motivate the client. Some clients will not be interested in individual body measurements, but for those who are, it is important that the measurements are accurate. Do not pull the tape measure too tight, but ensure it fits snugly over the area. Again, wearing minimal clothing is preferable. All measurements must be taken from a fixed point so that records are accurate (for example, so many centimetres above or below the navel; or so many cms above a point at the top of the patella when measuring thighs).

Distribution of fat

There are different types of body fat or **adipose tissue:** hard and soft adipose tissue and cellulite. The type and location on the body should be noted.

Hard adipose tissue

This type of fatty tissue is quite solid and well established. It can be difficult to distinguish from muscle as it is similarly hard to pick up and it can be found over well-toned muscle. Care should be taken to correctly identify hard adipose tissue, as it will impact on the massage movements you choose. Hard fat is more difficult to shift than soft fat.

Soft adipose tissue

This type of fatty tissue is easier to pick up and feels quite separate from the muscle layer beneath. Soft adipose tissue is relatively easy to shift by following a suitable diet and exercise regime.

Trapped adipose tissue

Deposits of fat are sometimes found trapped between bundles of muscle fibres. This is more common in people who have done a lot of regular training in the past and no longer do so, such as former athletes or dancers. Trapped fat is slow to respond to diet or exercise.

Cellulite

Cellulite is more common in women than men and can be present on slim figures as well as those who are overweight. It is easily recognised and often described as having an 'orange peel' appearance, where the skin appears lumpy and dimpled. This rippling of the tissue is caused by water retention and the stagnation of toxins and waste products in adipose cells. Because these cells have poor blood circulation, toxins are not efficiently removed from the area, causing the 'orange peel' effect.

If the skin ripples and looks like orange peel when the tissue is pressed between the palms of both hands, it is cellulite. In more advanced stages, the dimpling is sometimes noticeable without applying any pressure.

The areas subject to cellulite are the following:

- inner, upper and backs of the thighs
- buttocks
- hips
- stomach
- lower back
- inside and back of upper arms
- inside the knees
- ankles.

Some factors that contribute to the formation of cellulite include:

- insufficient water intake
- lack of proper exercise
- poor circulation
- sluggish digestion
- poor eating habits
- poor breathing
- sedentary living
- tension
- fatigue
- constipation.

Muscle tone

It is possible to obtain some indication of muscle strength by applying manual resistance to muscle action and feeling the degree

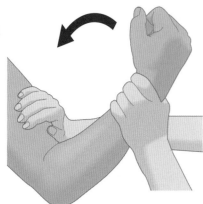

Figure 3.13 Testing biceps tone

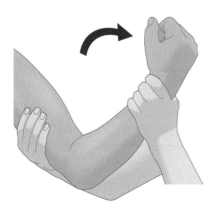

Figure 3.14 Testing triceps tone

of tone within the muscle. This will only provide a rough guide, as it is not possible to quantify the strength but only to categorise it as poor, moderate, good, very good or excellent. Muscles that are easily tested this way are the biceps and triceps, the abdominals, gluteus maximus and the hip abductors and adductors.

The following tests can be performed on the couch to give an initial guide to the client's strength and general mobility. Assess and record the outcome as poor, moderate, good, very good or excellent.

Biceps

The client bends the elbow to the mid-point of the range. Place one hand over the biceps on the anterior aspect of the upper arm. Grasp the wrist with the other. Instruct the client to bend the elbow while you stop the movement. Feel the increased tone with the hand placed over the muscle.

Triceps

With one hand, cover the triceps on the posterior aspect of the upper arm. Keep the other hand around the wrist. Instruct the client to straighten the elbow against resistance. Feel the increased tone with the hand placed over the muscle.

Abdominals (particularly rectus abdominus)

With the client lying supine (face up) on the couch, the strength of the abdominal muscles can be determined by the following sequence. This test can be split into three phases. Only clients with good muscle tone will be able to progress to phase three.

- Phase one: Place your hand on the abdominal area to feel the strength of the muscle, ask the client to breathe in, and on the out breath to lift the head with chin towards chest to look at their toes. For some clients this test may be all they can manage, due to poor muscle tone.

- Phase two: Place your hand on the abdomen with the other hand ready to support the client's back, if needed. Ask the client to breathe in, and on the out breath to lift the head and shoulders with chin towards chest to look at their toes.

- Phase three: Ask the client to bend their knees, feet flat on the couch. Place your hand on the abdomen with the other ready to support their back. Ask the client to breathe in and on the out breath to lift head, shoulders and vertebrae gently off the couch to perform a curl up.

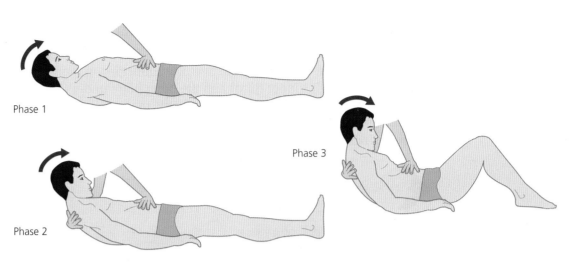

Phase 1

Phase 2

Phase 3

Figure 3.15 Testing abdominals tone

Gluteus maximus

With the client lying prone (face down), place one hand over the gluteus maximus on the left and the other on the back of the left leg (gastrocnemius). Instruct the client to raise the leg while you apply resistance. Feel the increased tone in the buttock. Repeat for the right side.

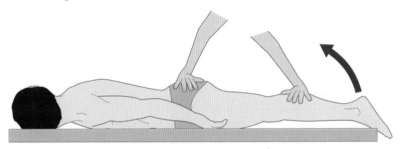

Figure 3.16 Testing gluteus maximus tone

Abductors

With the client lying supine (face up), legs straight, place one hand over the abductors on the outer aspect of the thigh above the greater trochanter and the other hand under the ankle to cup it. Instruct the client to 'push out' towards you. Resist the movement, using the hand at the ankle to push inwards. Feel the increased tone in the abductors. Repeat for the other side.

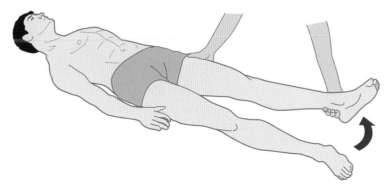

Figure 3.17 Testing abductors tone

Adductors

With the client lying supine (face up), legs straight and with one leg pushed outwards, place one hand over the adductors on the inner aspect of the thigh (upper third) and the other hand under the ankle. Instruct the client to pull the leg inwards towards the other leg. Resist the movement, using the hand at the ankle to pull outwards. Feel the increased tone in the adductors. Repeat for other side.

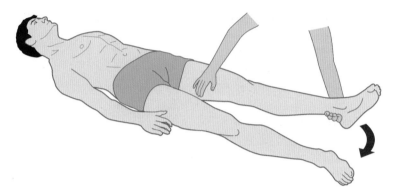

Figure 3.18 Testing adductors tone

Fluid retention

A client with puffy or swollen ankles, and sometimes hands, may be suffering from fluid retention. This puffiness is referred to as oedema. There are a number of possible causes: not drinking enough water, eating too much salt or eating lots of processed foods can all lead to fluid retention. Also, people who stand for long periods of time, such as those working in shops, can suffer from gravitational oedema. Fluid retention is also common before menstruation, when it can affect the abdomen and breasts. To test for fluid retention, press the client's skin in the oedematous area. If it remains indented and does not immediately spring back, this is a sign of fluid retention. Massage will help the lymphatic system to drain away the excess fluid.

Skin types

Because the treatment will include facial massage, it is important to assess the skin type and condition in order to decide on the most appropriate massage medium for the face.

Skin type	Explanation	Pores	Texture	Oil	Moisture	Additional notes
Normal (Balanced)	A normal skin type is referred to as a balanced skin as there is sufficient oil and moisture produced to keep the skin soft and supple.	small	fine	balanced	balanced	This is the ideal skin type.
Dry	A dry skin lacks oil and moisture. The sebaceous glands do not secrete sufficient sebum to lubricate and form a protective layer over the skin to prevent the loss of moisture from the upper layers. There may be signs of premature ageing, with fine to deep lines around the eyes, mouth and neck as dry skin tends to age more quickly than other skin types. Causes of dry skin include: hormone imbalance, central heating, sunbathing, crash diets, smoking and medication.	small to large	fine to coarse	insufficient	insufficient	Large pores and a coarse texture could be present on a dry skin as the client may have had a greasy skin when younger, resulting in the pores losing their elasticity.
Oily	An oily skin produces too much sebum in the ducts and hair follicles, which causes enlarged pores that are prone to comedones (blackheads) and blemishes. As the sebum builds up on the surface of the skin it affects the natural shedding of skin cells, causing the skin to look thick, dull and sallow. The overproduction of sebum is due to hormone imbalance.	large	coarse	over-production of sebum	usually good, as sebum helps to keep moisture within the skin	This skin type may become dehydrated if unsuitable products are used that strip the skin's protective acid mantle.
Combination	This can be a combination of two different skin types. The most common is an oily T-zone on the forehead, nose, inner cheeks and chin, while the outer region is drier.	medium to large	coarse on the T-zone, finer on the outer region	over-production of sebum in the T-zone	good in the T-zone if the correct skin care routine is followed	There are many more sebaceous glands located in the T-zone area. This is where the majority of comedones are found.

Table 3.1 Skin types

Skin conditions

The following are referred to as skin conditions. They can accompany any of the skin types.

Sensitive skin

A sensitive skin flushes very easily and reacts quickly to temperature change. It is also prone to allergic reactions. Common substances can cause irritation, leaving the skin red and blotchy. Dilated capillaries may be present on the cheeks and around the nose.

Dehydrated skin

This is characterised by a lack of moisture in the skin. It can be due to incorrect skin care routine, such as using too harsh a product, over-exposure to the sun and central heating or insufficient fluid intake. The skin may feel taut and itchy, with superficial flaking of the skin and a loss of plumpness.

Moist skin

This is skin that feels slightly wet or damp to the touch. It is usually an indication that the body is perspiring too much.

Oedematous skin

This is an accumulation of fluid in the tissues, which is a sign of an underlying problem that may need to be referred to another professional.

Ageing skin

The natural ageing process occurs over a period of time and is predetermined by genetic make up. Changes take place for the following reasons:

- Muscles lose their tone and those that are attached directly to the skin cause the overlying skin to stretch, producing lines.
- The loss of underlying fat will cause hollowed cheeks and eye sockets.
- The protein fibres in the dermis, collagen and elastin degenerate, causing the skin to loose its plumpness and elasticity.
- Cellular activity and desquamation decrease, leaving the skin looking dull and causing skin tags and uneven pigmentation, for example liver spots.

Contra-indications to massage

Understanding contra-indications

Massage must always be given to bring about improvement, either of specific conditions, or the general well-being of each client. Clients should always feel that the treatment is beneficial, helping them to achieve their desired results. Massage should never be given if there is any risk of harming the client or making any condition worse.

You have a legal responsibility under the health, safety and welfare legislation to protect yourself and the clients from harm. Remember that if the client is harmed in any way, they may make a claim against you. You must therefore ensure that you have not been negligent in any way, that you have selected the appropriate treatment and that you have a written record of the consultation, the treatment and the homecare advice given.

During the consultation you must decide whether massage is appropriate, safe and suitable for the client. If the client is suffering from any condition that could be aggravated or made worse by massage then obviously the treatment must not be carried out. These conditions are known as **contra-indications** to massage. Knowledge of the potential harmful effects of inappropriate massage is extremely important and so is the ability to recognise contra-indications.

Contra-indications can be divided into three categories:

- *total* contra-indications
- *local* contra-indications
- *caution*.

Total contra-indications

Massage should *not* be carried out on a client if any of the following conditions are present. This is out of concern for the client, whose condition could be adversely affected by massage, to protect you from possible infection and, in some circumstances, to protect you from possible legal action. If a massage is performed with due care and sensitivity, there are very few situations when it could cause a deterioration in a medical condition or aggravate symptoms. However, for the following conditions it is best not to carry out a treatment without first seeking medical advice. Doctors are unlikely to have time to respond to enquiries from therapists, therefore you must instruct your client to seek medical advice where appropriate.

Local contra-indications

Also referred to as contra-indications that restrict treatment, this refers to the areas of the client's body that must not be massaged as it may be uncomfortable for them, it could aggravate the condition or there are risks of cross-infection.

Massage with caution

These conditions are not contra-indicated but you may need to adapt massage techniques to ensure that you give an effective treatment. For example, you may have to modify the depth of pressure or omit some massage movements, such as percussion, to suit the condition.

In the workplace
Don't be embarrassed about telling the client of any abnormalities you find. It is always better to get them checked by a doctor and the client may not have been aware of them.

Condition	Brief description
Acne vulgaris	This is a chronic inflammatory condition of the skin. It usually appears at puberty, but it may also be seen in adults. It can be painful. Avoid massaging the area as it will cause discomfort and increases the risk of spreading infection. Also, the medium used may aggravate the condition.
Acquired Immunodeficiency Syndrome (AIDS)	The Human Immunodeficiency Virus (HIV) causes AIDS. Following infection with HIV, there may be no immediate symptoms and the incubation period may be up to eight years. Sufferers may not know they have the disease. The first symptoms are fatigue, fever, swollen glands and headaches. The next stage of the disease is chronically swollen glands in the armpits and groin. Because it attacks the immune system, the body is left defenceless against a wide variety of diseases. The virus can be transmitted by direct contact with bodily fluids (blood, semen and vaginal secretions). Massage may be carried out but avoid open cuts, abrasions and wounds. Check own skin and where necessary, cover injured areas with appropriate dressings. Follow strict hygiene procedures. Ensure linen is washed at a suitable temperature.
Acute infectious disease and fever	If the client feels hot, feverish, is perspiring and generally unwell, treatment is likely to be uncomfortable and you may be at risk of infection.
Acute urinary tract infections	Acute or chronic renal failure, acute stages of gout or a kidney stone attack are contra-indicated due to an overload on the urinary system from the increased amount of toxins produced.
Adrenal glands	**Cushing's syndrome** is a condition caused by high levels of the hormone cortisol secreted by the adrenal cortex. The function of cortisol is to help the body deal with stress. Symptoms include excess fat on the upper body, a large round face and slender arms and legs. **Addison's disease** is undersecretion of the hormones cortisol and aldosterone by the adrenal cortex. Aldosterone helps maintain blood pressure and salt and water balance. Symptoms include chronic fatigue, weight loss and muscle weakness. Adapt massage to suit client's needs.
Anaemia	The most common type of anaemia is due to iron deficiency. There is a reduction of red blood cells because the body does not have sufficient iron to form haemoglobin, the substance found in red blood cells that transports oxygen around the body. This type of anaemia can be caused by insufficient iron in the diet, inability to absorb the iron in the diet, or as a result of blood loss due to injury. Severe anaemia is contra-indicated because it may be a sign of a serious underlying medical condition.
Angina	This occurs due to a reduced blood supply to the heart by the coronary arteries. Fatty patches or plaques develop on the lining of these arteries, causing them to narrow. Symptoms may include breathlessness, tightness across the chest, fatigue and dizziness. Massage can be beneficial as it will help the client to relax, relieving stress and tension. Obtain medical consent.

Table 3.2 Contra-indications to massage

Condition	Brief description
Arteriosclerosis	This is the hardening (sclerosis) of the arteries as the arterial walls become thicker and lose their elasticity. Massage could cause a build-up of plaque in the arteries leading to the formation of clots. Obtain medical consent.
Asthma	This is an inflammatory disease of the bronchi, caused by coming into contact with allergens and irritants that trigger asthma symptoms. The airways produce more mucus as the muscles tighten around the airways, causing the tubes to narrow. Symptoms include coughing, wheezing, shortness of breath and tightness in the chest. Massage can be beneficial as it has a calming effect on the body. Spend time massaging the muscles involved in breathing. Consider placing your client in a semi-inclined or side-lying position with additional supports for ease of breathing during treatment. Ensure client has their inhaler within easy reach.
Basal cell carcinoma	This type of cancer originates in the epidermis. It is usually found on the head and neck where the skin has been exposed to sunlight or other forms of ultraviolet radiation, e.g. tanning equipment. It may appear as a skin growth or a raised area that looks pearly or waxy, flesh-coloured or brown; or a sore that never seems to heal. It can invade the surrounding area but does not usually spread to other parts of the body (metastasise). This is treated as a local (restricted) contra-indication to massage. Advise client to seek medical advice.
Bedsores/pressure sores	These are caused by sitting or lying in a certain position for too long. The blood supply to the area becomes restricted resulting in damage to the skin and underlying tissues and in severe cases the muscles and bones, too. Those at risk are individuals who are immobile. Do not massage the area as it will cause discomfort.
Blisters	These occur due to friction on the skin, e.g. from wearing shoes that are too tight, or as a result of sunburn or contact with chemicals. Fluid accumulates beneath the outer layer of skin and the area becomes slightly raised. As the skin heals beneath the blister the fluid slowly absorbs into the tissues. Massage will be uncomfortable in this area.
Bone fractures	These need to heal completely before it is safe to massage. Other areas may be massaged.
Bronchitis	This occurs in the bronchi of the lungs when the mucus membrane lining becomes inflamed. Coughing is a reflex action that helps to expel the build-up of inflammatory fluid and mucus in the airways. The cause of this condition can be viral or bacterial. Symptoms include a cough, shortness of breath and tightness in the chest. Avoid massage during the acute stage. Seek medical advice.
Bruising (recent or extensive)	Avoid these areas, especially if the discolouration is dark, purple, blue or black as it may be uncomfortable and could affect the healing process. Work around smaller bruises.
Burn, sunburn or wind burn	Avoid the area as it may be uncomfortable for the client.

Table 3.2 *Continued*

Condition	Brief description
Carbuncle 	This is a collection of boils, which can be very painful and must be referred for medical treatment. Do not massage over the area.
Chlamydia	Chlamydia is a sexually transmitted, bacterial infection. Often there are no initial symptoms until the disease develops, when these include a burning sensation during urination, bleeding after sexual intercourse and pain in the lower abdomen. Massage is not contra-indicated but omit the abdominal massage if uncomfortable.
Cirrhosis of the liver	This develops over a period of time when healthy tissue is replaced by scar tissue. This affects the normal functioning of the liver. The main causes are excess alcohol and infection of Hepatitis C virus. Do not massage if the condition is in an advanced stage. Seek medical advice.
Crohn's disease	This is an inflammation of the lining of the digestive system. It occurs mainly in the ileum, the last section of the small intestine, and also the large intestine. The walls of the intestines become thick and cause blockages. Symptoms include abdominal pain, tiredness and diarrhoea. Avoid deep abdominal massage, but gentle massage movements over the abdominal area will have a soothing effect.
Cuts, abrasions and wounds	With these there is a risk of infection and blood contamination. Avoid the area or cover with an appropriate dressing if possible.
Cystitis	This is an infection of the bladder that causes pain or burning sensation when passing urine. Other symptoms include wanting to pass urine more frequently, pain or tenderness in the lower back and blood in the urine. It may cause back pain over the kidneys. Adapt the massage to suit client's needs.
Dermatitis	This is inflammation of the skin and has many causes. It may be due to contact with a substance to which the person is sensitive. It may be caused by a reaction to specific drugs or exposure to irritants. Consider using hypoallergenic medium. Avoid the area if the skin is weeping.

Table 3.2 *Continued*

Condition	Brief description
Diabetes	This occurs when the blood sugar in the body is higher than normal due to insufficient insulin, the hormone produced by the pancreas, or when body cells do not respond to the insulin available. Symptoms include increased thirst, frequent urination, poor circulation, thin skin and possibility of itching skin and yeast infections. Some sufferers can be massaged but, as tissue healing is impaired in these clients, great care must be taken not to damage tissues particularly of the lower leg and foot. Some sufferers experience a loss of sensation and so deep massage should be avoided as clients will not be able to tell if pressure is too great. Blood sugar levels can drop following massage, so diabetic clients should be made aware of this. Check symptoms client has, avoid area if recently injected and be alert for any changes during treatment. Seek medical advice before treatment if unsure.
Diverticulitis	This affects the large intestine. It is the result of abnormal pouches protruding outwards from the inner lining of the large intestine, which become inflamed. Perform soothing massage movements over the abdomen but avoid deep abdominal massage as it may cause discomfort.
Drink or drugs	Massage must not be given to anyone under the influence of drink or drugs, as such clients may not be in control of their faculties.
Dysfunction or disorders of the nervous system	For example: multiple sclerosis, strokes, Parkinson's disease. Muscles may exhibit increased tone (spasticity), which may be made worse by massage. These clients should be treated under medical supervision.
Eczema	This is an allergy that forms red, itchy, scaly patches on the skin, which may ooze. Avoid the area if the skin is weeping.
Emphysema	This is classified under a group of diseases called Chronic Obstructive Pulmonary Disease (COPD). The alveoli in the lungs involved in the exchange of oxygen and carbon dioxide are impaired or destroyed. This results in difficulty with breathing. The causes of emphysema include smoking, and long-term inhalation of chemical fumes, pollution and dust. Obtain medical consent.
Endometriosis	Abnormal cells grow outside the uterine cavity, usually on the ovaries. It affects women during their reproductive years. Symptoms include pelvic pain, painful, irregular or heavy periods and pain experienced during sex. Omit the abdominal massage as it can be extremely tender.
Epilepsy	This is a brain disorder that causes fits, attacks or convulsions. These occur when the electrical activity in the brain is disrupted. It is safe to massage controlled epilepsy, but it is always advisable to seek medical consent. Do not leave anyone suffering from epilepsy unattended in a cubicle or on the couch.

Table 3.2 *Continued*

123

Condition	Brief description
Fibroids	These are benign tumours that consist of muscle and fibrous tissue that can grow in the womb. Symptoms include heavy and painful periods, bloating or pain in the abdomen and pain during sexual intercourse. Many women do not experience any symptoms. Omit the abdominal massage if the client feels any discomfort in this area.
Fleas	These jumping insects suck blood and their bites appear as a collection of red pimples, which are very itchy. If you suspect that a client is infested, advise them to seek medical advice. Massage is contra-indicated to prevent cross-infection. Any linen the client has been in contact with should be boil-washed.
Fragile skin	Older clients with thin, crepey skin and poor muscle tone must be massaged with great care. Pressure should be kept light to moderate and plenty of lubrication must be applied to prevent further stretching of the skin. All percussion movements, i.e. hacking, cupping, beating and pounding, should be avoided.
Furuncle or boil	This is an abscess under the skin, filled with pus, which is caused by bacteria entering the skin, usually through a hair follicle. Boils can be painful and should be medically treated. Do not massage over the area.
Gallstones	These develop in the gallbladder. In the majority of cases they do not cause any symptoms. However, if a gallstone becomes trapped in a duct it affects the flow of bile, which can cause abdominal pain, vomiting and jaundice. If the client does not have any symptoms, continue with the massage.
Gout (acute)	This is a form of arthritis caused by excess uric acid in the body. The kidneys produce uric acid as a by-product of metabolism. This can accumulate in the kidneys if they are not working efficiently, or in the blood supply if too much uric acid is produced, causing crystals to form in the joints, especially the big toe. Massage stimulates the release of toxins and so can aggravate the condition. Avoid massaging the area.
Haemophilia	This is a condition of diminished or absence of blood clotting. Anyone suffering from this condition will bruise and bleed easily, and should not be massaged.
Haemorrhage – recent	Medical advice should be sought as it will depend on the cause of the condition. If it is an internal condition, such as haemophilia, the client should not be massaged. However, if it is a known condition that will not be aggravated by massage, treatment may continue.

Table 3.2 *Continued*

Condition	Brief description
Heart attack (myocardial infarction)	This is a blockage of the coronary artery that supplies the heart with oxygen. It can be due to ateriosclerosis (see above) where plaques of cholesterol develop on the artery walls causing the lumen of the artery to narrow. It may be further exacerbated by blood clots forming on the surface of these plaques. The blood supply to the heart is severely disrupted causing damage to the heart muscle, which may result in disability or death. Warning signs include severe pain in the chest that lasts more than a few minutes; the pain spreads to the neck, shoulders and arms; the patient experiences nausea, sweating and breathlessness. Avoid massage for at least three months. Obtain medical consent after this period.
Heartburn	This occurs when the sphincter muscle between the stomach and the oesophagus is not working efficiently and the acid in the stomach flows back up the oesophagus, referred to as 'reflux'. Whether it is indigestion or heartburn, recommend that the client does not eat for three hours before the treatment.
Heart conditions	Because massage is thought to affect the rate of blood flow it may have an undesirable effect if there is a heart condition. Always seek medical advice if a client has heart problems. Relaxing massage may help stress-related heart problems.
Hepatitis	This is a viral infection causing inflammation of the liver. Chronic hepatitis lasts six months or more but it is the acute hepatitis that lasts six months or less that is infectious, so avoid massaging a client during this period to avoid cross-infection.
Hernia – abdominal area	This is when an organ in the abdomen pushes through a weak area in the inner lining of the abdomen wall. Omit the abdomen massage and spend more time on another area dependent on the client's needs.
Herpes simplex/ cold sore	This is caused by a virus living in the skin of the lips. It produces an eruption around the mouth that starts as an itchy red patch and develops into vesicles or a weeping blister, which then form a crust. It is very contagious. Do not treat the face of a client with cold sores to avoid cross-infection.
Hiatus hernia	This is when the stomach pushes through the diaphragm into the chest. Some clients suffer with heartburn, while others do not have any symptoms. During the massage clients with this condition will feel more comfortable in a half-lying/sitting position.
High blood pressure	Blood pressure varies with age, weight and fitness, but some people have consistently high blood pressure. Massage can frequently help, especially if the condition is stress-related. Medical advice should be sought if such people request massage; especially if they are not currently on medication.

Table 3.2 *Continued*

Condition	Brief description
Hyperthyroidism	This is over-activity of the thyroid, speeding up the body's metabolism and in some cases causing a goitre (swelling in the neck) as the gland enlarges. Other symptoms include palpitations, nervousness, insomnia and warm moist skin. Adapt the massage to suit client's needs.
Hypothyroidism	This is under-secretion of the hormone thyroxine by the thyroid gland. The function of thyroxine is to stimulate cell metabolism, growth and development. It can cause the condition myxoedema. Symptoms include weight gain, tiredness and puffiness of the face. Adapt the massage to suit client's needs.
Impetigo	This is a highly contagious bacterial infection of the skin. Usually located around the mouth, it begins as an itchy red patch that develops into pustules and further into flaky crusts. It is usually found in children, but adults may also be affected. This condition should be medically treated. Do not carry out massage if sores are weeping or client is being treated by their doctor. Treat as a local contra-indication if sores are not weeping.
Incontinence	This occurs when the muscles controlling the external sphincter of the urethra lose tone and elasticity. This can be a result of childbearing or can occur with age. Heavy pressure over the bladder will be uncomfortable and should be avoided.
Indigestion	This is also known as dyspepsia. Pain is experienced in the upper abdomen, usually after a meal. The acid produced in the stomach irritates the mucosa, the lining of the oesophagus, stomach and intestine. Causes include too much alcohol, stress and smoking. The symptoms are pain, sickness and flatulence. Suggest the client has a massage before eating.
Inflammatory disease	When the client is in the active phase of any inflammatory disease such as rheumatoid arthritis or when any area is red, hot and swollen, massage will be uncomfortable and will aggravate the inflammation
Joints – swollen, hot or painful	Do not massage over these areas as it may be uncomfortable for the client.
Kidney stones	These develop from substances that form urine in the kidneys. The majority of stones pass through the urinary system without causing problems. However if a stone becomes lodged in the ureter or urethra it can cause considerable pain in the abdomen or back. Other symptoms include blood in the urine, nausea and fever. Contra-indicated in the acute stage (see Gout).
Laryngitis	This is an inflammation of the larynx (voice box), usually due to a viral infection. Symptoms include hoarseness, loss of voice, sore throat, other flu-like symptoms may develop. Massage is contra-indicated during the acute stage to avoid cross-infection of the virus.

Table 3.2 *Continued*

Condition	Brief description
Leukaemia	This is cancer of the blood. The white blood cells, which form part of the body's immune system, fight infection. In leukaemia, too many abnormal white blood cells develop in the bone marrow and enter the bloodstream, outnumbering and disrupting the work of healthy blood cells. Seek medical consent.
Low blood pressure	A client may feel dizzy or faint if they sit up or get off the couch too quickly following treatment. Always supervise and give assistance if necessary. Low blood pressure is not usually considered a problem unless it is very low and the client is not on medication. Adapt the massage according to client's needs.
Lumbago	This is the term used to describe lower back pain, a common musculo-skeletal problem. The pain can range from mild to severe. Causes of this condition vary but can include sprain or strain of the lower back muscles and soft tissues. Symptoms include limited flexion and extension of the spine, poor posture and back pain. Adapt manipulations and pressure for the back area. Refer client to a health care professional, e.g. osteopath, chiropractor, physiotherapist.
Lung cancer	These malignant tumours grow aggressively and invade other tissues of the body via the blood and lymphatic systems. Causes of this disease include smoking and coming into contact with asbestos or radon gas. Symptoms are breathlessness, continued coughing (with blood-stained phlegm) and weight loss. Always liaise with the client's GP before offering treatment.
Lymphoedema	This is a long-term condition that causes swelling, usually in the arms or legs, due to damage of the lymphatic system. It can be a result of surgery or radiotherapy. Refer client to a health professional trained to deal with this condition, e.g. a physiotherapist or person trained in Manual Lymphatic Drainage (MLD).
Melanoma	This is a malignant tumour of melanocytes, the cells found in the basal layer of the skin that produce the pigment melanin. Symptoms to note are any moles growing bigger, changing colour, becoming more irregular, having a combination of different shades of brown to black, itching or bleeding. This type of cancer can metastasise. Seek medical advice.
Meningitis	This is caused by a bacteria or virus that infects the membranes that protect the brain and spinal cord, the meninges. Massage is contra-indicated due to risk of cross-infection.
Menstruation	Forms part of the menstrual cycle when the body sheds the lining of the uterus. Omit the abdomen during the first three days of a period as it may cause a heavier blood flow. Gently massage the lower back if the client experiences dull aching pain in this area.

Table 3.2 *Continued*

Condition	Brief description
Metal pins or plates	Metal pins and plates are sometimes inserted to support fractured bones. The metal implants may have sharp angles or edges (e.g. on screws) that can cause irritation to the surrounding tissues, particularly as residual inflammation never totally goes away. This can be aggravated by external pressure so massage over these areas should be avoided.
Migraine	This is a severe headache that can last a few hours or days. Symptoms include nausea, sensitivity to light, irritability and tiredness. Avoid massage during this time. However, massage on a regular basis will be beneficial as it helps to reduce stress and tension, which can cause migraine.
Moles – large, lumpy or inflamed	Work around these types of moles. Be aware of any changes in appearance particularly on the back of the body that would be difficult for the client to monitor. If a mole is asymmetric, the border is uneven, it changes colour or if the diameter extends recommend the client seeks medical advice.
Multiple sclerosis (MS)	This is a condition affecting the nerves in the brain and spinal cord. Each nerve fibre is protected by a myelin sheath, which ensures messages are transmitted effectively. The body's immune system that usually attacks bacteria and viruses attacks the myelin sheaths causing inflammation and scarring and inefficient transmission of messages. Symptoms include loss of balance and co-ordination, muscle weakness and spasms and fatigue. Seek medical consent.
Muscles – weak with poor tone	Effleurage and gentle kneading movements may be used but wringing and all percussion movements must be avoided as they will be uncomfortable for the client.
Myalgic encephalomy-elitis (ME)	This is also known as Chronic Fatigue Syndrome and is a condition that affects primarily the nervous and immune systems. Symptoms include severe fatigue after physical and mental exertion; problems concentrating; muscle and joint pain. Adapt manipulations and pressure to meet the client's needs.
Nausea	If the client is feeling sick, massage is likely to aggravate the condition. Nausea could also be symptomatic of an underlying condition.
Neuritis	This is the inflammation of a nerve or a group of nerves. The severity of the condition will depend on the areas involved. Symptoms include tingling and stabbing pain in the affected nerves and in severe cases the muscles around the nerve will lose the ability to contract. Use light movements to soothe the area.
Oedema	This is a medical term to describe fluid retention. The cause may be associated with high blood pressure, kidney problems or other systemic problems. Seek medical advice to establish the cause. If the oedema is recent, soft and due to gravitational effects, massage may be carried out.

Table 3.2 *Continued*

Condition	Brief description
Operations (recent)	Massage could irritate the area, increase the risk of infection and slow down the healing process. Avoid the area. If unsure, seek medical advice.
Osteoporosis	Great care must be taken when massaging anyone with this brittle bone disease. Plenty of lubrication and light pressure must be used. Light effleurage stroking and kneading are suitable but all percussion manipulations must be avoided. There is risk of accidental breaking of bones in severe cases.
Parkinson's disease	This is a long-term neurological condition caused by a shortage of dopamine, a chemical in the brain. It affects the way the brain co-ordinates body movements, for example posture and balance, walking and talking. Seek medical consent.
Pediculosis capitis	This is an infestation of the head: the louse obtains nourishment through blood sucking, causes intense irritation and lays eggs called nits among the hair. Massage is contra-indicated to avoid cross-infection.
Pediculosis corporis	This is infestation by the body louse. It lives in clothing and sucks blood for nourishment. It causes intense irritation of the body. Massage is contra-indicated to avoid cross-infection.
Pediculosis pubis	This is an infestation of the pubic hair by crab lice. It causes intense irritation and sucks blood. Massage is contra-indicated to avoid cross-infection.
Pelvic inflammatory disease (PID)	This is a bacterial infection, usually caused by chlamydia or gonorrhoea, which affects the reproductive organs. Symptoms include vaginal discharge, heavy periods, pain during sexual intercourse, infertility and pain when urinating. Many women do not experience any symptoms until the infection develops. Omit the abdominal massage as it may be uncomfortable and could aggravate the condition.
Phlebitis and thrombosis	Phlebitis is a painful condition where the lining of the vein becomes inflamed and may result in a clot forming on the vein wall, known as thrombosis. Any pressure applied to the vein or increase in the force of the circulation may dislodge the clot with potentially fatal consequences. Do not treat for six months after diagnosis then seek medical permission.

Table 3.2 *Continued*

Condition	Brief description
Pineal gland – imbalance	Hyper-secretion of the hormone melatonin causes Seasonal Affective Disorder (SAD), a type of depression that is referred to as the 'winter blues' or 'winter depression' as it usually occurs from September to April, when the amount of daylight is decreased. Symptoms include low mood, lack of energy, putting on weight and tiredness. Regular massage will help to relieve depression and uplift the client.
Pleurisy	This is the inflammation of the pleural membrane that lines the inside of the chest wall and the lungs. Between the layers is a fluid that acts as a lubricant to enable the lungs to move during expansion and contraction. The disease is caused by a viral infection. The sharp stabbing pain can be severe, resulting from friction as the pleura rub over each other. Symptoms include coughing, shortness of breath, rapid and shallow breathing and fever. Massage will have a soothing effect especially on the upper back and chest area.
Pneumonia	This is inflammation of the lung(s) when the alveoli become inflamed and fill up with fluid. The cause maybe viral, bacterial, or from fungi or parasites. These micro-organisms can enter the lungs via small droplets of water in the air; or via exposure to corrosive chemicals or through toxic smoke inhalation. Symptoms include a cough, pains in the chest, fever, breathing problems. Once the acute stage has passed massage can be carried out.
Pregnancy	In the late stages of pregnancy, or if the client is experiencing any problems with her pregnancy, seek medical advice. Avoid massage to the abdomen and deep tissue massage. Also be aware of the medium used, as certain blended oils are contra-indicated.
Prolapsed uterus/ vagina	This can be caused by a difficult childbirth, or by the ageing process. The muscles and ligaments holding the uterus in place weaken and may collapse, causing part of the uterus to sag into the vagina. Omit the abdominal massage as this will be too uncomfortable and may aggravate the condition.
Prostate cancer	This cancer develops in the prostate gland, which is part of the male reproductive system. It is a slow-growing cancer that can spread to other parts of the body if not treated. Mostly affects men over the age of 50. The main symptom is difficulty with urination. Massage is not contra-indicated but be aware that the treatment may be interrupted if the condition affects the client's bladder.
Psoriasis	This is a chronic skin disease that may affect small areas behind the knees or elbows, or it may be found over the entire body. It results in reddish patches covered with silvery scales that continually flake away. It is not infectious but avoid the area if the skin is broken.

Table 3.2 *Continued*

Condition	Brief description
Pustule 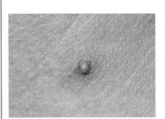	This is an elevated lump of skin containing pus: pustules often develop when hair follicles are infected by bacteria. Do not massage the area to avoid infection spreading.
Ringworm (Tinea): 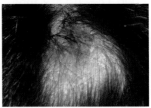 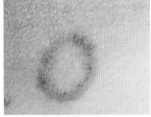 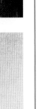 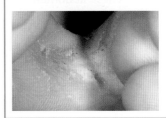	This is a fungal infection and has different names according to the part of the body affected: ***Tinea capitis*** *Tinea capitis* is ringworm of the scalp caused by a fungus. It infects the scalp and the hair shaft as it emerges from the scalp causing greyish, scaly areas with short, broken hairs. Do not massage to avoid cross-infection. Advise client to seek medical advice. ***Tinea corporis*** *Tinea corporis* is ringworm of the body caused by a fungal infection. It infects the skin all over the body. Red, round, scaly patches that spread outwards can appear anywhere on the body. Do not massage to avoid cross-infection. Advise client to seek medical advice. ***Tinea pedis (Athlete's foot)*** *Tinea pedis* affects the skin around and between the toes, forming red, itchy, scaly patches on the soles and between the toes. The skin may become sore, soggy and white. It is highly contagious. Do not treat the feet and cover them with disposable socks when treating other areas.
Rosacea 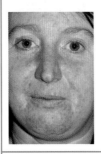	This is a chronic inflammatory condition found on the face. The skin is flushed and red due to dilation of blood vessels and appears coarse. Papules and pustules may develop. It is thought to be caused by intolerance to certain food or drink or over exposure to extremes of climate. Tea, coffee or alcohol may exacerbate the condition, as will exposure to sun and wind. The client will usually be under medical supervision: if they are not, suggest medical referral. Do not massage over the area as it could aggravate the condition.
Scabies 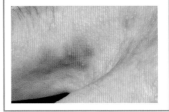	This is an infestation by itch mites. These are parasites that burrow into the skin around the wrists and fingers. It produces extreme irritation and is very difficult to eradicate. Do not massage to avoid cross-infestation. Advise the client to seek medical advice.

Table 3.2 *Continued*

Condition	Brief description
Scar tissue – recent	There is a danger of breaking down recently formed scar tissue. However, when the scar is completely healed (after about six months) massage may be given and is useful for stretching and loosening old contracted scar tissue.
Sciatica	This is caused by the compression or irritation of the sciatic nerve, the longest nerve in the body, which runs from the pelvis through the buttocks, down the legs to the feet. The pain can be mild to severe. An underlying cause can be a slipped disc. Avoid the area, although massage would be beneficial at non-acute times.
Sebaceous cyst 	This is a swelling of the sebaceous glands under the skin. They usually appear as small lumps on the scalp, neck or back. Do not massage over the area because it may be painful and uncomfortable for the client.
Severe headaches	These can be associated with more serious underlying conditions for example meningitis, stroke and brain tumours. If this is an unusual occurrence for the client seek medical advice.
Shingles or Herpes Zoster 	This is caused by the same virus that causes chicken pox. It infects the nerve and the area of skin that the nerve supplies. Symptoms include a tingling sensation followed by pain and a rash usually around the chest, abdomen or face. It is possible for someone who has not had chicken pox to catch it from contact with a person with shingles. Massage should be avoided to reduce the risk of cross-infection.
Sickle cell anaemia	This is an inherited condition that most commonly occurs in people of African or Caribbean descent. The red blood cells are sickle-shaped (crescent) instead of the flattened discs that are normal. These cells are rigid and sticky binding together and blocking small arteries with the potential to damage organs and tissues. Symptoms include fatigue, palpitations, pain and swelling of hands and feet. Severe sickle cell anaemia is contra-indicated. Seek medical consent.
Sinusitis	This is inflammation of the lining of the sinuses in the forehead and behind the cheekbones. Usually caused by viral or bacterial infections. Symptoms include runny nose, pain and tenderness in the area and a high temperature. Avoid the area if too tender.

Table 3.2 *Continued*

Condition	Brief description
Skin tags	A skin tag is a small flap of tissue that hangs off the skin by a connecting stalk. Skin tags are not dangerous. They are usually found on the neck, chest, back, armpits, under the breasts, or in the groin area. Skin tags appear most often in women, especially with weight gain, and in more mature people. Skin tags do not usually cause any pain. However, they can become irritated if anything rubs on them, such as clothing or jewellery. For this reason, avoid massaging them or massage with care.
Sprains – recent or muscle strains	Be aware that there may be damage to ligaments, tendons and muscle fibres, which must be allowed to heal before massage of the affected area. Focus on other areas of the body, which will benefit from massage.
Squamous cell carcinoma	This type of cancer originates in the epidermis and can spread to other parts of the body (metastasise). It is a relatively slow-growing cancer that is found on the skin exposed to sunlight or other forms of ultraviolet radiation, e.g. tanning equipment. The cancer appears as a growing lump with a rough, scaly surface and reddish patches that can develop into sores that do not heal. Changes in an existing mole or wart may manifest itself into a squamous cell carcinoma. This is treated as a local (restricted) contra-indication to massage. Advise client to seek medical advice.
Stretch marks	These are narrow streaky lines, usually red or purple, before fading to a silvery white colour. They are found on the abdomen, breasts, upper arms, buttocks and hips. They are caused by sudden stretching of the skin, e.g. in pregnancy, weight gain, growth during puberty and muscle building. Avoid deep massage or friction movements.
Stroke	This occurs when the blood supply to the brain is restricted or stopped causing damage to brain tissue. Do not massage. Seek medical advice.
Swellings, painful or inflamed areas of unknown origin	While massage is used to prevent or alleviate oedema (swelling in the tissues), medical advice must be sought if there is doubt as to the cause of the oedema and whether massage is suitable.
Thrombosis	See Phlebitis.
Thrush	Thrush is a fungal infection caused by candida albicans. Symptoms include itching, erythema and pain. Massage is not contra-indicated.
Transient ischaemic attack (TIA)	This is a mini stroke where the blood supply to the brain has been temporarily disturbed. Seek medical advice as there could be a risk of another attack.
Trigeminal neuralgia	This is a condition involving the Trigeminal, or 5th Cranial nerve. Symptoms include a stabbing, shooting pain, similar to an electric shock that affects the face and can last from a few seconds to minutes each time. Usually, just one side of the face is affected. Avoid the area during acute episodes.

Table 3.2 *Continued*

Condition	Brief description
Tuberculosis (TB)	This is a bacterial infection that affects the lungs but it can also affect other parts of the body via blood circulation from the lungs. The disease is carried via droplets of saliva from an infected person when they cough, sneeze or speak. Symptoms include a cough with blood in the sputum, fever, chills, night sweats and weight loss. Once the acute stage has passed, seek medical consent to confirm the client can have treatment.
Ulcerative colitis	This affects the lining of the large intestine or colon. It is a chronic disease that flares up and then disappears. The lining of the large intestine becomes inflamed, ulcers form and produce blood, mucus and pus. As the lining is damaged the large intestine cannot absorb water and this can cause diarrhoea. Other symptoms include abdominal pain, weight loss, nausea and tiredness. Gentle massage movements over the abdomen will help to soothe the area.
Ulcers	These can occur on different parts of the body. The term describes an open wound. They can be in the mouth or on the skin (e.g. bed sores). One common type is a peptic ulcer found in the stomach or upper part of the intestine, the duodenum. If the mucus does not work properly the acid in these areas will penetrate the lining and cause an ulcer. Symptoms include heartburn, regurgitating food, pain in the abdominal area and blood in vomit and bowel movements. Gentle massage movements over the abdomen will help to soothe the area.
Unstable angina	The symptoms are similar to angina, but with this type the pain can continue even when resting, lasts more than five minutes and does not respond to treatment. Under these circumstances obtain medical consent. Keep the client warm as cold can exacerbate the symptoms.
Urticaria (nettle rash or hives)	These are itchy, red, raised weals formed on the skin that can be caused by an allergic reaction to certain foods such as shellfish, strawberries etc. It is usually widespread. Do not massage as it could aggravate the condition.
Varicose veins, varicose ulcers	Any obvious, protruding varicose veins must be avoided. Manual massage proximal to the veins can help relieve the pressure.
Warts	These result from a virus that causes rapid cell division. Common warts are raised with a rough surface and are usually found on the hands. Plantar warts (verrucae) are found on the soles of the feet and grow inwards. They are painful upon pressure and should be referred for medical treatment. Warts are very contagious: avoid touching them and avoid working on clients if you have a wart. Do not massage over the area to avoid infection.

Table 3.2 *Continued*

Contra-actions

During the consultation, the client should be made aware of the reactions or responses that may be experienced either during or after treatment. A client's reaction to treatment will depend on their physical and emotional state.

The expected outcomes of the treatment are pleasant responses and include a feeling of relaxation, calm, peace and contentment and increased energy levels. Occasionally, however, adverse effects may occur during treatment. Always be alert to any abnormal changes happening to the client.

An allergic reaction to the medium

Action: Stop the treatment. Cleanse the skin with a hypoallergenic product and apply a cool compress to soothe the area. Record details on the consultation record for future reference.

Heightened emotional state due to the release of suppressed feelings and emotions

Action: liaise with the client to find out if they would like to:

- carry on with the treatment
- have a glass of water
- have a chat
- have a tissue
- stop the treatment and have some personal space.

Profuse sweating

Action: place the client in a semi-reclining position; offer a glass of water to help hydrate the body; remove excess sweat from the area; check the room temperature is suitable; allow client to rest for a few minutes. Liaise with the client about their thoughts on the rest of the treatment.

Nausea

Action: place the client in a semi-reclining position; offer water to sip slowly; allow them to rest and discuss options to continue, cut down or stop the treatment.

Headache

Action: place a cool compress on client's forehead; offer a glass of water and discuss options to continue, cut down or stop the treatment.

Area becoming very hot and red

Action: remove the medium and place a cool compress over the area and discuss options to continue, cut down or stop the treatment.

In the workplace

If the reaction occurs during the massage when you already have a lot of the medium on the body, recommend a shower, where feasible, to remove the medium. If there is no shower then cleanse the area as described above and apply a cool, damp towel.

Be aware

If a client usually reacts to products, carry out a skin test 24–48 hours prior to treatment. Apply a small amount of product by the elbow crease or behind the ear. A positive response includes tingling, erythema, inflammation and swelling. If any of these occur instruct the client to cleanse the area thoroughly. A negative response will be no reaction at all to the product. Record details on the consultation record for future reference.

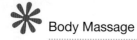

Restlessness and irritability

Action: stop the treatment while you talk to the client about how they feel and what they want to do.

Feeling faint

Action: place client in supine or recovery position; apply a cool compress to the forehead; make sure there is sufficient fresh air in the room; offer a glass of water and allow client to rest for 5–10 minutes. Discuss what they want to do in terms of treatment.

See Chapter 6 for contra-actions that may occur after treatment.

Preparation for massage

Preparation for massage involves the physical and mental preparation of you and the client as well as the preparation of the working area or room. The highest standards of health, safety and hygiene must be practised at all times. You carry a heavy responsibility for protecting yourself and your clients from the risk of cross-infection, infestation or any contamination by micro-organisms that cause disease. You must be aware of, and practise, all the precautions and procedures necessary for protecting health and preventing the spread of disease.

Preparation of working area

Ensure that the working area affords the client total privacy to change and receive treatment without being overlooked by others. The area may be a curtained section in a large salon, an individual walled cubicle or a small massage room. You should ensure there is enough space to walk around the couch and work from all sides.

- The area must be spotlessly clean and tidy.
- Items required during the massage must be neatly arranged on the trolley shelf and protected with clean paper tissue or a small sheet.
- A plentiful supply of clean laundered towels and linen should be to hand.
- Extra pillows, small support pillows or rolled towels should also be to hand.
- Shower and toilet facilities for the client's use should be accessible and regularly cleaned.
- A hand basin or sink should be available for you to wash your hands. Disposable towels or hot air dryers should be used to dry the hands. These must all be scrupulously clean.
- A lined bin with a lid should be to hand for disposal of waste.

Environment

The atmosphere created in the working environment should be quiet and calming. The area must be private, warm, well ventilated and free from distracting noises. Lighting should be soft or dimmed. The client must be positioned in a comfortable, well-supported position and must feel safe and secure.

The following factors affect the client's experience of the treatment and should be addressed before the client arrives. Always check that the client is comfortable and make adjustments where necessary and possible.

Lighting	Too bright	Too dim	Ideal
Lighting is an easy and immediate way to affect environment and mood	Client won't relax	Health and safety – you could trip	Soft lighting, e.g. from up-lighters, wall lights, battery operated tealights
	Could cause headaches	You could spill oil	Dimmer switches
	Could cause eye strain	Could cause eye strain	Corner lighting with uplighting shades
	Could cause temporary blind spots	Could cause sense of claustrophobia	Softly coloured shades
	Atmosphere is spoilt	Could make client feel insecure (especially where you and client are of opposite sex)	Directional lamps. All these will encourage the client to relax.
Temperature	**Too hot**	**Too cold**	**Ideal**
	You will get hot and sweaty	Your hands will be cold, making the client tense	Room temperature should be maintained at around 21°C
	Could cause fatigue or feeling of faintness	Could make concentration difficult	Thermostatically controlled heating is desirable
	Saps your energy	Misdirects your energy	Additional blankets or towels or a lightweight duvet should be available
	Client will sweat, making the skin moist and difficult to massage	Client will not want to undress	Appropriate medium should be warmed in your hands before applying to the client's skin
	Client will feel sticky and uncomfortable	Will cause dissatisfaction	
	Vasodilation will cause erythema	Vasoconstriction will cause client's skin to go pale and feel cold	

Table 3.3 Creating the right environment

	Could cause agitation and irritation and prevent relaxation	Could cause agitation and irritation and prevent relaxation	
Ventilation	**Too stuffy**	**Too draughty**	**Ideal**
	Causes headaches	Client will not want to undress	Windows which can be opened and closed are desirable.
	Build up of CO_2 causes feelings of lethargy and lightheadedness	Effects as for 'Too cold'	Natural ventilation is best but air conditioning is an alternative.
	Could cause agitation and irritation and prevent relaxation		Free-standing fans can aid flow of air but they can be hazardous.
Sound	**Too quiet**	**Too loud**	**Ideal**
	No sound can cause you and the client to feel self-conscious	Will cause irritation and prevent relaxation. This can also occur if the client doesn't like the music	Select appropriate music for the type of massage, e.g. soothing music for a relaxing massage, upbeat music for an invigorating massage.
	Emphasises bodily noises which can cause embarrassment		Alternatively background music can relax the client and enhance their enjoyment of the treatment.
	Can prevent relaxation		
Aroma			A pleasant but not overpowering aroma is conducive to relaxation, such as subtle oils. These can be placed in containers over a heat source.

Table 3.3 *Continued*

Besides these physical factors, other things contribute to the atmosphere of the workplace. The client will pick up any tensions between colleagues. Personal presentation, attitude and body language will all impact on the client's confidence. The look and presentation of the workplace also affects the client's first impressions.

Selection of massage couch

Selecting and purchasing a massage couch can be difficult as there is a wide choice available. Selection is often based on the cost of the couch, but there are other important points to bear in mind when buying. Consider the following points:

- It must be wide enough for the clients to turn over easily and to feel safe and secure.
- It must be long enough to support the length of the body.
- It must be robust, secure and firm. It must not move or rock with the massage nor grate nor squeak as this will disturb the client and prevent them from relaxing.
- It must be at the correct height for working. If it is too high you will have to stretch to reach certain areas. You will not be able to use body weight correctly to apply the required pressure. If it is too low you will have to bend over too much. This will cause shoulder and back problems. When standing upright next to the couch with the arms by the side, the couch should be just below the level of the wrist.
- The covering should be of smooth, washable material that is easy to wipe over and keep clean.
- If you need a couch that you can move from room to room or take on home visits then select the portable folding variety. Ensure that the legs are sturdy and that the hinges are secure and firm. Apply pressure sideways and to the top and bottom to test whether it shakes, rocks or stays firm.

If you are using the couch for other treatments, select from the multi-purpose varieties. The most useful couches are the adjustable height hydraulic varieties, but these are expensive and may be outside your budget. However, they are ideal for massage as the height can be adjusted to accommodate all types of client, from small and thin to large and obese. Some couches have a hole for the face to make positioning and breathing easier when lying prone.

Preparation of massage couch

Prepare the couch before the client arrives, as follows:

- Cover the entire surface with a towelling or cotton sheet – the fitted types are best, as they stay neat and tidy.
- Cover this with a large bath towel or cotton sheet. This must be removed and washed at a minimum of 60°C after each client and a clean one reapplied. Many salons and colleges use disposable paper sheets (couch roll) to save on the laundry.

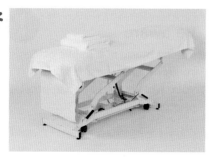

Figure 3.19 Prepared massage couch

These are quite acceptable, but they can tear and crumple during the massage and may interfere with some movements.

- Use one or two pillows for the head. Cover these with pillow slips and then a towel.
- Fold two large towels and place them at the foot of the bed. These will be used to cover the client.
- Place extra pillows, large and small, and a rolled towel on the trolley for use if extra support is required during the massage.

Preparation of trolley

- Select a trolley with a hard, smooth surface, free of cracks and easy to clean. Ensure that it is robust and sturdy so that it cannot be pushed over. Lockable wheels are an advantage as the trolley may be pulled or pushed into a convenient position.
- Place the trolley near the massage couch so that all items will be to hand when required.
- Wipe the shelves with disinfectant of the correct dilution.
- Cover the shelves with paper sheets, folding under all edges for neatness.
- Arrange cleaned bottles and bowls neatly on this sheet. Always place commodities in the same order to ensure that they are easy to identify and reach when needed. Plastic baskets may be used to hold the bottles neatly. Clean these with disinfectant before loading.

The following items should be laid out on the top shelf of the trolley:

- a suitable product for cleansing the face
- mitts and a warm bowl of water to which you have added an appropriate solution or product to wipe over the feet, to cleanse the feet if the client has not showered or had a hydrotherapy treatment
- a good quality oil, lotion or cream to use as a medium for the massage
- talcum powder to use instead of oil or cream as a massage medium for very hairy clients
- a bowl containing tissues and cotton wool.

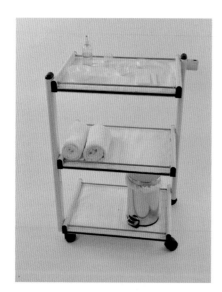

Figure 3.20 Prepared trolley

At the end of each day, strip the trolley down. Wipe the shelves with disinfectant, clean all the bottles and bowls, then either store the commodities in a cupboard ready for use the following day or re-lay the trolley and cover.

Lubricants used for massage

Manufacturers produce a wide variety of oils, creams, lotions, gels and powders that are suitable for massage. The cheapest products are not always the most cost-effective, as you may need to use more of the product: the more expensive may go further. The massage medium should be selected to suit the needs of the client, and with experience you will develop your own preferences. It is important to try different types of lubricant when you are practising massage routines and also to try them on your own skin so that you know how it feels for the client.

Oils tend to offer the highest level of lubrication and are suitable for all skin conditions, especially thin skin. Lotions and creams tend to be more nourishing and may have additives that are beneficial for a variety of skin conditions. Powders may be more suitable for oily skins because powder helps to absorb sebum and sweat, but if sweating is excessive, the powder, sebum and sweat may congeal to form a tacky mess. (If this happens, clean the area and use a more suitable medium.) Gels are usually light textured and non-sticky, leaving no residue on the skin. These can be cost-effective as not so much medium is needed to cover an area. The moisturising properties help to nourish and soften the skin. There are gels available to suit a range of skin conditions.

Massage can be performed without lubrication and many manipulations where the tissues are grasped and lifted, such as picking up and wringing, are more effective when there is no lubrication and so less slippage.

Neuro-muscular techniques are performed without lubrication because friction is required between your fingers and the skin in order to move underlying tissues.

Reasons for using lubricants

Using lubricants helps to:

- reduce friction between your hands and the body part you are massaging
- improve the gliding movement of your hands over the part
- increase client comfort
- prevent dragging and pulling hairy skin
- prevent stretching loose, fragile skin
- nourish dry, scaly skin
- produce psychological and therapeutic benefits if pre-blended oils are used.

>
> **Be aware**
> The use of essential oils is restricted to those qualified in aromatherapy, as different blends have specific therapeutic effects and some are contra-indicated for certain conditions.

Types of massage lubricants

Vegetable oils are the most widely used as these are absorbed into the skin and nourish it. They include almond oil, apricot oil, sunflower oil, grapeseed oil, olive oil, avocado oil, and coconut oil. Each has slightly different properties.

Almond oil

Almond oil is extracted from the nut of the ancient almond tree of the *Rosaceae* plant family. The botanical name is *Prunus communis*. It is a light yellow colour with a slight nutty odour. The oil is rich in nutrients as it contains unsaturated fatty acids, protein and vitamins A, B, D and E.

Uses:

- beneficial for any skin type but especially dry skins as it absorbs easily and helps to moisturise
- helps to warm the body reducing muscle pain and stiffness
- lubricates the skin combating itching and inflammation.

Apricot kernel

The apricot tree belongs to the *Rosaceae* plant family. The botanical name is *Prunus armeniaca*.

The oil extracted from the kernel is rich in essential fatty acids and vitamin A. It has a fine-textured oil, usually colourless but sometimes with a tinge of yellow. It easily absorbs into the skin to nourish and lubricate. The oil is particularly beneficial in skin care.

Uses:

- beneficial for dehydrated, mature and sensitive skins
- soothes inflammation
- helps to relieve skin conditions such as eczema.

Sunflower oil

Sunflower oil belongs to the *Asteraceae* family. The botanical name is *Helianthus anuus*. It is extracted from sunflower seeds rich in linoleic acid, an essential fatty acid that contributes to a healthy skin. The oil also contains a high percentage of vitamin E. It is a fine oil that does not leave a residue on the skin.

Uses:

- ideal for dry skins as the composition of the oil is similar to sebum
- helpful for respiratory problems.

Grapeseed oil

Grapeseed oil belongs to the *Vitaceae* plant family. The botanical name is *Vitis vinifera*. Extracted from grape seeds, this oil is light, fine and non-greasy with little or no odour and is slightly astringent on the skin. It contains a high level of linoleic acid, an essential fatty acid that is beneficial for the skin.

Uses: beneficial for all skin types especially oily and acne.

Olive oil

Olive oil belongs to the *Oleaceae* plant family. The botanical name is *Olea europaea*. It is extracted from the flesh of olives and is dark green to yellow in colour. The consistency is thick and has a rather oily odour, so mix with another oil.

Uses:

- beneficial for mature skins as it is nourishing
- soothing properties help damaged or inflamed skin
- relieves sprains and muscular aches and pains.

Avocado oil

Avocado oil belongs to the *Lauraceae* plant family. The botanical name is *Persea Americana*. This is a very rich and nourishing oil, extracted from the flesh of the avocado fruit. Cold pressed oil is rich green in colour. The oil contains saturated and monounsaturated fatty acids and vitamins A, B and D. It is one of the oils that has the ability to penetrate deeper into the skin.

Uses:

- nourishing for all skin types, especially dry and mature skins
- helps prevent premature ageing of the skin
- healing properties for eczema and psoriasis.

Coconut oil

Coconut oil belongs to the *Arecaceae* plant family, the botanical name is *Cocos nucifera*. The oil is extracted from the dried flesh of the coconut and contains nourishing properties. It may cause a reaction on some skins.

Uses:

- moisturising properties for the skin
- conditioning properties for the hair.

Jojoba (ho-ho-ba) oil

Jojoba oil belongs to the *Simmondsiaceae* plant family. The botanical name is *Simmondsia chinensis*. It is extracted from the crushed seeds of the jojoba evergreen shrub and is a liquid wax, not an oil. The composition of jojoba resembles sebum and it also contains antibacterial and anti-inflammatory properties. Jojoba is usually mixed with another carrier oil.

Uses:

- soothing for sensitive and irritated skins
- beneficial for oily and acne skins and blocked pores
- useful for a dry scalp, eczema and psoriasis
- helps rheumatism and arthritis due to anti-inflammatory properties.

Mineral oils are sometimes used, for example: baby oil, liquid paraffin, cold cream, but they are not recommended as they are not absorbed easily and may block the pores in the skin. Less mineral oil is needed because it tends to lie on the surface of the skin for longer. (Remember to pour less mineral oil into the palm before massage.)

Lanolin (from sheep's wool) is used as a base for some products as it has beneficial moisturising properties.

Precautions

Lubricants may produce an allergic reaction in some clients. These reactions may range from abnormal reddening of the skin,

> **Learning point**
> Some vegetable oils can turn rancid and have a short shelf life: check this before you buy, and buy small quantities only. Lubricants must be stored in containers with small apertures to prevent contamination by micro-organisms that could be transferred to you and the client. Self-dispensing plunge containers are the best.

> **Be aware**
> During consultation, check if the client is allergic to lanolin. If in doubt, carry out a skin test 24 to 48 hours before the treatment or use an alternative product.

raised wheals or a rash to very serious shock with fatal consequences. The client may not be aware that they are allergic to a product. It is therefore safer to carry out a skin test 24 to 48 hours prior to treatment.

Preparing yourself to give a massage

Before carrying out a treatment you must prepare yourself physically, paying due consideration to high standards of professionalism and hygiene. You must also prepare psychologically and give due thought to the type of massage required.

Personal hygiene

- A daily bath or shower should be taken to maintain cleanliness of the skin, hair and nails, and to remove stale sweat odours.

- An antiperspirant should be used to prevent excessive sweating and the odour of stale sweat.

- Hair should be clean and neat; it should be kept short or tied back from the face. Hair must never fall forward around your face and shoulders or touch the client.

- Nails must be well manicured and kept short; they should not protrude above the fleshy part of the finger tip. Massage movements cannot be correctly performed if the nails are long, and long nails may harbour dirt or bacteria. Nail polish should not be worn as some clients may be sensitive to the product and an allergic reaction may result.

- Hands must be well cared for; they must be smooth and warm for massage. You should protect the hands with rubber gloves when doing chores. A good-quality hand lotion should be used night and morning. Gloves should be worn in cold weather. You should not massage with open cuts or abrasions on the hands: cover them with an appropriate dressing.

- Jewellery should be removed or kept to a minimum of wedding ring and small ear studs. Rings, bracelets and watches can harbour micro-organisms or can injure the client if dragged on the skin. Long earrings and necklaces may jangle, producing a noise that is disturbing to the client.

- Uniform should be crisp, well laundered and changed frequently (at least every other day). The style should allow free, unrestricted movement of the arms during massage.

- Well-fitting low-heeled or flat shoes without holes or 'peep toes' will protect the feet and avoid pressure points. Support tights will help prevent tired legs and varicose veins.

- If you are suffering from colds or infections, it is preferable that you should not treat clients. The wearing of a surgical mask will, however, greatly reduce the risk of cross-infection.

- You must wash your hands before touching a client and after cleaning the feet prior to the massage.

Be aware

Many clients may be allergic to nut oils: some may even have severe allergies that can quickly result in anaphylactic shock. This presents as a rapid pulse, difficulty in breathing, profuse sweating and collapse. Check whether the client suffers from any allergies, during consultation and before massage.

Be aware

Read the manufacturer's instructions and list of ingredients before deciding on a product. Ask for samples to try before you buy.

Learning point

Wash your hands before pouring the lubricant into the palm of one hand. Do not pour too much and take care not to spill any, as this is wasteful and will make the floor slippery. Spread the lubricant between the palms of both hands to warm it before applying to the client.

Best practice

Ideally, working uniform should not be worn out of the workplace to prevent micro-organisms being brought into the workplace. It is best to change at work.

Psychological preparation

Preparing the mind enhances concentration and co-ordination and contributes to expertise and effectiveness of the massage.

- Develop a calm, tranquil and positive attitude. It is important to feel secure, confident and relaxed yourself as this is transmitted to the client both by your attitude and through your hands.

- Develop co-ordination between mind and body. The hands and body must move as a whole. Think of your foot position, posture, arm/hand positions, speed, pressure and rhythm. Remember that massage is a skill that must be learned and requires constant practice to perform it well. It is very similar to learning to play a musical instrument.

- Develop sensory awareness, i.e. the ability to sense and visualise structures through the hands. Through the sensory receptors in the hands you learn to identify bony points, degrees of tone or tension in muscles, and variations found on different tissues and different clients. This ability only comes through practice and the experience of treating a variety of different types of client, e.g. young, old, thin, obese, toned, with poor muscle tone, tense or relaxed.

- Learn to synchronise speed, rhythm and depth so that these remain consistent throughout the treatment. These will vary depending on the effects required (see Chapter 6). Maximum effectiveness of the treatment will occur only if these factors are co-ordinated.

Preparing the client

- Speak to the client in a polite and friendly manner.
- Maintain client privacy at all times.
- Take the client's outdoor clothes or show them where to hang them.
- Show the client the treatment area.
- Give client instructions of how to prepare and leave the room.
- Ask the client to remove all jewellery and to place it somewhere safe.

Positioning the client

- Position the client correctly on the couch. A correct, well-supported position will ensure that the client is comfortable and will aid muscle relaxation. If the client is not well supported and comfortable, the muscles will be tense and will contract to hold the body parts. They will become restless and unable to relax and the massage will be ineffective. The position of the client must also allow you to reach all areas easily without stooping or over-stretching.

- When positioning client in the **supine** lying position (face up) offer the client one or two pillows under the head for support.

> **Be aware**
>
> The client is responsible for the safekeeping of their own possessions. Do not offer to store valuables.

Another pillow placed under the knees will help to flatten the lumbar spine. Some clients like this knee support and it is particularly beneficial for those with back pain. This pillow must be fairly small and firm so that it does not hinder the leg massage.

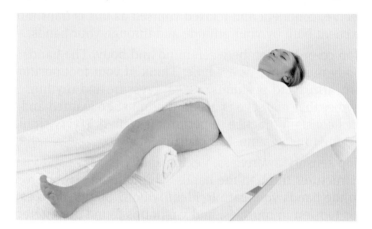

Figure 3.21 Supine lying position

- When positioning client in the **prone** lying position (face down) the head is usually turned to one side, with or without a pillow under the head depending on client preference. A pillow placed under the abdomen will round out the lumbar spine, which will make those clients with lordosis more comfortable. A small, firm pad or tightly rolled towel can be placed under the ankles. This ensures that the anterior tibial tendons are not over-stretched. Alternatively, the feet may just hang over the edge of the couch. The arms may be placed down along the body or bent and placed on either side of the head. If the treatment includes the scalp it will not be necessary to protect the hair.

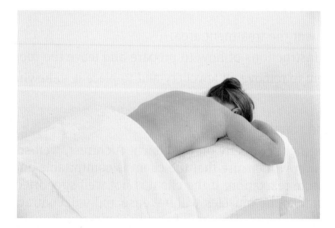

Figure 3.22 Prone lying position

- Cover the client with two towels: one placed across the upper trunk from neck to waist, the other placed lengthways from the waist to the feet.

- Each part is uncovered when being worked on and then re-covered as the massage moves on.
- Always ask if the client is warm and comfortable.

Sitting

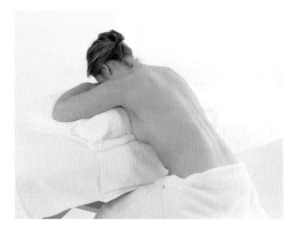

Figure 3.23 Client sitting at the couch

Massage of the neck and upper back is frequently done with the client sitting. It is also a comfortable position for a pregnant client who requires a relaxing back massage.

- Place a stool, without wheels, to the side or the end of a couch. Cover with a towel.
- Place one or two pillows on the couch and cover with a towel.
- Ask the client to undress, sit on the stool and lean forward onto the pillows.
- Ensure that the client is comfortable and well supported, with the arms and head resting on the pillow.
- Cover with a towel until the massage begins.

Use of heat prior to massage

Heating the tissues prior to massage enhances the effect of the massage. The application of heat will dilate the superficial blood vessels, and increase the circulation and metabolic rate. The warmth will relieve pain and tension, thus promoting relaxation. These factors will increase the effect of the massage that follows.

- Mild, gentle heat may be given for 15–20 minutes.
- Any form of heating may be used, depending on client preference, suitability and availability, for example infra-red, radiant heat, steam bath, sauna bath, hydrotherapy, hot pack/hot towels.

Be aware

Heat should not be used if contra-indicated, nor in the treatment of oedema or acute injury.

Questions

1. It is important the client signs the consultation record to confirm that they:

   a. agree to pay at the end of the treatment

   b. understand the details discussed and recorded

   c. agree to the conditions under the Data Protection Act 1998

   d. will attend the appointments or pay a cancellation fee.

2. A person described as an endomorph will be:

   a. tall and long-limbed with fat deposits around the hips

   b. slim and slightly muscular

   c. curvaceous with small hands and feet

   d. muscular with broad shoulders and slim hips.

3. During a postural assessment you note the client's shoulders are rounded. This may indicate muscle imbalance in the:

   a. pectorals and sterno-cleido-mastoid

   b. levator scapulae and upper fibres of trapezius

   c. rhomboids and levator scapulae

   d. middle fibres of trapezius and rhomboids.

4. If a client had the condition lordosis the muscles that will require strengthening are:

   a. rectus abdominus and the hamstrings

   b. erector spinae and ilio-psoas

   c. quadratus lumborum and gluteus maximus

   d. external obliques and ilio-psoas.

5. A client who has winged scapulae will have weak:

   a. rhomboids and levator scapulae

   b. intercostals and upper fibres of trapezius

   c. serratus anterior and lower fibres of trapezius

   d. pectoralis major and latissimus dorsi.

6. To be able to calculate the client's Body Mass Index (BMI) you will need to know their height and:

   a. figure measurements

   b. weight

   c. distribution of fat

   d. dress size.

7. An oily skin can look dull and sallow due to:

   a. a build up of sebum on the surface preventing desquamation

   b. poor circulation

   c. a hormone imbalance

   d. too much sebum in the pores, which causes them to enlarge.

8. Which of the following is a protein found in the dermis?

   a. Keratin.

   b. Antibody.

   c. Melanin.

   d. Collagen.

9. Which of the following is a contra-action to treatment?

   a. Dermatitis.

   b. Headache.

   c. Indigestion.

   d. Sinusitis.

10. Impetigo is caused by:

    a. bacteria

    b. yeast

    c. virus

    d. fungi.

11. Which of the following conditions is caused by too much uric acid in the body?

    a. Heartburn.

    b. Hernia.

    c. Osteoporosis.

    d. Gout.

12. Seasonal Affective Disorder (S.A.D) is caused by an imbalance of the:

    a. adrenal glands

    b. pineal gland

    c. thyroid gland

    d. thymus gland.

13. A condition recognised by reddish patches covered with silvery scales is called:

    a. an allergic reaction

    b. eczema

    c. psoriasis

    d. dermatitis.

14. A condition that affects the alveoli of the lungs is called:

    a. asthma

    b. emphysema

    c. pleurisy

    d. bronchitis.

15. If a client had the condition herpes zoster, what should you do?

    a. Do not give a treatment.

    b. Avoid the area and spend more time elsewhere.

    c. Adapt the pressure to suit the client's needs.

    d. Omit tapotement.

16. The condition Crohn's disease affects the:

    a. liver

    b. bladder

    c. stomach

    d. lining of the intestines.

17. Myalgic encephalomyelitis (ME) is thought to be a condition that mainly affects the:

    a. muscular and nervous systems

    b. cardiovascular and lymphatic systems

    c. nervous and immune systems

    d. endocrine and immune systems.

18. If a client had the condition *tinea pedis*, what should you do?

    a. Advise them to rebook when the condition has cleared.

    b. Offer them waterproof plasters to cover the area.

    c. Carry out the massage as usual but with lighter pressure.

    d. Keep the area covered and spend more time elsewhere.

19. A dehydrated skin is characterised by:

    a. superficial flaking and a loss of plumpness

    b. an accumulation of fluid in the skin

    c. moist areas that feel cold when touched

    d. open pores and excess sweat.

20. As the skin ages, cellular activity in the basal cell layer decreases, causing:

    a. a lack of plumpness

    b. hypersensitivity

    c. uneven pigmentation

    d. loss of elasticity.

4 Classification of massage and the five massage groups

After you have studied this chapter you will be able to:

1. list the five main groups of massage and the manipulations that belong to each group
2. describe the different techniques for each movement
3. explain the effects of each movement
4. perform each movement.

Classification of massage movements

The terminology used to describe the massage movements in each group has evolved over the centuries. There are differences in terminology from country to country and from school to school. The terminology used today is based on the Swedish remedial massage devised in Sweden by the physiologist Per Henrik Ling, and Dr Johann Mezgner of Holland. This has been modified over the years with input from French, German and British physicians and practitioners.

The names of the groups describe the action of the hands on the tissues. The five main groups are:

- **Group 1 Effleurage:** where the hands skim over the surface of the tissues
- **Group 2 Petrissage:** where the hands press down or lift and squeeze the tissues
- **Group 3 Percussion or tapotement:** where the hands strike the tissues
- **Group 4 Vibration:** where the hands vibrate or shake the tissues
- **Group 5 Friction:** (sometimes included with petrissage) localised manipulations performed with the fingers or thumb.

Each of these groups may be further broken down into different manipulations that have their own technique and specific effects.

Massage has several *physiological effects* on clients and *benefits* for them. Physiological effects are what happens within the body, for example, stimulation of lymphatic drainage. Benefits often arise from these physiological effects, for example increased lymphatic drainage will prevent or relieve oedema.

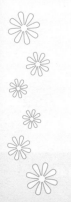

Group	Manipulations
1 Effleurage	Effleurage Stroking
2 Petrissage	Kneading Wringing Picking up Skin rolling
3 Percussion or tapotement	Hacking Cupping or clapping Beating Pounding
4 Vibration	Vibration Shaking
5 Friction	Circular or transverse

Table 4.1 Classification of massage movements

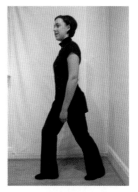
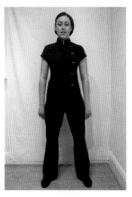

Figure 4.1 Walk standing and stride standing positions

It is important to ensure that you are standing correctly in order to perform these movements effectively. Protect yourself from strain and injury by adopting the correct posture. Two standing positions are used in massage:

- **walk standing** (i.e. with one foot in front of the other) is used when massaging up and down the length of the body
- **stride standing** (i.e. with the feet apart) is used when working across the body.

Always keep the back straight and the shoulders relaxed. Allow the knees to bend when necessary to apply body weight and to reach all areas. Increased depth and pressure must come from body weight transmitted through the arms, but not by pushing with the arms. Use a slight swaying body movement to achieve this. Keep the feet apart – this improves balance and provides stability, as it gives a wider base.

The effleurage group

The word effleurage comes from the French verb *effleurer*, which means to skim over. There are two manipulations within this group:

- effleurage
- stroking.

Although the two manipulations are similar, in that the relaxed hands move over the surface of the body, there are important differences to note. These differences lie in the direction of the strokes and in the differences in the pressure applied.

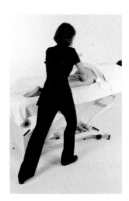
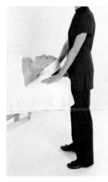

Figure 4.2 Walk standing and stride standing position when performing a treatment

Differences between effleurage and stroking

- Effleurage must always follow the direction of venous return back to the heart and the direction of lymphatic drainage towards the nearest group of lymphatic nodes. Stroking may be performed in any direction.

- The pressure during effleurage may be light, moderate or heavy, but always increases at the end of the stroke towards the lymphatic nodes. The pressure of stroking is selected at the commencement and is maintained throughout. It also may be light, moderate or heavy pressure depending on the type of massage given.

- When performing effleurage, hand contact is maintained during the return of the stroke, although little pressure is applied. When performing stroking, the hands may maintain contact or may lift off the part on return.

Be aware !

Always ensure that sufficient oil (or other appropriate medium) is used to avoid dragging the skin and causing discomfort.

Effleurage

As explained earlier, effleurage is a manipulation where one or both hands move over the surface of the body, applying varying degrees of pressure according to the type of massage being given. Effleurage will produce superficial effects when the pressure is light to moderate, but will produce deeper effects if the pressure is heavy.

Effleurage – technique (leg)

Ensure that the client is warm and comfortable.

↓

Take up a *walk standing* position with the *outside foot forward*: make sure you can reach all parts.

↓

Remember to *bend* the *front knee* as the movement progresses and *use body* weight to apply pressure (pressure must not be applied through the arms and shoulders alone). Keep your *back straight* (see Figure 4.1).

↓

Ensure that your hands are warm, relaxed and supple – they must *mould* and adapt to the *body contours*.

↓

The hands must move in the *direction of venous return* back to the heart, beginning distally and working proximally.

↓

The strokes must be directed towards, and *end* at, a group of **lymphatic nodes** wherever possible.

↓

Learning point

Distal means a structure that is further away from the root or origin, i.e. further away from the trunk.
Proximal means a structure that is towards the root or origin, i.e. nearer the trunk.

The *pressure* should *increase slightly* at the end of the stroke.

↓

The hands *maintain contact* on the return of stroke but apply little pressure.

↓

The movement must be *smooth and rhythmical*, with continuous flow and even pressure.

↓

The whole of the palmar surface of the hand, fingers and thumb should *maintain contact* with the body in a relaxed manner.

↓

The hands usually work together with even pressure and rhythm. However, the hands may be used alternately when care must be taken to maintain an even pressure under each hand and to *synchronise the flow and rhythm*.

Learning point
Do not extend, abduct or link the thumbs, and do not spread the fingers out, as these habits will give uneven pressure.

Remember
On small areas, one hand may work while the other supports the tissues. On very small areas such as the face, fingers or toes, the thumbs only may be used in a sweeping action.

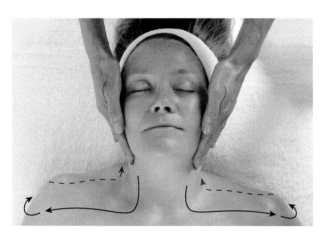

Figure 4.3 Effleurage to sternum

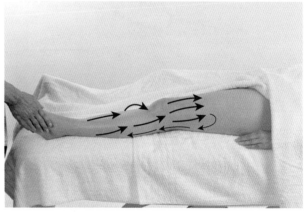

Figure 4.4 Effleurage to leg

Deep effleurage

Heavier pressure is sometimes required to affect the deeper tissue and muscles. This does not mean the use of greater force but rather the more effective use of body weight. Deep effleurage is used for promoting relaxation in deep muscles and improving the local circulation. The manipulations are also used for athletic well-toned clients with muscle bulk.

Deeper effleurage movements include reinforced hand manipulations where one hand is placed on top of the other to reinforce the pressure applied.

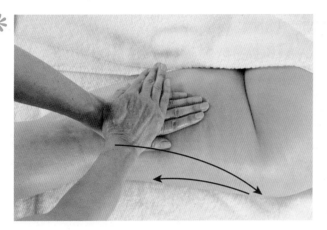

Figure 4.5 Deep effleurage to the hamstrings using one hand to reinforce

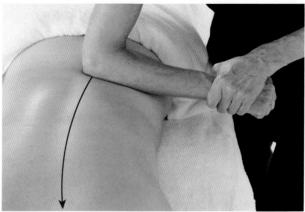

Figure 4.6 Deep effleurage using the forearm over the back

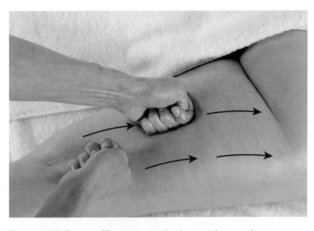

Figure 4.7 Deep effleurage to the hamstrings using clenched fists alternately

Effleurage with the forearm is another deep technique that is particularly effective over the large sheet-like muscles of the back.

Effleurage using the clenched fists can be effective for particularly dense areas, for example the back and upper leg.

These techniques are also used to treat musculo-skeletal problems.

Effleurage – physiological effects and the resulting benefits

- As the hands press on the tissues and move along they push the blood in the veins onwards. This speeds up the removal of deoxygenated blood and waste products from the tissues.
- Deep effleurage performed over muscles after exercise or any athletic performance will hasten the removal of lactic acid and relieve pain and stiffness. Effleurage will help the muscles to recover and return to normal function.
- As a result of increased venous drainage the blood flow through the capillary beds is speeded up. This increases the arterial blood flow, bringing oxygen and nutrients to the tissues more quickly. These factors improve the condition of the tissues.
- The increased blood flow will increase the metabolic rate of the tissue cells, which also will improve their condition.
- Effleurage stimulates venous drainage and a sluggish circulation, which will help to prevent varicose veins and varicose ulcers.
- The increased blood flow and friction of the hands on the part will warm the area. This will aid relaxation and relieve pain.
- Lymph removes large protein particles and tissue fluid from tissue spaces. Speeding up the drainage of lymph prevents stagnation of fluid in the tissues leading to swelling (oedema). Effleurage and squeezing are manipulations that help to prevent and relieve oedema.

- The increased blood flow and dilation of capillaries in the skin will produce an erythema, which improves skin tone. The increased blood flow also nourishes the skin, improving its condition.
- The cells of the stratum basale are stimulated and mitosis (cell division) increases. As more cells are produced they move upwards to the surface, improving the condition of the skin.
- The movement and friction of the hands over the skin removes the dry, flaking cells of the stratum corneum, so desquamation is speeded up and the condition of the skin improves.
- The sebaceous glands are stimulated and produce more sebum, which keeps the skin soft and supple.
- The warmth generated by massage stimulates the sweat glands, increasing the elimination of waste products.
- Slow rhythmical effleurage has a soothing effect on sensory nerve endings in the skin, which will promote relaxation.

Effleurage – benefits
- Relieving oedema.
- Improving the condition of muscle tissue.
- Improving the condition and suppleness of the skin (also aided by massage medium).
- Promoting relaxation.
- Invigorating an area using rhythmical, fast movements with deep pressure.
- Relieving pain and promoting quick recovery following exercise, sport or athletic performance.

Stroking

Stroking is very similar to effleurage in that one or both hands move over the surface of the body applying varying degrees of pressure, but there are differences, as explained earlier.

Stroking – technique

> The therapist's stance depends on the direction of movement – **walk standing** (one foot in front of the other) if working top to bottom; **stride standing** (feet apart) if working from side to side.

↓

> The hands must be *warm, relaxed and supple*; they may mould and adapt to the contours of the body but this is not always so.

↓

> The *wrists* must be very *flexible and loose*.

Be aware !

If the pressure is very light or barely touching, the nerve endings will be irritated. If the pressure is very deep the pain sensors will be stimulated. Both these effects will increase tension and should be avoided.

Learning point

As the first manipulation, effleurage is used to spread the massage medium (the oil or cream). This also enables the client to become accustomed to the therapist's hands, which aids client relaxation. Effleurage can be used as a linkage movement to provide continuity and smooth transition between other massage groups.

Remember

The hands may or may not be lifted off the part at the end of the stroke.

Learning point
Pressure may be light to moderate for a relaxing massage, or firm and heavy for a vigorous massage.

The movement can be *performed in any direction*.

The *pressure* is selected at the commencement of the stroke and *maintained throughout the stroke*.

The movements must be *rhythmical* with *continuous* flow.

The whole of the palmar surface of the hand, fingers and thumb may remain in contact with the part, *or* the fingers only may be used.

Learning point
Stroking is frequently performed from the nape of the neck to the base of the spine, or transversely across the abdomen, back or thigh.

The hands usually *work alternately*, one hand commencing a stroke as the other reaches the end.

The hands *may* work in *opposite directions* if working across the back; one beginning on the right side, the other on the left side, then crossing the back.

Remember
Psychological effects (effects on the mind) also result from massage. Soothing stroking produces feelings of *deep relaxation*, which may induce sleep and help insomnia.

Learning point
Using deep digital stroking of the abdomen in the direction of movement of the contents of the colon (clockwise starting on client's right side) may stimulate peristalsis and general movement of the contents of the colon.

Stroking – physiological effects and the resulting benefits

Soothing stroking, performed slowly with light pressure:
- Soothes sensory nerve endings in the skin, which promotes relaxation.
- Produces contraction of superficial capillaries, which will cool down an area, for example where there is oedema.

Stimulating stroking, performed vigorously with pressure:
- Stimulates sensory nerve endings, which counteracts feelings of lethargy and tiredness.
- Produces dilation of superficial capillaries, increasing the circulation to the skin, giving an erythema, which improves skin tone.
- Stimulates the sebaceous glands to secrete more sebum, which keeps the skin soft and supple.
- Stimulates the sweat glands to produce more sweat, improving elimination.

Soothing stroking – benefits
- Relaxing a tense, nervous client.
- Helping insomnia.

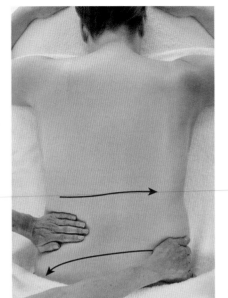

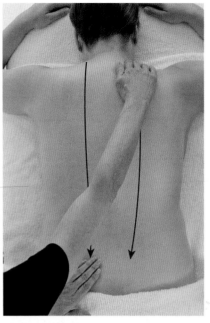

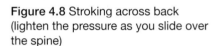

Figure 4.8 Stroking across back (lighten the pressure as you slide over the spine)

Figure 4.9 Stroking down erector spinae (keep an even rhythm throughout the movement)

Stimulating stroking – benefits

- Stimulating a lethargic or tired client.
- Warming up an area.
- Easing constipation.

> **Activity** ✳ ✳ ✳
>
> Practise effleurage and stroking on each other giving feedback on depth, speed, rhythm and continuity. Adapt for a relaxing massage and for a vigorous, stimulating massage. Always consider stance, posture and using your body weight.

The petrissage group

The word 'petrissage' comes from the French verb *pétrir*, meaning 'to knead'. There are four manipulations in this group but some can be further subdivided. The main four are:

- kneading
- picking up
- wringing
- skin rolling.

All the manipulations in this group apply pressure to the tissues, but each manipulation differs in technique. The true kneading manipulations apply pressure to the tissue and move them over underlying bone in a circular movement. However, other manipulations have evolved where the tissues are lifted away from the bone, squeezed and then released. Some of the manipulations in this group are quite difficult to perform and much practice is needed to perfect them.

Kneading

There are many forms of kneading. The terminology used for each one will tell you what should be done, so study them carefully.

- Palmar kneading: this is kneading with the palmar surface of the hand. There are different forms of palmar kneading.
- Digital kneading: this is kneading with the digits (i.e. the fingers) – the index, middle and ring fingers are usually used.
- Thumb kneading: this is kneading with the thumbs.
- Ulnar border kneading: this is kneading with the ulnar border of the hand (ulnar bone or little finger side).

Palmar kneading

Palmar kneading applies pressure to the tissues through the palmar surface of the hands and fingers, and moves the superficial tissues over the deep tissues.

The hands work in a circular motion, applying pressure on the upward movement over the first half of the circle and releasing slightly as the hand comes down to complete the circle. This ensures that the pressure is applied in the direction of venous return to the heart and lymphatic drainage to the lymph nodes.

A variety of methods of palmar kneading may be used – selection depends on the area being treated.

- Single-handed kneading: one hand performs the kneading while the other supports the tissues. This is useful on smaller muscles such as triceps and biceps in the arm.
- Alternate palmar kneading: one hand works slightly before the other, resulting in alternate upward pressure. The hands are placed on either side of a limb (e.g. one on the abductors and one on the adductors of the leg) or they may be placed on the right and left side of the spine if kneading the back from the nape of the neck to the sacrum. One hand starts, then after half a circle the other hand begins producing alternate pressure upwards. This produces excellent mobilisation of the tissues. Avoid working over the femoral triangle as vital structures main arteries, veins, lymph nodes and nerves pass through it just below the skin. This is also a sensitive area that may stimulate a client in an inappropriate way (sexually).
- Reinforced palmar kneading: one hand lies directly on top of the other, reinforcing its movement. This produces very deep pressure, which is useful on large muscle groups such as the quadriceps, hamstrings, posterior tibials, and also on areas of dense adipose tissue over the hips, waist and sides of the trunk.

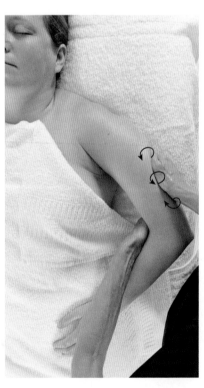

Figure 4.10 Single-handed kneading to triceps

● Double-handed kneading: the hands work side by side, moving the tissues in a large circle with the pressure upwards. This is useful when covering large areas, e.g. from one side of the back to the other. It is also used over the quadriceps and hamstrings on very large thighs.

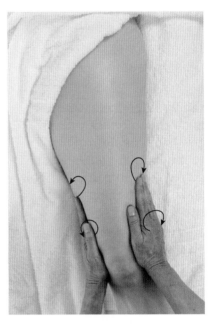

Figure 4.11 Alternate palmar kneading to abductors and adductors

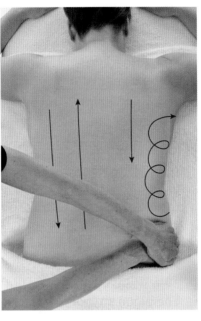

Figure 4.12 Reinforced palmar kneading to lateral aspect of back (work across the back in four lines. Do not massage beyond the inferior angle of the scapula)

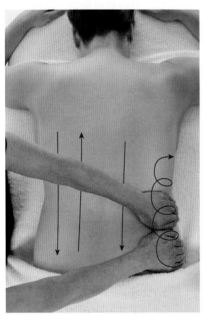

Figure 4.13 Double-handed kneading to lateral aspect of back (as you move across the back ensure you do not apply pressure on the spine)

Palmar kneading – technique

Stand in walk or stride standing, depending on the direction of work.

↓

The hands must be *warm, relaxed and supple* – they must *mould* to the contours of the body.

↓

The *pressure* must be directed *upwards* through the palms and fingers in the *direction of venous return* to the heart and the lymphatic drainage.

↓

The *pressure* is applied *upwards* on *each half circle* and then released slightly to complete the circle while maintaining contact.

↓

Learning point
The hands may work upwards and downwards in continuous sequence, or they may work in one direction and slide back, maintaining contact.

The *pressure* must be *firm* enough to prevent skin rubbing. The flesh should move under the hands.

The heel of the hand *must not* dig into the part.

The movements must be *smooth*, *rhythmical* and with *continuous flow*.

Palmar kneading – physiological effects and the resulting benefits

- The alternate pressure and relaxation of the hands as they move over the area exert a pumping action on the underlying capillaries and veins. This speeds up the flow of blood through the vessels so that waste products are removed and fresh blood delivers nutrients and oxygen more quickly. This will improve the condition of the tissues and help prevent varicose veins and varicose ulcers.

- The flow of lymph through the lymphatic vessels and towards the lymph nodes is speeded up in the same way. Thus, large particles of waste and tissue fluid are removed more quickly. This will reduce or prevent oedema.

- The blood supply to muscles is improved. The waste products of fatigue are removed more quickly, which will reduce pain and stiffness, particularly following exercise or sport.

- Fresh blood brings nutrients and oxygen to nourish muscle cells. This improves the tone and condition of the muscles.

- Slow, deep, rhythmic kneading will increase the blood supply and raise the temperature of the muscle, giving a feeling of warmth that eases tension and promotes relaxation.

- Deep and vigorous kneading will warm and stimulate the muscles. Warm muscles contract more efficiently and are more elastic than cold muscles – they are therefore less likely to suffer injury.

- Deep kneading will press the tissues against the bone. This will stimulate the blood supply to the periosteum and the bone, resulting in an increase in delivery of nutrients to the bone.

- Palmar kneading also affects the condition of the skin in a similar way to effleurage. The circulation to the skin is increased, producing hyperaemia and erythema, therefore the condition and tone of the skin improves.

- Sebaceous glands are stimulated to produce more sebum, which keeps the skin soft and supple.

- The friction of the hands on the part and stimulation of mitosis increase the rate at which the cells of the stratum corneum are shed, which also improves the smoothness and condition of the skin.

- Sweat glands are stimulated and excrete more sweat.

Learning point
Hyperaemia is increase in blood flow. Erythema is reddening of the skin.

Learning point
Kneading over the abdomen in the direction of movement of the contents of the colon (clockwise starting on the client's right side) will stimulate peristalsis.

Palmar kneading – benefits

- Relieving oedema.
- Improving the condition of muscle tissue and maintaining tone and elasticity.
- Removing waste products of fatigue following exercise, sport or athletic performance, thus relieving stiffness and pain and promoting fast recovery.
- Promoting muscle relaxation.
- Producing a sedative and general relaxing effect.
- Mobilising tissues, which improves extensibility and loosens tight fascia and adhesions.
- Improving the condition of the skin (the massage medium also nourishes the skin).
- Relieving constipation.

> **Remember**
> Psychological effects (effects on the mind) also result from massage. Kneading helps to increase alertness and feelings of well-being and prevent lethargy, if the movements are performed briskly.

Digital and thumb kneading

Small circular movements are performed over small areas or small muscles using the pad of the thumb or the pads of the first, second and third fingers. Again, the pressure must be applied in an upward direction, on half the circle, and then eased as the fingers come round and down.

Suggested areas for digital movements include:

- over the upper and middle fibres of the trapezius muscle
- down the erector spinae
- around the colon (following the direction of movement of the contents of the colon)
- over the pectoral muscles
- around the malleoli.

Suggested areas for thumb movements include:

- over the upper and middle fibres of the trapezius muscle
- down the erector spinae
- around the patella
- over the anterior tibialis
- over the dorsum and sole of the foot
- over the flexors and extensors of the forearm
- between the metacarpals and metatarsals
- over the palmar and dorsal surface of the hand
- around the sacrum.

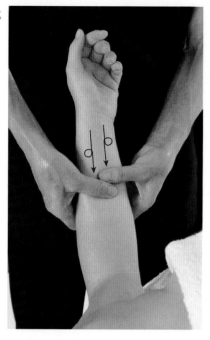

Figure 4.14 Thumb kneading on the flexors of the arm (bend the elbow so the muscles are not stretched)

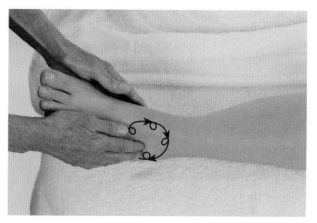

Figure 4.15 Digital kneading around malleoli

Digital and thumb kneading – technique

Select use of thumbs or digits depending on the area to be treated. Pressure may be applied alternately or together.

↓

Select the *depth of pressure* according to the *condition* of the tissues.

↓

Perform *small, circular* movements applying the pressure *upwards on each half circle* and then releasing slightly to complete the circle while maintaining contact.

↓

Each circular movement should move on smoothly and continuously to the next.

Be aware

Do not hyper-extend the thumbs or fingers as this could cause you to develop repetitive strain injury.

Ulnar border kneading – technique

This is similar in technique, effects and uses to digital kneading, However, the ulnar border of the hand is used to obtain greater depth. The ulnar border of the hand is placed on the part and moved in circles. It is used mainly over the soles of the feet and around the colon in abdominal massage. When performed around the colon the pressure changes: the pressure is upwards over the ascending colon (on the client's right side); the pressure is across over the transverse colon; and downwards over the descending colon (on the client's left side).

Digital, thumb and ulnar border kneading – physiological effects and resulting benefits

● The small kneading movements will increase the circulation to small, localised areas, thus improving the condition of tissues and loosening adhesions.

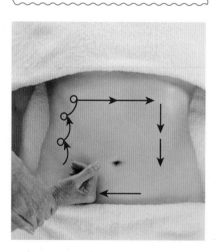

Figure 4.16 Ulnar border kneading to the colon (pressure is applied on the upward movement over the ascending colon; across on the transverse colon; and down on the descending colon)

- Lymphatic drainage will be increased in sluggish areas such as around the ankles, which may help relieve oedema.

Digital, thumb and ulnar border kneading – benefits

- Relieving pain and tension, especially over the trapezius and sacrum.
- Reducing fatigue and pain in the feet following prolonged standing.
- Breaking down or loosening adhesions.
- Promoting relaxation using slow, rhythmical movements.

Wringing

Wringing is a manipulation where the tissues are lifted away from the bone, and pushed and wrung from side to side as the hands move up and down. It must not be used on over-stretched muscles as it can aggravate the condition. On muscles with poor tone it may pinch causing discomfort to the client.

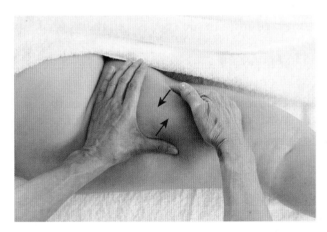

Figure 4.17 Wringing to the hamstrings

Wringing – technique

The stance is usually *stride standing*.

↓

The hands must be *warm, relaxed and supple*.

↓

The tissues are *grasped in the palm* of the hand and held between the *fingers and thumb* (taking care not to pinch).

↓

The tissues are *lifted away* from the bone.

↓

> **Be aware** ❗
> *Do not* pinch with the thumbs and fingers of the same hand.

> **Remember**
> The fingers of the right hand work with the thumb of the left hand to lift the flesh diagonally, then the fingers of the left hand move towards the thumb of the right hand.

> **Learning point**
> The hand may work upwards and downwards in continuous sequence, or it may work in one direction and slide back. Use the other hand to support the tissues.

The tissues are *moved diagonally* from side to side by pushing the fingers of one hand *towards the thumb of the opposite hand*.

Keeping the tissues in the palm and *lifted away* from the bone, the hands *move up and down* along the length of the part, *pushing* the flesh from side to side.

The hands *work up and down* until the area is well covered and *return to starting point*.

Wringing – physiological effects and the resulting benefits

- The alternate squeezing and releasing action of the hands on the tissues again increases the circulation to the area, removing waste products and bringing oxygen and nutrients to the area, thus improving the elasticity and extensibility of the muscles.
- Tissue fluid is squeezed from tissue spaces and the flow of lymph is speeded up.
- The increased blood flow will increase metabolism and help to soften areas of adipose tissue.
- The increased blood flow will raise the temperature of the area slightly, which will aid relaxation and relieve pain.
- It has a sedative effect on nerve endings when performed in a slow, rhythmical relaxing manner. When performed briskly and vigorously, it stimulates the area.

Wringing – benefits

- Easing tension and relieving pain.
- Improving the elasticity of skin and muscles.
- Softening areas of adipose tissue.
- Mobilising one tissue over another.
- Promoting relaxation if performed slowly and rhythmically.
- Stimulating and invigorating if performed briskly.

Picking up

Picking up is also a manipulation where the tissues are lifted away from the bone, squeezed and released. It may be performed with one hand or with both hands. It must not be used on stretched muscles or those with poor tone because it could cause pinching of the tissues.

Single-handed picking up – technique
This method is performed with one hand grasping the muscle.

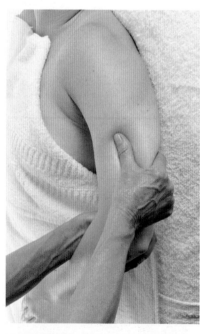

Figure 4.18 Single-handed picking up triceps (note the position of the client's arm).

The stance is *walk standing*.

Spread the thumb *away* from the fingers, i.e. *abduct the thumb*.

Place the *thumb on one side* of the muscle or group and the *fingers* together *on the other side.*

Grasp and lift the muscle in the palm of the hand, *squeezing* with the thumb and fingers (do not pinch).

Release the muscle and move the hand forward, *pushing upward* with the *palm and web* of the abducted thumb. Slight flexion and extension of the wrist accompanies this movement.

The hand moves upwards in this manner, *picking up, squeezing, releasing and moving on.*

Reinforced picking up – technique

The stance is *walk standing*.

Place one hand (right if you are right-handed) on the part, as explained in single-handed picking up.

Place the other hand over the top, with the thumb *over* the index finger of the underneath hand.

The hands then work together (like the wings of a bird) with the fingers of the right and left hand *lifting, squeezing and releasing.*

The arms need to be fairly straight for this manipulation, as body weight is applied *through the arms.*

Double-handed picking up – technique

This is performed by two hands working in a synchronised manner up and down, usually on the large muscle groups of the leg or on adipose tissue at the sides of the trunk and hips.

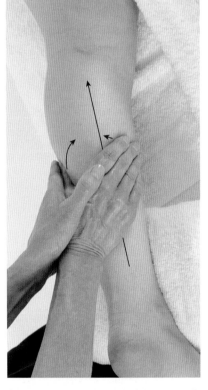

Figure 4.19 Reinforced picking up of gastrocnemius

Be aware

Make sure the pressure of the movement comes from the fingers of each hand, not the underneath thumb.

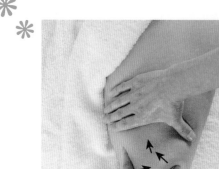

Figure 4.20 Double-handed picking up of quadriceps

Stance is usually *stride standing*.

↓

The hands are placed on the area with the *web* of each *abducted thumb* facing towards each other, with the thumbs and fingers placed around the part and *elbows out* (abducted).

↓

One hand starts *lifting and squeezing* the tissues (as before). On release of the tissues by this hand, the other performs the same action slightly above, maintaining the *rhythm*.

↓

In this way the hands move up over the area in *synchronised chugging* movements.

↓

The pressure upwards is emphasised by the hand that is *pointing and working upwards* in the direction of venous return.

Picking up – physiological effects and the resulting benefits

The effects and benefits of picking up are as for wringing.

Skin rolling

This manipulation presses and rolls the skin and subcutaneous tissues against underlying bone, therefore it can only be performed where there is a bony framework underneath to work against.

It is particularly effective when used transversely across the back, over the ribs or across the limbs.

Skin rolling – technique

The stance is *stride standing*.

↓

Place the *hands flat* over the area with the thumbs abducted.

↓

Lift and *push* the flesh with the fingers towards the thumbs.

↓

Roll this flesh, using the thumbs moving across *towards* the fingers.

↓

Move smoothly onto a lower area and then work back.

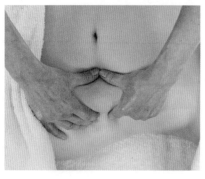

Figure 4.21 Skin rolling to the abdomen (beneficial for stimulating and softening areas of subcutaneous fat)

Skin rolling – physiological effects and the resulting benefits

These are mainly on the skin and subcutaneous tissue.

- Skin rolling increases blood flow to the skin, thus producing an erythema.
- The increased blood flow delivers nutrients and oxygen to the skin cells and removes waste products more quickly, thus improving the condition of the skin.
- The friction of the hands on the skin aids desquamation.
- The increased blood circulation increases metabolism and softens areas of subcutaneous fat.
- It stimulates sebaceous glands to produce more sebum helping to lubricate the skin.
- It stimulates sweat glands to excrete more sweat.

Skin rolling – benefits

- Improving suppleness and elasticity of the skin (the massage medium also helps to nourish the skin).
- Softening and stimulating areas of subcutaneous fat.
- Softening and mobilising scar tissue.
- Inducing relaxation if performed slowly.
- Stimulating and invigorating if performed briskly.

The percussion (tapotement) group

As their name suggests, all the manipulations of this group strike or tap the part. The hands are used alternately to strike the tissues with light, springy, rhythmical movements. When performing these manipulations, particular care must be taken to avoid bony prominences, ridges or areas where the bone is not well covered.

There are four manipulations in this group, named according to the position of the hands and the way in which they strike the part:

- hacking
- cupping
- beating
- pounding.

Hacking

This manipulation uses the ulnar border of the hand and the little finger, ring and middle fingers to strike the tissues in a light, springy, brisk manner. The forearm must alternately pronate and supinate to allow the fingers to strike the part. The hands strike alternately.

> **Learning point**
> As the skin is moved over underlying tissues, its elasticity and suppleness is improved. This will help to soften established scar tissue.

> **Be aware**
> Percussion group
> They must not be performed on old or very thin clients, or those with loose, poorly toned muscles and little adipose tissue.

> **Learning point**
> These manipulations are never used in a relaxing massage because they are too vigorous and stimulating.

> **Be aware**
> It is important to avoid flexion and extension of the elbow joint as the resulting 'chopping' action is too heavy and powerful.

Body Massage

Activity ✻✻✻

This is a difficult manipulation to master and much practice is needed to perfect it. Practise initially on a pillow and perfect the technique on your peers before performing on a client.

Hacking – technique

The stance is usually *stride standing*.

Place the hands together with the *fingers straight* as in prayer, (thumbs against chest).

Take the *elbows away* from the sides, i.e. abduct the shoulder joint. The wrists should now be extended at an 80–90° angle.

Place the *arms parallel* and just *above* the part to be worked on.

Pronate and supinate the forearm so that the little fingers *strike* the part *lightly* and then *lift* away.

Part the hands and strike the area *alternately* (remember to keep the elbows out and wrists extended).

Relax or *softly flex* the fingers and, keeping the same action, strike the part alternately with the *ulnar border* of the *little, ring and middle* fingers.

Strike *lightly, briskly and rhythmically* with alternate hands.

Work up and down or across an area – cover thoroughly.

The hands may also diverge – the heels of the hand stay close but the fingers diverge forming a 'V' shape. This is useful over the upper fibres of the trapezius, below the nape of the neck.

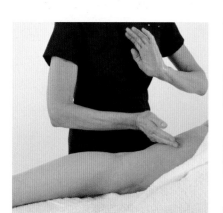

Figure 4.22 Hacking to back of the leg (hamstrings)

Learning point

Pronation and **supination** are movements that occur between the radius and ulnar. Pronation turns the hand backwards or downwards. Supination turns the hand forwards or upwards.

Be aware

Hacking over sensitive or painful areas of cellulite must be very light, or omitted.

Hacking – physiological effects and the resulting benefits

The effects are similar for all the percussion manipulations, except that beating and pounding are heavier manipulations and produce deeper effects.

- Increases the circulation to the area, producing hyperaemia and erythema.
- Stimulates and softens areas of adipose tissue and is very effective on areas of hard fat and cellulite.
- Stimulates reflex contraction of muscle fibres and may increase muscle tone.
- Increased blood flow warms the area and increases the metabolic rate.
- Stimulates spinal nerves when performed down each side of the spine, producing an invigorating effect.

Learning point
Hacking must be performed lightly and briskly to produce the most beneficial effect on muscle fibres. Other manipulations are not as brisk and sharp, and so they do not produce as great an effect.

Hacking – benefits

- Warming an area.
- Softening areas of fat.
- Invigorating and giving a feeling of glow and well-being.
- Stimulating muscles with poor tone.

Cupping (clapping)

Cupping (also known as clapping) is performed using the cupped hands to strike the part alternately. The movements are light and brisk, producing a hollow sound.

Cupping – technique

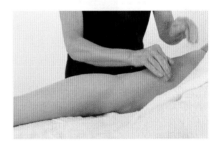

Figure 4.23 Cupping to the back of the leg (hamstrings)

The stance is usually *stride standing*.

↓

Make a *hollow shape* with the hand by *flexing* the metacarpophalangeal joints (knuckle joints). Keep the thumb in contact with the index finger.

↓

Straighten the elbows – they may *flex and extend* slightly with the movement.

↓

Place the hands on the part.

↓

Flex and extend the wrist as the hands *lift up and down* alternately; keep the wrists *loose and flexible.*

↓

Strike the part *lightly and briskly* with the fingers, part of the palm and heel of the hand.

↓

The hands should *clap* the area, making a hollow sound.

↓

Be aware
Avoid a slapping noise, which will occur if the hands are too flat. This will sting and be uncomfortable for the client.

Work up and down or across the area. Cover it thoroughly *four to six times*, until an erythema is produced.

Cupping – physiological effects and benefits

The effects and benefits of cupping are similar to those of hacking, but cupping is not as effective for stimulating muscle contraction.

Beating

This is a heavier percussion movement that is useful on very large heavy areas of adipose tissue, particularly over the buttocks and thighs. The manipulation is performed by striking the area with a loosely clenched fist. The back of the fingers and heel of the hands strike the part as the hands alternately drop heavily onto the area.

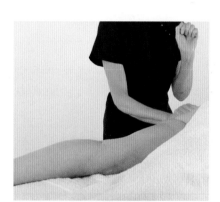

Figure 4.24 Beating to the gluteal area

Beating – technique

The stance is usually *stride standing*.

Loosely clench the fingers; keep the thumb against the hand.

Place the loosely clenched hands on the part so that the back of the fingers and heel of the hand lie in contact with the part.

Extend and flex the wrist and **lift** the arms slightly so that the hands fall alternately and *heavily* on the part.

Work up and down or across the area and ensure that you cover it thoroughly *four to six times*.

The movement should be *brisk and rhythmical*. The pressure can vary from *light to heavy*, depending on the required outcome and the type of tissue being worked on. Well-toned, bulky muscles or a depth of adipose tissue (fat) will be suitable for heavier pressure.

It is usual to work with both hands *striking* the part alternately, but it is possible over small or awkward areas to use one hand only, supporting the tissues with the other.

Beating – physiological effects and benefits

These are similar to hacking, but beating is heavier and is particularly effective in stimulating and softening adipose tissue on the buttocks and hip areas.

Pounding

This, again, is a heavy percussion movement, performed by the ulnar border (little finger side) of the loosely clenched fist. The side of the hands strikes the part alternately. As it is a heavy movement it is usually used on the buttocks and hip areas.

Pounding – technique

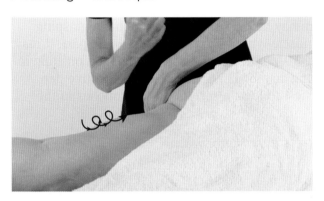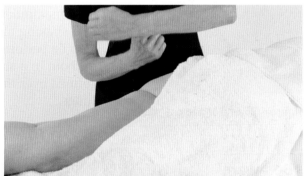

Figure 4.25 Pounding to the gluteal and hip area

The stance is usually *stride standing*.

↓

Loosely clench the fingers.

↓

Place the ulnar border of the hands on the part, with one hand *slightly* in front of the other.

↓

Lift the front hand and *strike* behind the back hand, as the back hand *lifts* off the part.

↓

Continue to *circle* the hands *over* each other, *striking* the part *alternately* with each hand.

↓

The movement should be *brisk and rhythmical*. The pressure can vary from *light to heavy*, depending on the desired effect and density of tissue.

↓

Cover the area thoroughly *four to six* times, or until the desired erythema reaction is achieved.

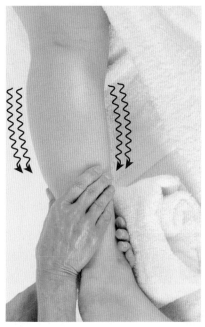

Figure 4.26 Shaking to gastrocnemius

Be aware

Shaking of the chest to loosen secretions requires the correct positioning for drainage of lung secretions and is not covered in this book.

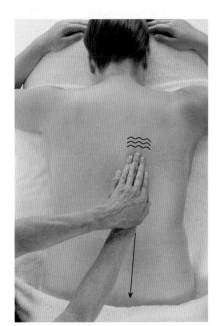

Figure 4.27 Vibration to the back

Pounding – physiological effects and benefits

The effects and benefits of pounding are as for beating, cupping and hacking.

The vibration group

There are two manipulations in this group: shaking and vibration. Both produce vibrations or tremors within the tissues. Shaking is a much bigger, coarser movement and produces shaking of the muscle, while vibrations are fine movements that merely produce a tremor.

Shaking

This manipulation may be performed with one hand grasping and shaking the muscle while the other supports the part. It may also be performed with both hands working together, pushing in and out in a shaking action. This is particularly effective performed over the chest to loosen secretions and mucous in the lungs.

Shaking – technique

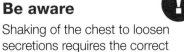

The stance is usually *walk standing*.

↓

Support the part with the other hand so that the muscle is *relaxed*.

↓

Grasp the muscle, usually towards its *distal* end. Lift it between the thumb and fingers, being careful not to pinch.

↓

Shake the muscle *gently* from side to side. As the muscle relaxes, a greater degree of movement will be possible.

Shaking – physiological effects and the resulting benefits

Increases blood circulation to the area, warming the tissues, which will reduce pain and stiffness in the muscle.

Shaking – benefits

Relieving pain and stiffness in muscles, particularly after exercise or athletic performance.

Vibration

This manipulation is usually performed with one hand. However, on large areas both hands can be used. The hand is placed over the area and vibrated either up and down or from side to side. The action produces vibrations in the underlying tissue.

Vibration – technique

The stance is *walk standing* or *stride standing*.

↓

Support the part with one hand (depending on the area).

↓

Keep the fingers *straight* and the thumb *adducted*.

↓

Vibrate the hand (or fingers) up and down or from side to side to produce a tremor in the tissues. The *hand maintains contact* throughout.

↓

The vibrations may be *static* and performed in one area only, or they may *run or move* over the part.

Vibration – physiological effects and the resulting benefits

- Stimulates sluggish lymphatic drainage aiding absorption of tissue fluid.
- Soothes superficial nerves, relieving tension and promoting relaxation.
- When performed along the colon, it will help relieve flatulence.

Vibration – benefits

- Relieving tension and aiding relaxation.
- Relieving flatulence.

The friction group

These are very localised manipulations performed with the fingers or thumb. They may be applied transversely across muscle fibres or in a circular movement. They are deep movements performed with much pressure. The pressure may be selected at the commencement and kept constant throughout, as is usual with transverse frictions, or the pressure may get progressively deeper, as with circular frictions. The pressure must, however, be completely released before moving on to a new area.

Circular frictions – technique

These are small circular movements performed by the fingers or thumb.

Learning point
Vibrations can be produced using the fingers or the whole hand, depending on the area being worked on and on personal preference.

Remember
Adduct means: movement towards the mid line. **Abduct** means movement away from the mid line.

Be aware
Avoid tension developing in the working hand, arm and shoulder.

Learning point
Frictions are usually performed on dry skin, free of oil or talcum powder, so that the fingers/thumb move the skin and do not slip over it. During the course of a massage treatment, however, it is not always necessary to remove the medium from the area prior to commencing frictions as long as the fingers/thumb do not slip.

Remember
These are specialised movements, used when localised depth and pressure is required. They should not be confused with digital or thumb kneading, which applies constant upward pressure using a circular movement.

Learning point
Fast stroking is also sometimes referred to as brisk friction because the hands do apply friction to the area, but this covers a large area and is not localised.

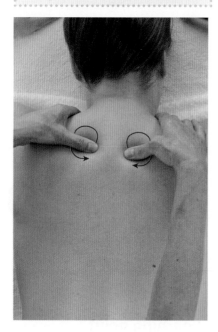

Figure 4.28 Circular frictions to tension nodules in trapezius

Be aware !
For circular and transverse frictions do not hyper-extend the thumbs or fingers as this could cause you repetitive strain injury. This is so easily done when pressure is applied.

Learning point
The fingers or thumb should not slide or rub over the surface of the skin, but the superficial tissues should move with the fingers over the deeper tissues.

Be aware !
Areas requiring circular or transverse frictions may be tender and care must be taken not to cause unnecessary pain through excessive pressure.

The stance is usually *walk standing*.

Identify nodules, adhesions or areas of tension requiring frictions e.g. the back, around joints and over ligaments.

Use the thumb or the fingers: the middle finger is usually used to reinforce the index and ring fingers.

Circular frictions are performed in *small circles*, moving *deeper and deeper* into the tissues to a maximum depth, then *released*. Repeat *three or four* times over the same spot and then move to another area as required.

Effleurage or *stroke* the area frequently between friction manipulations and at the *end* of the treatment to drain and soothe the area.

Transverse frictions – technique

These are backward and forward transverse movements performed across ligaments or joints.

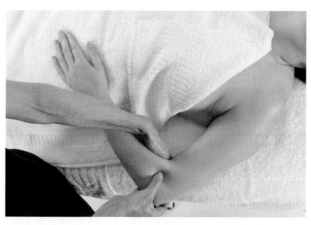

Figure 4.29 Transverse frictions to extensor tendon

The stance is *stride standing* or *walk standing*.

Identify nodules, adhesions or areas of tension requiring frictions e.g. the back, around joints and over ligaments.

Use the thumb or fingers as before.

↓

For transverse frictions, the *pressure* is selected at the *commencement* and is *maintained* throughout the movement – *it does not get deeper*.

↓

Place the thumb or fingers at *right angles* to the part, e.g. the ligament or muscle fibres, and move *transversely* across it, forwards and backwards *six to eight* times. Release and repeat.

↓

Effleurage or *stroke* the area frequently between friction manipulations, and at the end of the treatment, to drain and soothe the area.

Circular and transverse frictions – physiological effects and the resulting benefits

- Increases the circulation to localised areas, producing an erythema and promoting healing.
- Increases circulation when working over ligaments and around joints, improving their function.
- Movement of the tissues over one another will break down adhesions, mobilise fibrous tissue and improve the extensibility of old scar tissue.
- Deep frictions will break down and disperse fibrous nodules and ease fibrositic conditions.
- Stimulate spinal nerves, producing feelings of invigoration.

Circular and transverse frictions – benefits

- Promoting healing of joints and ligaments.
- Improving movement around joints.
- Stretching and loosening old scar tissue.
- Dispersing tension nodules, particularly in the upper and middle fibres of the trapezius.
- Increasing circulation and promoting healing of chronic tendon strains, such as tennis or golfer's elbow.
- Stimulating and invigorating lethargic clients when performed along each side of the spine.

Questions

EFFLEURAGE GROUP

1. The headings for the five main groups of massage are:

a. petrissage, hacking, digital kneading, effleurage, tapotement

b. tapotement, vibration, effleurage, petrissage, friction

c. vibration, cupping, wringing, effleurage, tapotement

d. effleurage, skin rolling, petrissage, tapotement, hacking.

2. The percussion group consists of the following manipulations:

a. beating, kneading, hacking, pounding

b. cupping, pounding, skin rolling, hacking

c. pounding, vibrations, cupping, hacking

d. hacking, beating, pounding, cupping.

3. The main difference between stroking and effleurage is that with stroking:

a. hand contact is maintained throughout the movement

b. the movement always follows the direction of lymph drainage

c. the pressure is increased at the end of the stroke

d. the hands are usually lifted off the area on the return stroke.

4. Which of the following would benefit an older client with poor muscle tone?

a. Effleurage applied with the forearm to stimulate the muscle fibres to relax and contract.

b. Deep effleurage movement to increase blood supply to the muscle fibres to increase tone.

c. Light to moderate effleurage to take into account the underlying bones and muscles.

d. Reinforced effleurage to increase venous drainage and remove waste products.

5. Effleurage movements should always be towards the heart to:

a. stimulate the skin and underlying tissues

b. improve the suppleness of the skin

c. follow lymph drainage and venous return

d. stimulate sweat and sebaceous glands.

6. Effleurage stimulates mitosis in the stratum:

a. spinosum

b. basale

c. granulosum

d. corneum.

7. Skin tone is improved by the:

a. dilation of superficial capillaries

b. stimulation of sebaceous glands

c. elimination of waste materials

d. stimulation of sensory nerve endings.

8. Soothing stroking:

a. stimulates sensory nerve endings

b. produces contraction of superficial capillaries

c. stimulates peristalsis

d. energises a lethargic client.

9. The sweat glands eliminate waste to help:

a. regulate body temperature

b. the drainage of tissue fluid

c. the skin shed dead cells

d. increase blood circulation.

10. The correct stance when performing effleurage movements to the back is to keep the:

a. front knee straight, back slightly curved and apply pressure using hands and arms

b. front knee bent, back slightly curved and apply pressure using upper body weight

c. front knee bent, back straight and apply pressure using body weight

d. front knee straight, back straight and apply pressure using body weight.

PETRISSAGE GROUP

1. Which of the following manipulations is part of the petrissage group?

   a. Frictions, cupping, wringing.

   b. Double handed kneading, shaking, skin rolling.

   c. Skin rolling, picking up, wringing.

   d. Wringing, vibrations, thumb kneading.

2. Kneading movements involve:

   a. grasping and lifting the tissues in the palm of the hand and squeezing with the thumb and fingers

   b. applying pressure to the tissues and moving them over the underlying bone in a circular movement

   c. applying pressure transversely across muscle fibres

   d. grasping the muscle and moving it from side to side.

3. Skin rolling is mainly used to:

   a. stimulate peristalsis

   b. nourish ligaments and joints

   c. promote healing

   d. soften and mobilise adipose tissue.

4. Which of the following manipulations is usually performed between the metacarpals?

   a. Reinforced kneading.

   b. Single-handed picking up.

   c. Thumb kneading.

   d. Ulnar border kneading.

5. The manipulation involving the fingers of one hand working with the thumb of the other hand to move the tissues diagonally from side to side (and vice versa) is:

   a. picking up

   b. kneading

   c. skin rolling

   d. wringing.

6. Ulnar border kneading is usually performed:

   a. on the sole of the foot

   b. down each side or the spine

   c. on the quadriceps

   d. on the flexors of the forearm.

7. Which movement could be used each side of the spine to stimulate spinal nerves?

   a. Skin rolling.

   b. Thumb kneading.

   c. Wringing.

   d. Picking up.

8. The petrissage group of manipulations is used mainly on:

   a. lymphoid tissue

   b. muscle tissue

   c. nervous tissue

   d. loose connective tissue.

9. Petrissage movements performed briskly will:

   a. increase alertness

   b. produce a sedative effect

   c. increase lethargy

   d. help insomnia.

10. Digital and thumb kneading are used to:

   a. break down adipose tissue

   b. stimulate the sweat glands

   c. loosen adhesions

   d. improve the elasticity of skin.

PERCUSSION GROUP

1. Which of the following movements are classified under the heading percussion group?

   a. Pounding and shaking.

   b. Shaking and vibrations.

   c. Cupping and vibrations.

   d. Beating and clapping.

2. When performing hacking, the forearms:

   a. pronate and supinate

   b. flex and extend

   c. laterally and medially rotate

   d. abduct and adduct.

3. Beating is performed by striking the area with the:

   a. fingers and palms of the hands

   b. metacarpo-phalangeal joints flexed

   c. back of the fingers and heel of the hands

   d. ulnar border and loosely clenched fists.

4. Cupping is a movement performed by striking the area with the:

   a. fingers and palms of the hands

   b. metacarpo-phalangeal joints flexed

   c. back of the fingers and heel of the hands

   d. ulnar border and loosely clenched fists.

5. The technique for pounding is to use the:

   a. fingers and palms of the hands

   b. metacarpo-phalangeal joints flexed

   c. back of the fingers and heel of the hands

   d. ulnar border and loosely clenched fists.

6. Which of the following movements produces a hollow sound?

   a. Cupping.

   b. Pounding.

   c. Hacking.

   d. Beating.

7. Percussion movements are beneficial on:

   a. bony areas to increase blood circulation to the periosteum

   b. poorly toned muscles to improve blood supply to the muscle fibres

   c. areas of adipose tissue to increase metabolic rate

   d. spinal processes to stimulate spinal nerves.

8. The most effective movement that stimulates the reflex contraction of muscle fibres is:

   a. hacking

   b. picking up

   c. cupping

   d. skin rolling.

9. Which of the following has the deepest effect on the tissues?

   a. Vibrations.

   b. Beating.

   c. Hacking.

   d. Cupping.

10. The definition of 'hyperaemia' is:

   a. vasoconstriction

   b. reddening of the skin

   c. overactive red blood cells

   d. an increase in blood flow.

VIBRATIONS AND FRICTIONS

1. Vibrations help to:

   a. invigorate the client

   b. soothe and cool the area

   c. soften adipose tissue

   d. relieve flatulence.

2. Shaking is used to:

   a. stimulate and soften adipose tissue

   b. increase sebaceous gland secretion

   c. relieve pain and stiffness in muscles

   d. improve reflex contraction of muscle fibres.

3. The technique for vibrations is to:

   a. keep the fingers straight and thumb adducted

   b. grasp the tissues between the fingers and thumb

   c. place loosely clenched fists on the area

   d. flex the fingers and abduct the thumb.

4. Frictions are usually performed:

   a. on adipose tissue

   b. on loose muscle fibres

   c. over the colon

   d. around joints.

5. Frictions are usually applied with the:

   a. fingers

   b. ulnar border

   c. palm of the hand

   d. forearm.

6. Which of the following movements should be used regularly when performing frictions?

   a. Skin rolling.

   b. Kneading.

   c. Effleurage.

   d. Picking up.

7. Frictions are usually performed without medium:

   a. as there is sufficient sebum on the skin

   b. as the pressure on the tissues produces too much sweat

   c. to move the superficial tissues over the deeper tissues

   d. to ensure the movement is comfortable for the client.

8. Which of the following movements is sometimes referred to as a brisk friction movement?

   a. Stroking.

   b. Kneading.

   c. Shaking.

   d. Picking up.

9. The technique for circular frictions is to apply:

   a. a constant pressure throughout the movement

   b. pressure that gets progressively deeper throughout the movement

   c. pressure that gets progressively lighter throughout the movement

   d. only gentle pressure.

10. The difference between frictions and thumb kneading is that frictions are:

   a. performed in a circular movement with pressure in the direction of venous flow

   b. performed in specific areas requiring depth and pressure

   c. performed over bony prominences

   d. helpful for stimulating lethargic clients.

5 Massage routines and relevant anatomy and physiology

After you have studied this chapter you will be able to:

1. give the approximate timing for each area when giving a general body massage
2. visualise the tissues in the areas being massaged
3. identify the principal bones, muscles, blood vessels and lymphatic nodes
4. discuss the importance of continuity, depth, speed and rhythm and how they should be varied
5. select an appropriate form of massage to suit different conditions
6. perform a variety of manipulations on all areas of the body.

Basic guidelines

Order and timing

The timing of a body massage is usually one hour but may be longer. Remember that for a first treatment you will need to allow time for a full consultation and assessment. In many workplaces, additional time is given for a first appointment. For subsequent treatments you will have to include in your treatment timing a few minutes to recap the client's record card and check with the client any changes in their details and any physical changes you should be aware of.

The suggested order of covering the body is usually:

1. right leg – 7 minutes
2. left leg – 7 minutes
3. left arm – 5 minutes
4. right arm – 5 minutes
5. décolleté – 5 minutes
6. abdomen – 5 minutes
7. back of legs – 6 minutes
8. back – 20 minutes.

Following these guidelines during training will get you used to working to deadlines and following a set procedure. This will help you learn how long to spend on each area and will enable you to develop a good rhythm and pace.

These timings are approximate suggested guidelines only, which you will use during your training. In the workplace, timings will vary to suit client needs, and depending on whether it is a first

treatment or part of a course of treatment. More attention may be required on some areas than others. For example, if there were oedema of the ankles then a longer time would be spent on the legs; tension in the upper back would require additional manipulations and a longer time spent on this area.

Scalp and face massage is now very popular, especially for reducing tension, and many workplaces offer this as part of a full body massage.

Massage of the abdomen is frequently omitted. During the client consultation ask the client whether they want the face and head massage included, and/or the abdomen left out. A woman who is in the first two or three days of her period or who is experiencing heavy periods should not have abdominal massage. Also, women from some cultures may consider abdominal massage to be too intimate. This must be decided before the treatment starts as it will affect the order and timing of the massage.

The conventional order of massage then changes so that the face and head massage conclude the treatment, so the order would be as follows:

- back
- back of left leg
- back of right leg
- **client turns**
- front of right leg
- front of left leg
- left arm
- right arm
- (abdomen)
- décolleté
- face
- head.

Again, this sequence is for guidance only; the length of time you spend on each area can be adapted to suit the needs of the client.

Key points for massage

The following ten key points should be considered every time you perform a massage to ensure that you meet the needs of the client and to maintain consistency in your technique. This will ensure repeat business and recommendations.

- **Comfort**: massage must always be comfortable. It must not hurt the client, even the vigorous and stimulating techniques.
- **Direction**: pressure must be applied in the direction of venous drainage towards the heart and the direction of lymphatic drainage to the nearest lymphatic nodes. (Do not pull back what you have pushed along as this is counter-productive.)
- **Order**: begin with effleurage, follow with applicable petrissage manipulations then percussion if suitable, and complete with

In the workplace

Every place of work within the Beauty Therapy industry will have its own treatment menu. These have usually been adapted from experience and knowing their clientele. Some will offer treatments of half an hour or 45 minutes (e.g. a back massage); others will be longer. You must be flexible enough in your approach to be able to adapt these timings appropriately or you may get a reputation for always running late or for rushing a client. This could lose you repeat business and recommendations.

Be aware

For a male client, omit the abdomen as this could be too stimulating and potentially embarrassing for both of you!

Remember

During training you should be aiming for even coverage all over the body, and balance between the right and left sides. The client must not feel that any part has been neglected.

effleurage. Effleurage and stroking may be interspersed among any of the other manipulations.

- **Continuity**: massage should be continuous – the transition between strokes should be barely perceptible. The hands should not be lifted off the area once treatment has commenced until that area is completed. Move smoothly from one stroke to another.

- **Speed**: this must be selected according to the type of massage required – slow for relaxing, moderate for a general massage, and faster for a vigorous, stimulating massage.

- **Depth**: this must be selected according to the type of massage, as described – moderate depth for a relaxing and general massage, deeper for a vigorous massage. Depth must also be adjusted to suit the client and the desired outcome of the treatment. For example, young, fit clients will take greater depth than older clients; well-toned clients will take greater depth than those with loose, flabby muscles or thin clients; obese clients or those with specific areas of hard adipose tissue will require greater depth. Those accustomed to massage generally prefer a deeper massage than new, nervous clients.

- **Rhythm**: this must be consistent regardless of the type of client. The rhythm is selected at the beginning of the massage and maintained throughout, e.g. slow rhythm for a relaxing massage, moderate for a general, and a faster rhythm for a vigorous massage.

- **Stance**: protect yourself from strain and injury by adopting the correct posture. There are two standing positions used in massage:

  a) **walk** standing (i.e. with one foot in front of the other) is used when massaging up and down the length of the body

  b) **stride** standing (i.e. with the feet apart) is used when working across the body

- **Concentration**: maintain your concentration throughout the massage. Although massage movements become semi-automatic as expertise develops, it is still important to concentrate fully on the task in hand. Continuity and rhythm will suffer if there is a lapse in concentration, and this is transmitted to the client.

- **Coverage**: cover the whole area thoroughly. Do not neglect small areas as this will result in uneven coverage.

Underlying structures

When performing massage it is important to visualise mentally the tissues that the hands are moving over and to sense variations in tension or abnormalities through the hands. A knowledge of the anatomical structure of the area is therefore essential.

The following text identifies the important structures, lists suggested massage routines and highlights areas where special care is needed. Refer back to the sections in Chapter 2 on the skeletal system, the cardiovascular system and the lymphatic system for diagrams of the joints, the main arteries and veins and main lymphatic nodes.

It is very important to learn the names of the muscles, bones and joints, as well as where they are in the body and/or what their function is. There is a lot to learn and it can be difficult information to retain, so it is important to set aside time to revise often.

> ### Activity ✳ ✳ ✳
>
> Prepare a set of cards: on one side write the name of the bone or muscle or joint, and on the reverse write its location and function as appropriate. You can use these cards in quizzes to reinforce your learning and for revision. Test yourself and other students whenever an opportunity arises.

The underlying structure of the legs

Bones

The leg contains the following bones:

- **femur**: thigh bone
- **tibia**: medial and larger bone of the lower leg
- **fibula**: lateral and thinner bone of the lower leg
- **patella**: small bone on front of the knee joint that allows the patella tendon of the quadriceps muscle to move smoothly over the knee joint
- **tarsals**, **metatarsals** and **phalanges** of the ankle and foot.

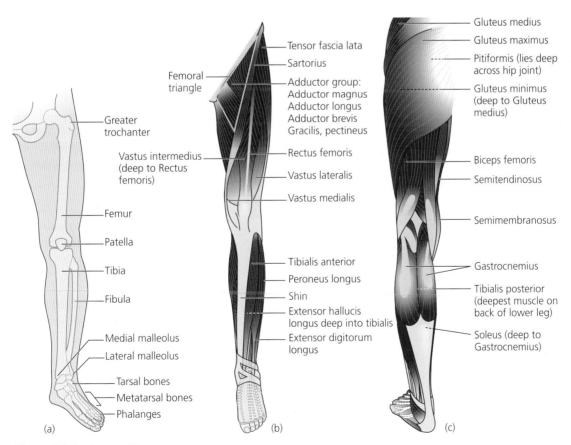

Figure 5.1 Anatomy of the leg

Joints

Name	Type	Movement
Hip	Ball-and-socket (synovial), formed by acetabulum of innominate bone and the head of the femur	Flexion, extension, abduction, adduction, rotation (medial and lateral) and circumduction
Knee	Hinge (synovial), formed by the condyles of the femur and the condyles of the tibia	Flexion and extension
Ankle	Hinge (synovial), lower end of tibia and fibula and talus	Dorsi flexion (foot up) and plantar flexion (point foot)
Intertarsal	Gliding (synovial) between tarsal bones	Inversion (turn foot in) and eversion (turn foot out)
Metatarso-phalangeal	Condyloid (synovial)	Flexion, extension, abduction, adduction and circumduction
Inter-phalangeal of toes	Hinge (synovial)	Flexion and extension

Table 5.1 Classification of leg joints (see Chapter 2 for diagrams of joints)

Muscles

Name	Position	Action
Thigh		
Sartorius	Diagonally across front of thigh	Flexes the hip and knee joint
Quadriceps group (4) Rectus femoris Vastus medialis Vastus lateralis Vastus intermedius	Front of thigh Front of thigh (superficial) Medial aspect of thigh Lateral aspect of thigh Front of thigh, deep	Large powerful group that extends the knee joint and keeps it straight when bearing weight
Hamstrings (3) Biceps femoris Semimembranosus Semitendinosus	Back of thigh	Work as a group to extend the hip joint and flex the knee joint
Adductors (5) Adductor magnus Adductor longus Adductor brevis Pectineus Gracilis	Medial aspect of thigh	Work as a group to adduct the hip joint (pull inwards) and rotate it laterally

Table 5.2 Classification of leg muscles

Name	Position	Action
Abductors (3) Gluteus medius Gluteus minimus	Outer buttock region	Work as a group to abduct the hip joint and rotate it medially
Tensor fascia lata	Upper outer thigh	(Also tenses the band of fascia on the lateral aspect of the thigh)
Gluteus maximus	Large superficial buttock muscle	Extends the hip joint
Piriformis	Lies deep, across the hip joint	Abducts and laterally rotates the thigh
Lower leg		
Anterior tibials (3) Tibialis anterior Extensor hallucis longus Extensor digitorum longus	Antero-lateral aspect of lower leg	All dorsi flex the foot and invert it Extends the big toe Extends other toes
Posterior tibials (5) Gastrocnemius Soleus Tibialis posterior Flexor hallucis longus Flexor digitorum longus	Superficial calf muscle Deep to gastrocnemius and in the calf Deep muscles of the calf	Flexes the knee joint; plantar flexes the foot Plantar flexes the foot Plantar flexes the foot Flexes the big toe Flexor digitorum flexes the other toes
Peronei (3) Peroneus longus Peroneus brevis Peroneus tertious	Lateral aspect of lower leg	Dorsi flex the foot and evert it
Numerous small muscles lie in layers in the sole of the foot and between the metatarsals		

Table 5.2 *Continued*

Blood supply
(See also 'The cardiovascular system' in Chapter 2.)

Main arteries
Blood is carried to the leg by the large femoral artery and its branches.

Main veins
Blood is carried from the legs by the great and small saphenous veins, the femoral vein and its branches.

Lymphatic drainage

There are two groups of nodes in the leg:

- **popliteal nodes:** behind the knee, into which the lymph from the lower leg drains
- **inguinal nodes:** in the groin, into which lymph from the leg drains.

(See also 'The lymphatic system' in Chapter 2.)

Points to consider

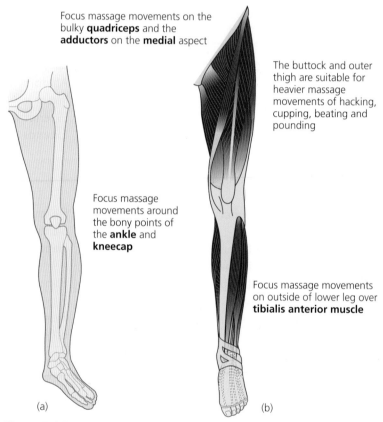

Focus massage movements on the bulky **quadriceps** and the **adductors** on the **medial** aspect

The buttock and outer thigh are suitable for heavier massage movements of hacking, cupping, beating and pounding

Focus massage movements around the bony points of the **ankle** and **kneecap**

Focus massage movements on outside of lower leg over **tibialis anterior muscle**

(a)

(b)

Figure 5.2 Areas to be massaged

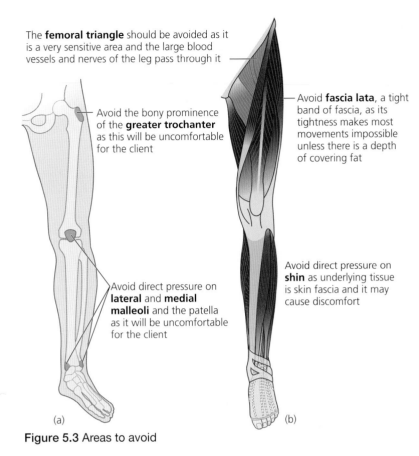

The **femoral triangle** should be avoided as it is a very sensitive area and the large blood vessels and nerves of the leg pass through it

Avoid the bony prominence of the **greater trochanter** as this will be uncomfortable for the client

Avoid **fascia lata**, a tight band of fascia, as its tightness makes most movements impossible unless there is a depth of covering fat

Avoid direct pressure on **lateral** and **medial malleoli** and the patella as it will be uncomfortable for the client

Avoid direct pressure on **shin** as underlying tissue is skin fascia and it may cause discomfort

(a)

(b)

Figure 5.3 Areas to avoid

Learning point

During the massage it may be necessary to use some form of support to ensure the client is comfortable, for example a bolster pillow(s) or rolled towel(s). Place above the popliteal space when massaging the front of the leg, above both knees when massaging the upper body especially if the client has back problems, and under the ankle joint when massaging the back of the legs and the back.

Massage routine for front of legs

The suggested massage routine for the leg is as follows:

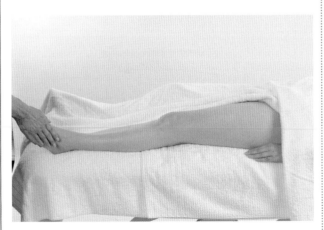

▲ 1. Effleurage (front and sides)

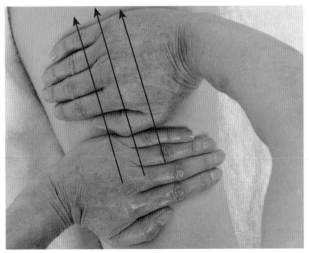

▲ 2. Deeper effleurage over thigh

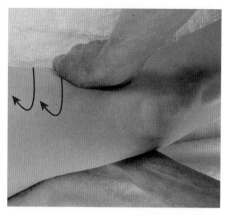

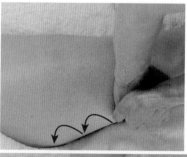
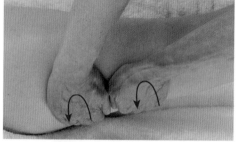

▲ 3. Alternate palmar kneading over abductors and adductors (avoid massaging over the femoral triangle)

▲ 4. Reinforced or double-handed kneading over thigh

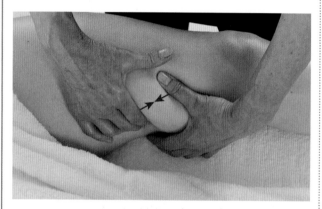

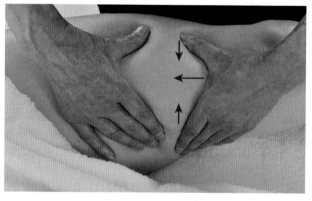

▲ 5. Wringing to thigh (medial to lateral and back)

▲ 6. Picking up – reinforced or double handed (double-handed picking up illustrated here; follow with tapotement if appropriate)

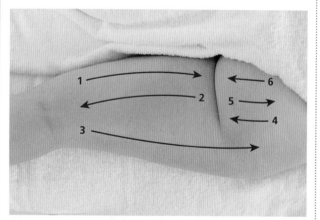

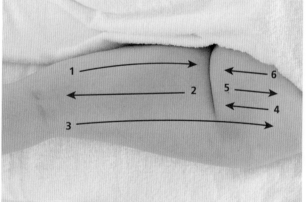

▲ 7. Tapotement (optional) – hacking. The movements in steps 7–10 will depend on the type of massage the client needs.

▲ 8. Tapotement (optional) – cupping

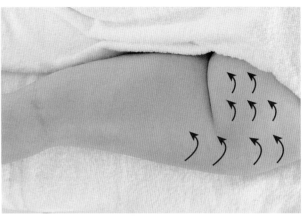

▲ 9. Tapotement (optional) – beating

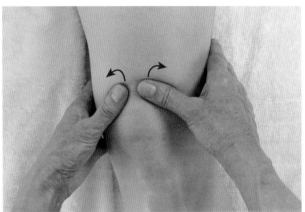

▲ 10. Tapotement (optional) – pounding

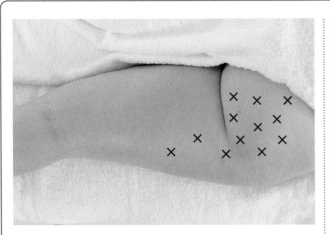

▲ 11. Deep effleurage to thigh

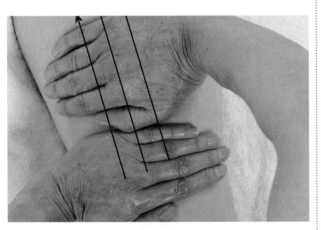

▲ 12. Thumb kneading around patella

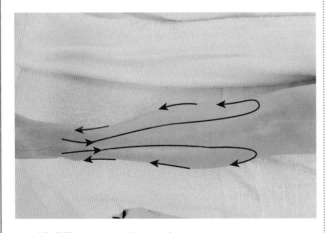

▲ 13. Effleurage to lower leg

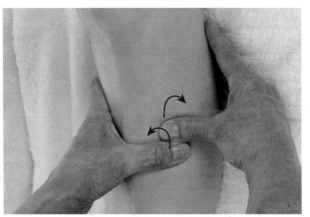

▲ 14. Thumb kneading to anterior tibials (lateral to shin bone)

189

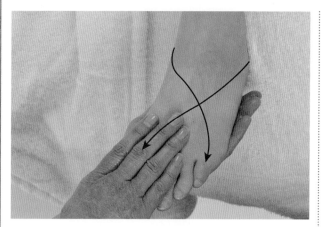

▲ 15. Stroking to dorsal surface of foot

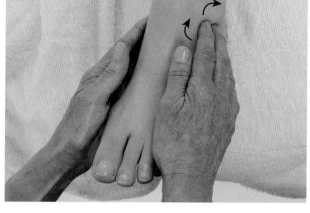

▲ 16. Digital kneading around malleoli

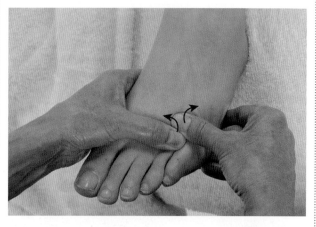

▲ 17. Thumb kneading between metatarsals

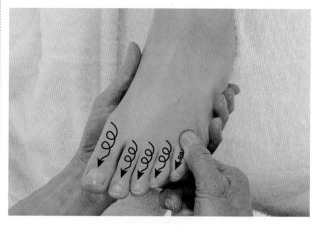

▲ 18. Thumb kneading to toes

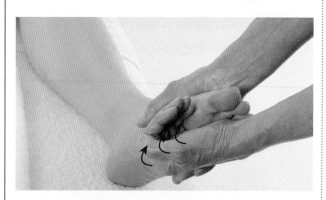

▲ 19. Ulnar border kneading to sole of foot

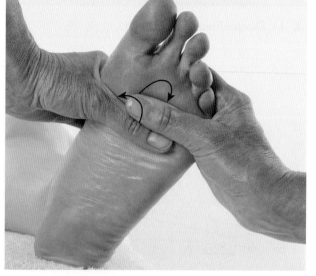

▲ 20. Thumb kneading to sole of foot

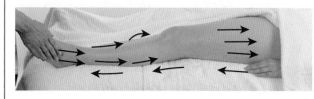

▲ 21. Effleurage to whole leg.

Learning point

Hacking and cupping are added to the thigh for a more invigorating massage, but not for a relaxing one.

Massage routine for back of legs

This is usually performed after the abdomen, when the client has turned over, and before the back routine.

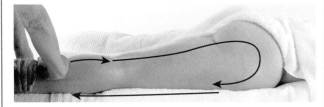

▲ 1. Effleurage to back of leg and buttock (lighten the pressure over the popliteal space)

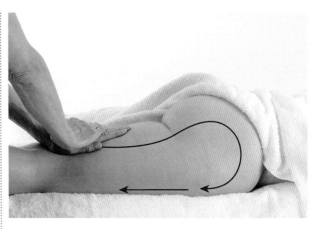

▲ 2. Deep effleurage to hamstrings and buttock

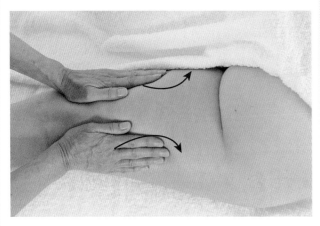

▲ 3. Alternate palmar kneading to hamstrings and buttock

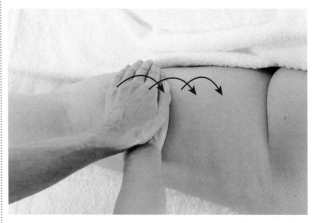

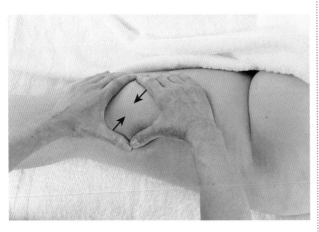

▲ 5. Wringing to hamstrings and buttocks

▲ 4. Reinforced or double-handed kneading to top of thigh and buttock

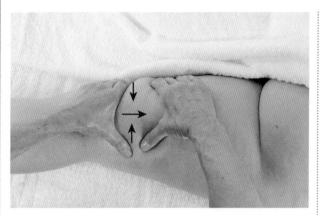

▲ 6. Double-handed picking up to hamstrings and buttocks

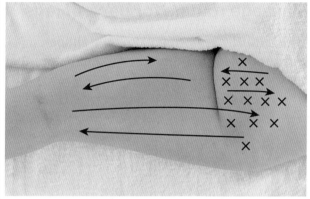

▲ 7. Hacking, cupping, beating and pounding

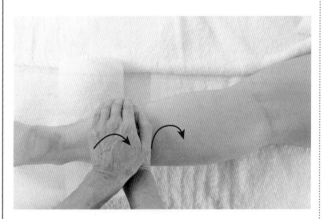

▲ 8. Deep effleurage to thigh and buttock

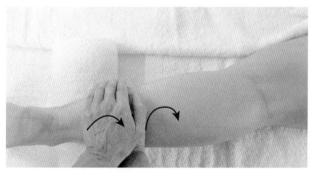

▲ 9. Effleurage to gastrocnemius

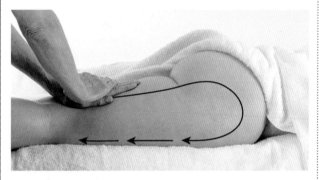

▲ 10. Reinforced kneading to gastrocnemius

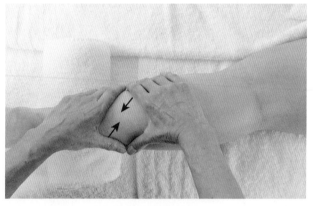

▲ 11. Wringing to gastrocnemius

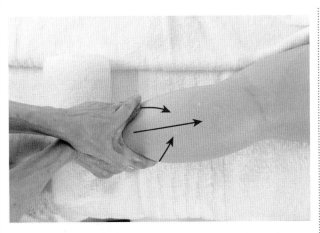

▲ 12. Reinforced picking up to gastrocnemius

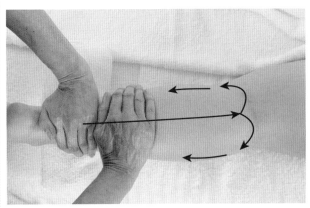

▲ 13. Effleurage to gastrocnemius

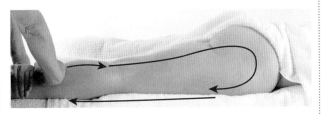

▲ 14. Effleurage to back of leg and buttock (lighten the pressure over the popliteal space)

Learning point
Hacking, cupping, beating and pounding are used on the buttock for an invigorating massage and for treatment of cellulite.

Underlying structure of the arms

Bones

The arm contains the following bones:

- **humerus**: bone of the upper arm
- **radius**: lateral bone of the forearm
- **ulna**: medial bone of the forearm
- **carpals**, **metacarpals** and **phalanges** of the wrists and hands.

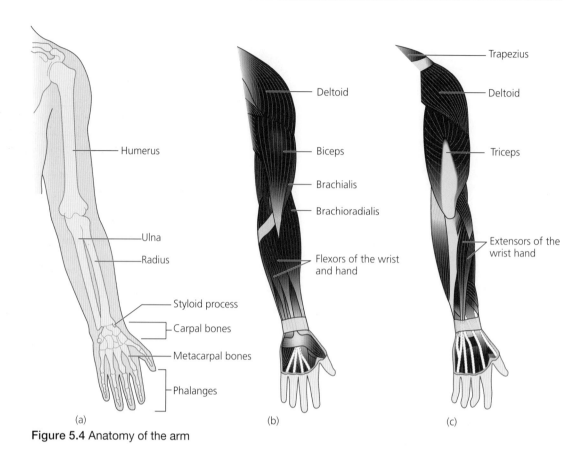

Figure 5.4 Anatomy of the arm

Joints

See also Figures 2.22 and 2.23 in 'The skeletal system' in Chapter 2.

Name	Type	Movement
Shoulder	Ball-and-socket (synovial), formed by the glenoid cavity of the scapula and the head of the humerus	Flexion, extension, abduction, adduction, rotation (medial and lateral) and circumduction
Elbow	Hinge (synovial)	Flexion and extension
Radio-ulnar joint	Pivot (synovial)	Pronation and supination
Wrist joint	Condyloid (synovial)	Flexion, extension, abduction, adduction and circumduction
Metacarpo-phalangeal	Condyloid (synovial)	Flexion, extension, abduction, adduction and circumduction
Interphalangeal	Hinge (synovial)	Flexion and extension

Table 5.3 Classification of arm joints

Muscles

Name	Position	Action
Deltoid	Covers the shoulder	Three sets of fibres: anterior fibres flex shoulder joint; middle fibres abduct shoulder joint; posterior fibres extend shoulder joint
Triceps	Posterior aspect of upper arm	Extends elbow joint
Biceps	Anterior aspect of upper arm	Flexes elbow joint
Brachialis and brachioradialis	Deep to biceps	Flex elbow joint
Flexors of the wrist and fingers	Many muscles lie in layers on the anterior aspect of the forearm	Flex wrist and fingers
Extensors of the wrist and fingers	Many muscles lie in layers on the posterior aspect of the forearm	Extend wrist and fingers

Table 5.4 Classification of arm muscles

The small muscles of the hand lie in the palm and also form the thenar eminence on the thumb side and the hypothenar eminence on the little-finger side. Other small muscles lie between the metacarpals.

Blood supply

Main arteries

Blood is carried to the arm by the axillary artery, the brachial artery, the radial artery and the ulnar artery.

Main veins

Blood is carried from the arm by the cephalic vein, the basilic vein, the brachial vein and the axillary vein.

Lymphatic drainage

There are two groups of nodes in the arm:

- supra trochlear: at the elbow, drains the forearm
- axillary: in the axilla (armpit), drains lymph from the arm.

Points to consider

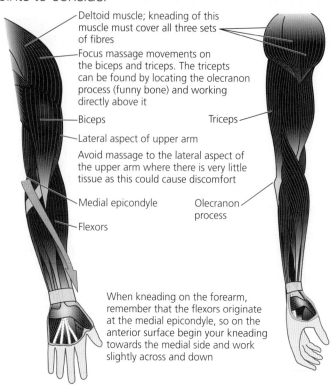

Deltoid muscle; kneading of this muscle must cover all three sets of fibres

Focus massage movements on the biceps and triceps. The tricepts can be found by locating the olecranon process (funny bone) and working directly above it

Biceps

Triceps

Lateral aspect of upper arm

Avoid massage to the lateral aspect of the upper arm where there is very little tissue as this could cause discomfort

Medial epicondyle

Olecranon process

Flexors

When kneading on the forearm, remember that the flexors originate at the medial epicondyle, so on the anterior surface begin your kneading towards the medial side and work slightly across and down

Figure 5.5 Flexors of the lower arm

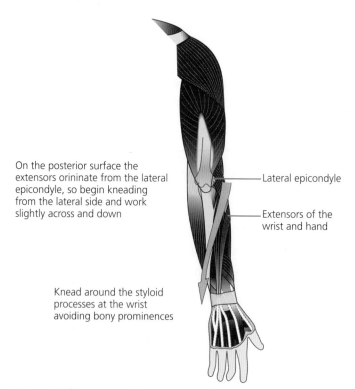

On the posterior surface the extensors orininate from the lateral epicondyle, so begin kneading from the lateral side and work slightly across and down

Lateral epicondyle

Extensors of the wrist and hand

Knead around the styloid processes at the wrist avoiding bony prominences

Figure 5.6 Extensors of the lower arm

Massage routine for the arms

The suggested massage routine for the arm is as follows:

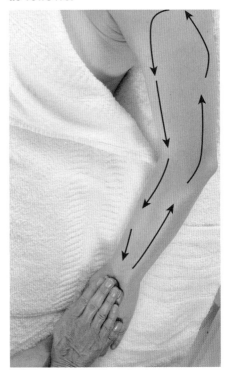

▲ 1. Effleurage to arm

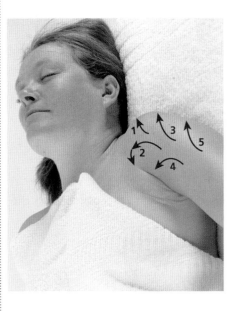

▲ 2. Alternate palmar kneading over deltoid. Work down the deltoid to the point of insertion on the anterior and posterior fibres, as shown above, then work up the middle fibres. Repeat the movement.

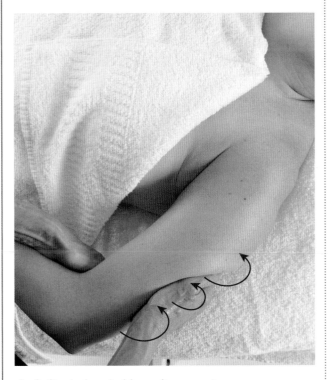

▲ 3. Single-handed kneading to triceps

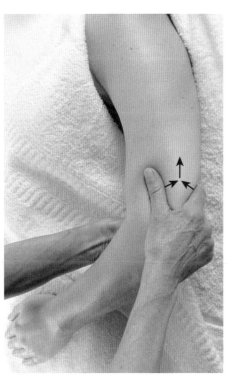

▲ 4. Single-handed picking up to triceps

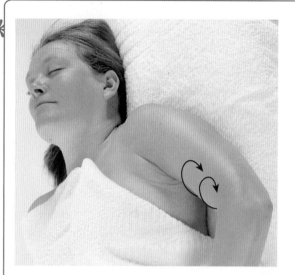

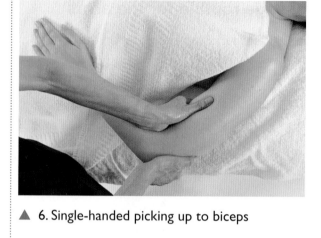

▲ 6. Single-handed picking up to biceps

▲ 5. Single-handed kneading to biceps (support the elbows as shown in 6)

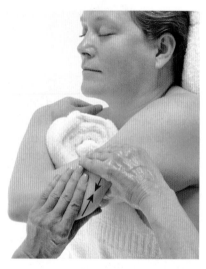

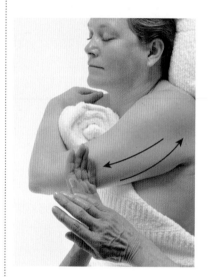

▲ 7. Wringing to triceps (if suitable). If the movements shown in steps 7–9 are suitable for your client, support the client's arm with a bolster pillow or rolled towel

▲ 8. Hacking

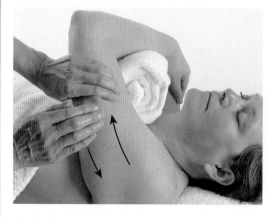

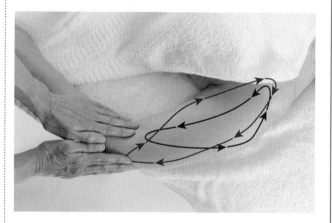

▲ 9. Cupping to triceps

▲ 10. Stroking to upper arm

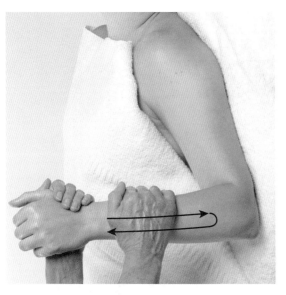

▲ 11. Effleurage to forearm. Change over hands and effleurage the flexors of the lower arm

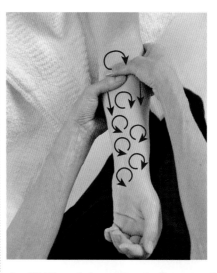

▲ 12. Thumb kneading to flexors of wrist (anterior aspect). Your hands support the client's arm. The client's hand should not rest against you

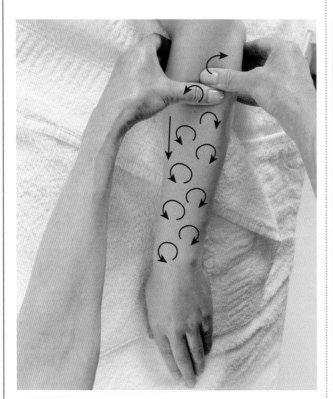

▲ 13. Thumb kneading to extensors of wrist (posterior aspect)

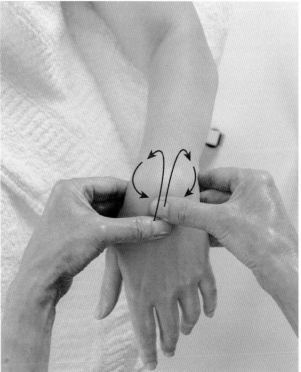

▲ 14. Thumb kneading around styloid processes

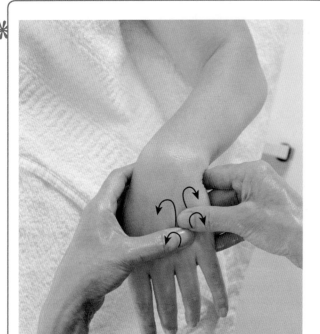

▲ 15. Thumb kneading between metacarpals (dorsal aspect)

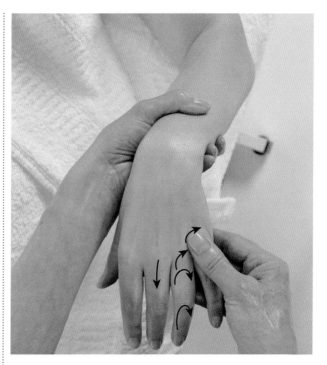

▲ 16. Thumb kneading to fingers (it is more comfortable for the client to support their arm below the styloid processes)

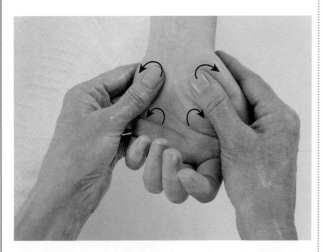

▲ 17. Thumb kneading to thenar and hypothenar eminences and palm

Learning point
Hacking and cupping may be performed on triceps for an invigorating massage.

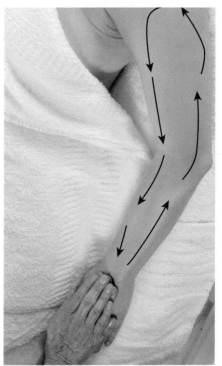

▲ 18. Effleurage to arm.

Underlying structure of the chest and abdomen

Bones

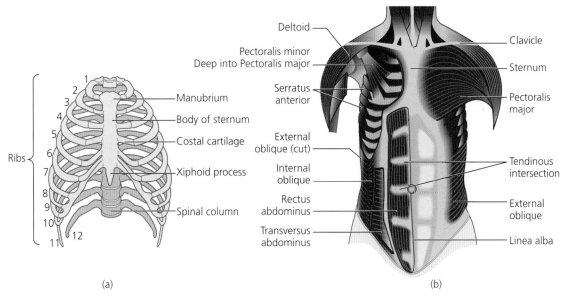

Figure 5.7 Anatomy of the chest and abdomen

The chest contains the following bones:
- **sternum**: breast bone
- **clavicle**: collar bone
- **ribs**: 12 pairs.

Joints

Name	Type	Movement
Sterno-clavicular	Gliding (synovial) between the clavicle and sternum	Accompanies shoulder joint and girdle movements
Acromio-clavicular	Gliding (synovial) between the clavicle and acromion process of scapula	Accompanies shoulder joint and girdle movements

Table 5.5 Classification of chest joints

The ribs join the sternum via the costal cartilages and form a cage that protects the heart and lungs. There is no bony protection for the abdomen and its contents.

Muscles

Name	Position	Action
Chest		
Pectoralis major	Covers the chest	Flexes the shoulder joint and medially rotates it. Protracts the shoulder girdle
Pectoralis minor	Smaller and deep to pectoralis major	Holds the tip of the shoulder down during arm movements
Abdominal wall		
Rectus abdominis	Column of muscle, one on each side of midline	Flexes the trunk; one side working, side flexes the trunk
External oblique	Flat sheet of muscle passing obliquely down and in from ribs to pelvis and midline	Rotates the trunk to the opposite side; one side working aids side flexion of the trunk
Internal oblique	Flat sheet of muscle passing obliquely upwards and in from pelvis to midline and ribs	Rotates the trunk to the same side; one side working aids side flexion of the trunk
Transversus abdominis	Flat sheet of muscle passing transversely across the abdomen	Compresses the abdomen; used in all expulsive actions

Table 5.6 Classification of muscles of the chest and abdomen

Blood supply

Main arteries

Blood is carried to the chest region via the subclavian artery and to the abdomen via the common iliac artery.

Main veins

Blood is carried from the chest via the superior vena cava. Blood is carried from the abdomen via the inferior vena cava.

Lymphatic drainage

See also Figures 2.33 and 2.34 in 'The lymphatic system' in Chapter 2.

There are three groups of nodes in the chest and abdomen:

- axillary nodes: in the axilla, into which lymph from the chest region drains
- inguinal nodes: in the groin
- abdominal nodes: into which lymph from the abdomen drains.

Points to consider

Avoid pressure over the clavicle as this is uncomfortable.

The clavicular glands that lie in the décolleté above and below the clavicle may become very tender in the pre-menstrual female and pressure should be kept very light.

If muscle tone of the abdominals is poor, or if they are loose and over stretched, then manipulation and pressure must be light. If the muscles are well toned or covered by layers of adipose tissue (fat) then deeper pressure may be used.

Heavy percussion movements should be avoided over the abdomen and chest.

Massage will stimulate peristalsis (the movement of alternate contraction and relaxation of the intestines) and is frequently used to aid movement through the colon. Appropriate pressure must therefore be applied in the direction of movement through the colon.

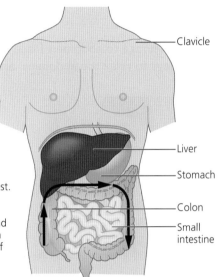

Clavicle

Liver

Stomach

Colon

Small intestine

Figure 5.8 Chest and abdomen: points to consider

Massage routine for the décolleté/chest area

This area may be massaged before the abdomen, or if the routine changes to include the face and/or head, then the décolleté area can be included before the face massage as suggested later. Your position will then change from the side of the couch to the head of the couch and the movements are adapted. It is much easier to perform massage to this area from the head of the couch but it is a matter of preference. See pages 204–5 for photographs of massage from the head of the couch.

Massage routine for the abdomen

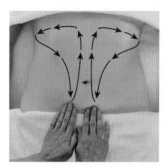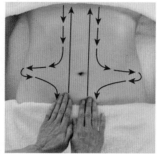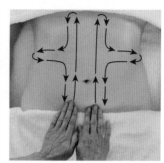

▲ 1. Effleurage to abdomen. Place a bolster pillow or a rolled towel under the upper legs to relax the abdominal area

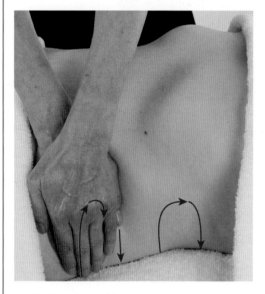

▲ 2. Reinforced kneading to the waist

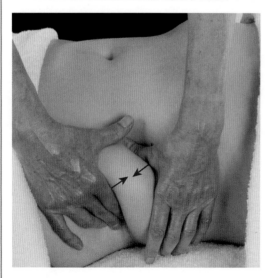

▲ 3. Wringing to the waist if suitable

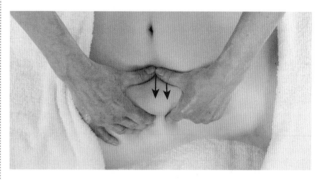

▲ 4. Skin rolling to the waist

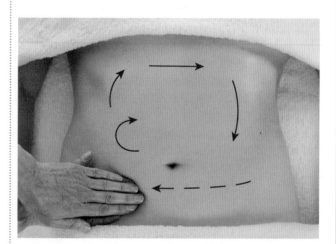

▲ 5. Digital kneading around colon. When working over the colon pressure is applied on the upward movement over the ascending colon; across on the transverse colon; and down on the descending colon

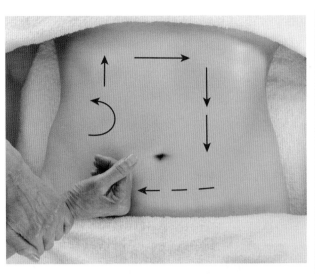

▲ 6. Ulnar border kneading around colon

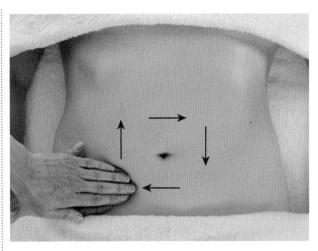

▲ 7. Reinforced stroking to colon

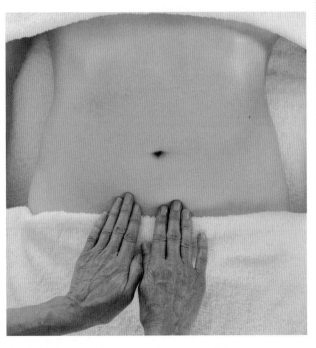

▲ 8. Effleurage (see step 1 on page 204)

Underlying structure of the back

Bones

The back contains the following bones:

- **vertebral column**: made up of 26 separate bones in five regions – cervical (7), thoracic (12), lumbar (5), sacral (5 fused), coccyx (4 fused)
- **ribs**: 12 pairs of ribs form the thorax and articulate with the spine behind and the sternum in front

- **scapulae**: these lie on the upper back, one on each side of the vertebral column
- **innominate** or **pelvic**: these articulate with the sacrum behind, forming a ring of bone known as the pelvis. They join to form a cartilaginous joint called the symphysis pubis in front.

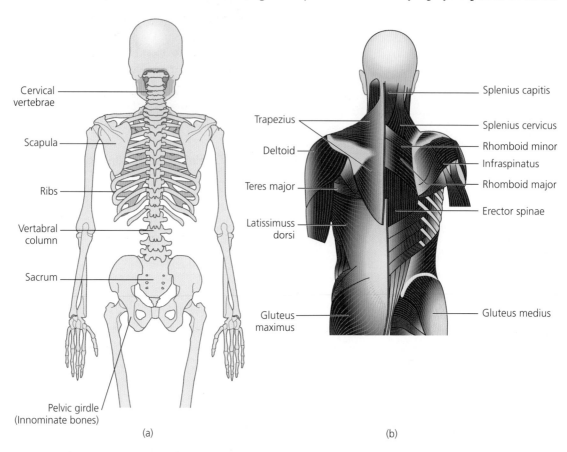

Figure 5.9 Anatomy of the back

Joints

See also Figure 2.21 in 'The skeletal system' in Chapter 2.

Name	Type	Movement
Intervertebral	Cartilaginous, between the vertebrae	Very little movement between each pair, but considerable movement when spine moves as a whole. Flexion, extension, side flexion and rotation
Sacroiliac	Gliding (synovial) between the sacrum and right and left innominate bones	Hardly any movement; slightly increases during pregnancy

Table 5.7 Classification of back joints

Muscles

Name	Position	Action
Trapezius	Covers the upper back	The upper fibres extend the head and elevate the shoulders. When one side is working it side flexes the head to the same side and elevates one shoulder. The middle fibres retract the shoulder girdle
Rhomboid major and minor	Lie deep to trapezius between the scapulae	Retract the shoulder girdle
Latissimus dorsi	Covers the lower back. From the lumbar region it passes upwards and outwards and inserts on the front of the humerus	Extends the shoulder joint and medially rotates it. Raises the trunk towards the arms as in climbing
Erector spinae	Lies deep to other muscles. Forms three columns from lumbar spine up along ribs to transverse and spinous processes to the cervical spine	Extends the trunk; one side working side flexes the trunk to the same side
Quadratus lumborum	Deepest muscle lying on either side of the lumbar spine	Extends the trunk; one side working side flexes the trunk to the same side
Splenius capitis	Deep to trapezius along the ligamentum nuchae into the occipital bone	Both sides working extends the head; one side working rotates the head to the same side
Splenius cervicus	Deep to splenius capitis	As above extends the head; rotates the head to the same side

Table 5.8 Classification of back muscles

Lymphatic drainage

See also Figures 2.35 and 2.36 in 'The skeletal system' in Chapter 2.

- The upper back drains into the axillary nodes.
- The lower back drains into the inguinal nodes.

- When working around the scapula, slide lightly over acromion process to avoid discomfort.
- An extra pillow may be required under the bust to improve contour and comfort where there is evidence of kyphosis.
- An extra pillow may be required under the abdomen to level out the lumbar spine and improve comfort where there is evidence of lordosis.

Points to consider

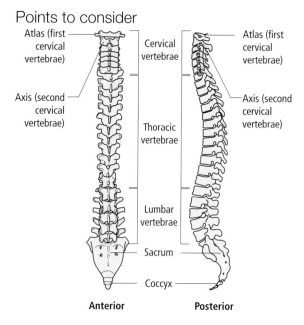

Figure 5.10 Back: points to consider

Massage routine for the back

The suggested massage routine for the back is as follows:

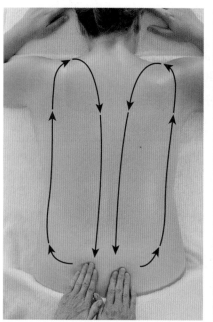 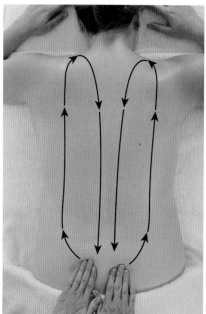 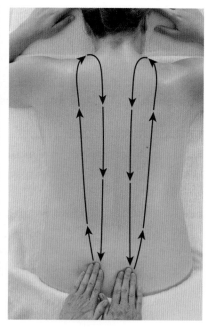

▲ 1. Stroking over the back. Use this movement to palpate and sense the tissues as you move over the area

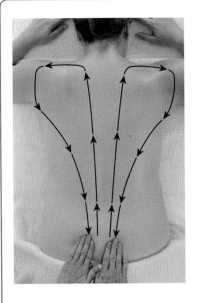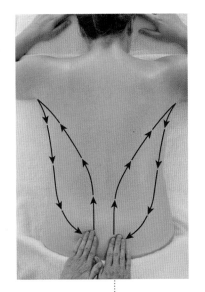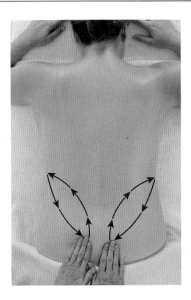

▲ 2. Effleurage over back

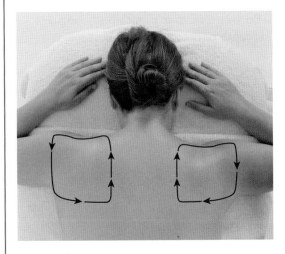

▲ 3. Effleurage over trapezius (neck and shoulders)

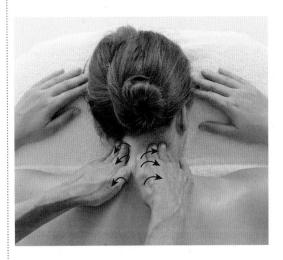

▲ 4. Finger kneading each side of neck

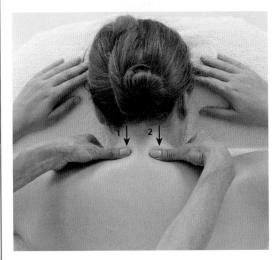

▲ 5. Thumb kneading either side of neck

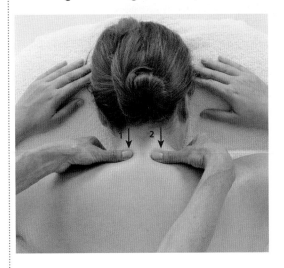

▲ 6. Alternate thumb stroking on neck area

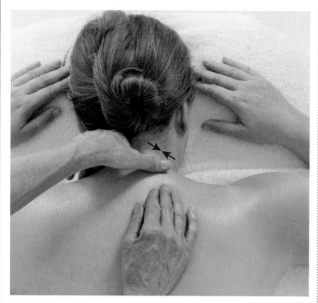

▲ 7. Picking up on the neck

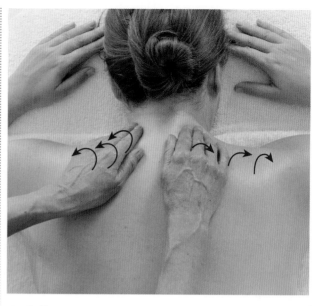

▲ 8. Digital or thumb kneading to upper fibres of trapezius. Be aware of your client's body language; ensure the depth of pressure is comfortable

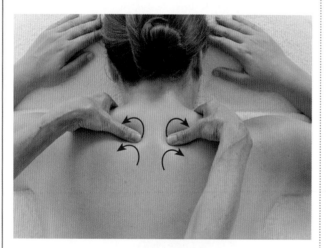

▲ 9. Digital or thumb kneading from neck down between scapulae

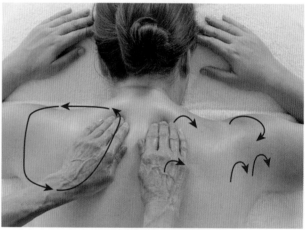

▲ 10. Finger kneading around scapulae

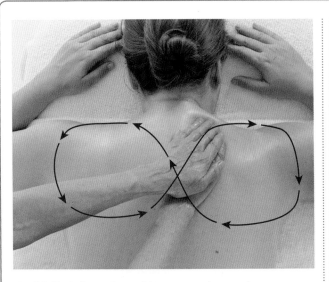

▲ 11. Reinforced stroking around scapulae (figure of eight)

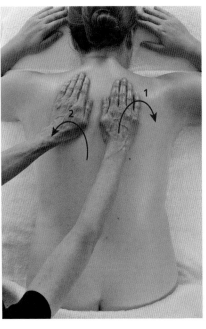

▲ 12. Alternate palmar kneading all over back: work down the back then on return stroke work up close to the spine.

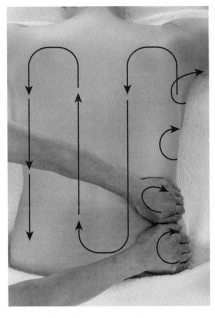

▲ 13. Double-handed kneading over back (one side to other and back in four strips)

Learning point
If the client has sufficient adipose tissue, wringing movements may be carried out moving up along the hip, waist and side of ribs.

211

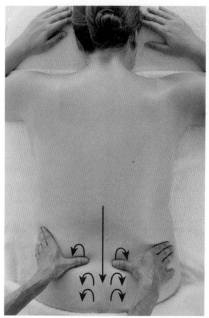

▲ 14. Thumb kneading to scarum and lumbar area

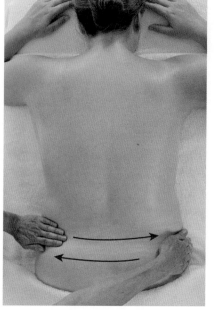

▲ 15. Transverse stroking over back

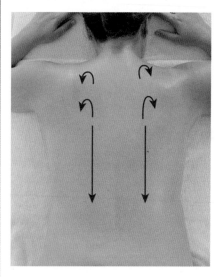

▲ 16. Alternate finger kneading down right and left erector spinae

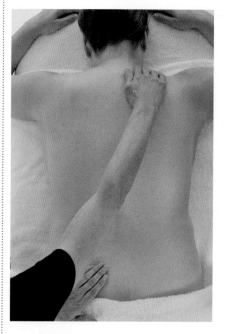

▲ 17. Stroking down right and left erector spinae

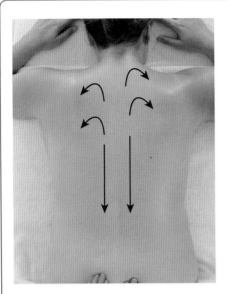

▲ 18. Effleurage over the back
(Repeat movement shown in step 2)

Learning point
Light hacking and cupping over the back may be included for an invigorating massage.

Underlying structure of the head and face

Bones of the skull
These include the cranial and facial bones.
The eight cranial bones are:

- one frontal bone
- two parietal bones
- two temporal bones
- one occipital bone
- one sphenoid
- one ethmoid.

The thirteen facial bones are:

- one maxilla (two bones fused)
- one mandible
- two zygomatic
- two nasal bones
- two lacrimal bones
- two inferior nasal conchae
- one vomer
- two palatine (not shown in diagram: these form part of the mouth; nasal cavity and the orbits).

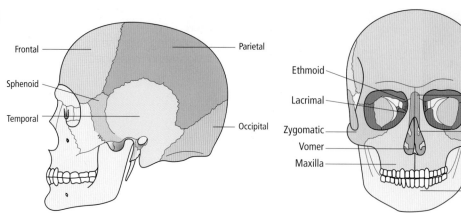

Figure 5.11 Bones of the skull

Figure 5.12 Bones of the face

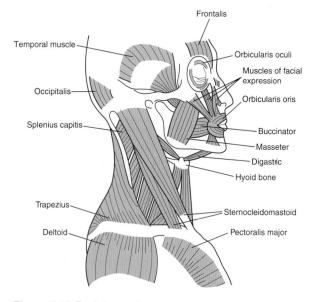

Figure 5.13 Facial muscles

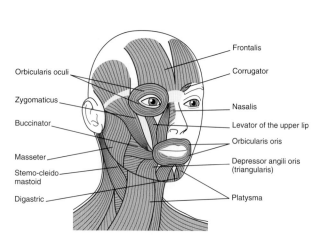

Figure 5.14 Muscles of the face and skull (side view)

Muscle	Position	Action
Frontalis	Covers top of skull	Raises the eyebrows (surprise); wrinkles the forehead (frowning); moves the scalp
Occipitalis	Covers back of skull	Moves scalp when raising eyebrows or wrinkling forehead
Corrugator	Between the eyebrows	Draws eyebrows inwards and down
Nasalis	Side of nose	Compresses the nostrils
Orbicularis oculi	Surrounds the eye	Closes the eye gently or tightly
Levators of the upper lip	Above the upper lip	Raises the upper lip
Zygomaticus	Above the corner of the mouth to zygmatic bone	Raises the corner of the mouth
Buccinator	Deep, horizontal in the cheek	Compresses the cheek; used in sucking and blowing
Temporalis	Side of the head	Moves mandible when chewing
Masseter	Between mandible and zygomatic arch	Raises the mandible to close the mouth
Depressor anguli oris (triangularis)	Below corner of the mouth	Draws corner of the mouth downwards
Orbicularis oris	Around the mouth	Closes and protrudes the lips
Digastric	Beneath the chin	Protrudes the jaw; depresses the mandible
Platysma	Covers the side and front of neck	Depresses the angle of the mouth; wrinkles the skin of the neck
Sternocleidomastoid	Covers side of the neck	Flexes the neck when both sides work together. When working independently, laterally flexes neck to the same side or laterally rotates head to opposite side.

Table 5.9 Classification of facial muscles

Blood supply

Arteries

Blood is delivered to the head via the external and internal carotid arteries.

Veins

Blood is carried from the head via the external and internal jugular veins.

Lymphatic drainage
- anterior and posterior auricular nodes
- occipital nodes
- submandibular nodes
- superficial and deep cervical nodes.

Massage routine for the décolleté/chest area from the head of the couch

1. Apply the lubricant to décolleté region and around the back over upper trapezius.

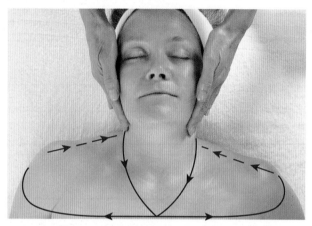

▲ 2. Effleurage. Place fingertips at the side of the neck. Slide under the clavicle onto the sternum, fingers overlapping above the breasts. Pull hands apart, apply suitable pressure towards the axilla, on and around the shoulders, over the trapezius, up the neck and stretch before reaching the occipital bone

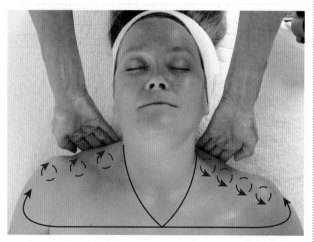

▲ 3. Repeat Step 2, using finger kneading over the trapezius, up the back of the neck, stretch before reaching the occipital bone

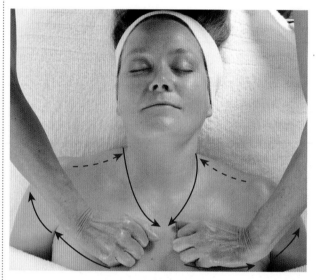

▲ 4. Knuckling. Place fingertips at the side of the neck. Slide under the clavicle onto the sternum, with fingers overlapping above the breasts. With knuckles facing, knuckle across the pectoral muscle in circular movements towards the axilla, slide around the deltoid, over the trapezius up the neck and stretch before reaching the occipital bone

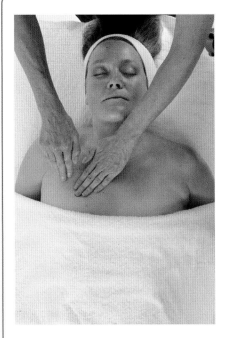

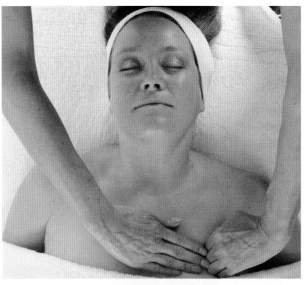

▲ 5. Alternate finger stroking. Place the fingertips at the side of the neck, slide around the clavicle onto the pectorals. Work on the right side, fingers of the left hand point to the axilla, fingers of the right hand point towards the sternum. Work across towards the right axilla with short overlapping strokes. Repeat movement three times. Work on left side three times

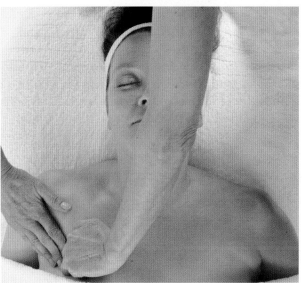

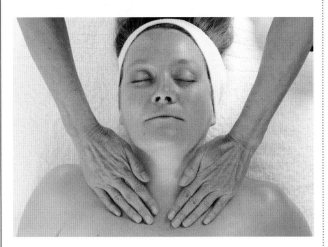

▲ 7. Repeat Step 2

▲ 6. Lymph drainage. Left hand in fist at axilla, fingers of right hand point towards the fist. Move fist lightly over pectorals on left side, apply pressure with fingers and fist as they move over pectorals on right side, draining lymph into right axilla. Change over right hand in a fist at right axilla, fingers of left hand point towards the fist. Move lightly over the right pectorals, increasing the pressure over the left pectorals, draining lymph into the left axilla.

Massage routine for the face

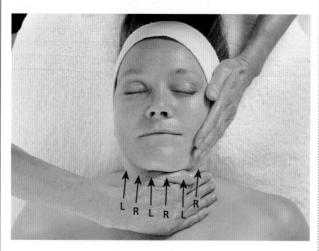

▲ 1. Effleurage. Place the right hand at the base of the neck on the left-hand side. Place the left hand on the jawline on the left-hand side. Six alternate strokes across the neck draining into submandibular submental lymph nodes. Left hand finishes at right-hand jawline. Slide along the jawline to the left-hand side and repeat movement. Position the fingertips under the chin area ready for the next movement

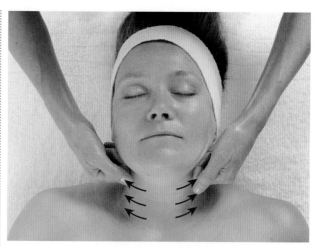

▲ 2. Knuckling across the neck in three rows, starting at the top of the neck either side of the windpipe, working out until in line with the ear lobes. Repeat with two more rows, working down to just above the base of the neck

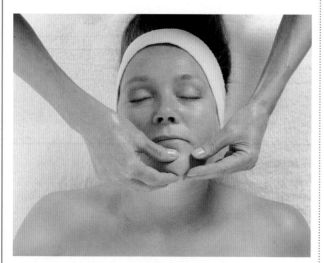

▲ 3. Double-handed picking up along the jawline – centre to left; left to right; right to centre

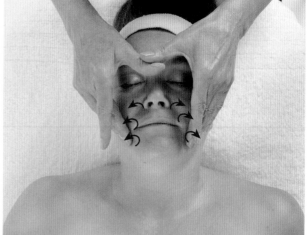

▲ 4. Finger kneading up the labial nasal folds – pressure on the upward movement. Repeat movement

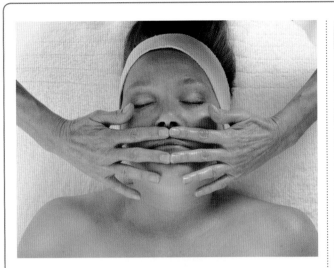

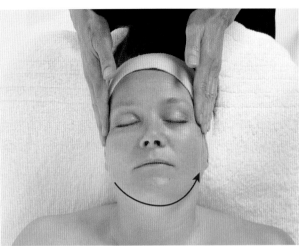

▲ 5. Levator lifts. Place the index fingers together (tips only) above the top lip and tips of the middle fingers under the bottom lip. Pull fingers apart beyond the corner of the lips. Turn and lift the index fingers, holding the muscle with the middle and ring fingers. Move up the sides of the nose without pressure and lift the corrugator. Move fingers still pointing downwards, across the forehead to the temples (avoid lifting the eyebrows). Slide down the face along the jawline with ring finger and repeat movement

▲ 6. Masseter lifts. Take the right hand down the side of the face along the jawline, on the left side, with the fingers pointing towards the ear and wrist above the chin lift the masseter muscle. Hold in position for a count of two; still in contact, turn hand so fingers are pointing down towards the neck. Hold in position for a count of two. Release muscle and slide hand up and over the forehead to the right temple. Repeat on right side

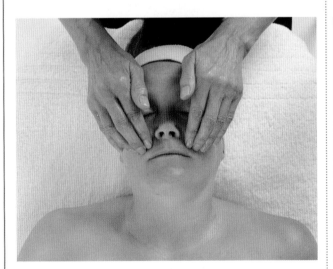

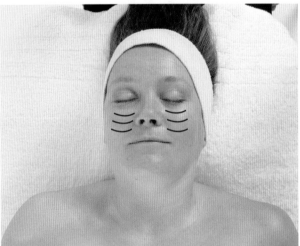

▲ 7. Finger pressures (index, middle and ring fingers) to cheek area in three lines. Starting either side of the nostrils work out, slide in. Repeat the movement under the zygomatic bone and ridge of eye sockets, following the lines as shown in step 8

▲ 8. Lymph drainage over cheek area. Place index, middle and ring fingers either side of nose under zygomatic bones. Slide out towards the parotid lymph node to drain area. Repeat on other two lines

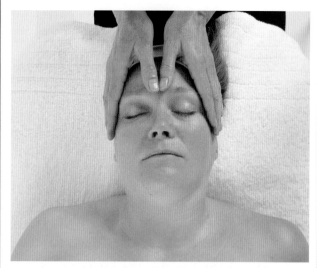

▲ 9. Lymph drainage over forehead. Place fingers at temples and thumbs side by side on the corrugator. Slide thumbs with pressure to the hairline and place overlapping hands on the forehead. Draw fingers outwards towards and drain to parotid lymph node. Repeat the movement

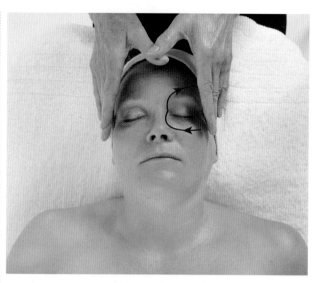

▲ 10. Eye circles. Place the fingers at the temples and slide the ring fingers under the eyes and in towards the nose; just above the corner of the inner eye lift the corrugator towards the eyebrow, release pressure and return to the temples. Repeat the movement

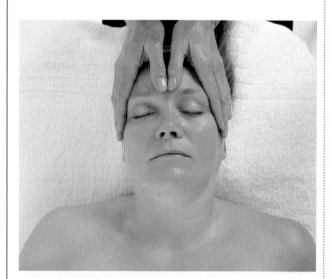

▲ 11. Thumb frictions. Place thumbs together just above the eyebrows and, working in a clockwise direction, apply pressure in a small circular motion, release and move up the forehead and repeat the movement

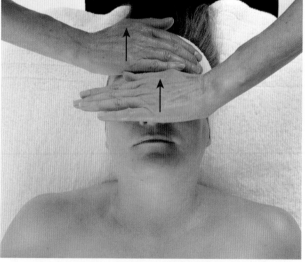

▲ 12. Forehead stroking. Position the hands horizontally, slide the right hand over the forehead closely followed by the left hand. Contour hand and fingers to the area. For the last movement, place one hand on top of the other and slide out to the temples

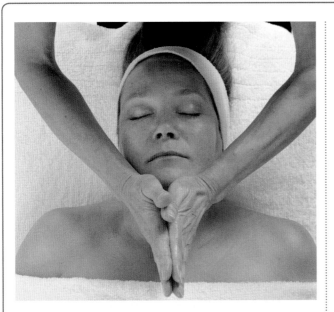

▲ 13. Effleurage. Slide index fingers down the jawline, heel of hands to stay in contact with the chin. Cup the chin by overlapping hands or linking fingers, pull apart, slide over the cheek area, up either side of the nose, pull up on the corrugator with the fingers and slide out to temples and apply pressure. Repeat movement

Massage routine for the scalp

This can be performed with or without medium. If using, spread medium on to the hands and stroke through the hair from the roots to the ends.

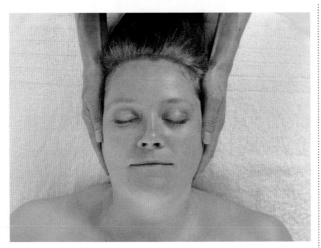

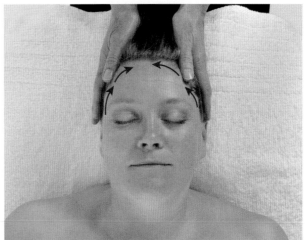

▲ 1. Stroking. Place thumbs in front of the ears and fingers lightly on top. The pads of the thumbs trace the hairline in a stroking movement to the centre of the forehead. Draw the fingers of both hands through the hair from roots to tips; pull at the roots to stimulate hair growth. Repeat the movement

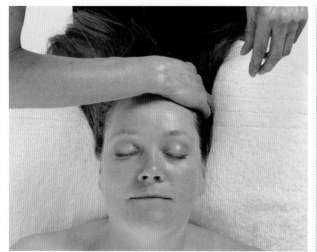

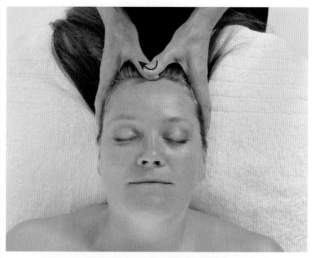

▲ 3. Reinforced thumb frictions. Circles in a clockwise direction down the centre of the scalp from hairline to crown. Ensure thumbs move the scalp and do not move over the scalp

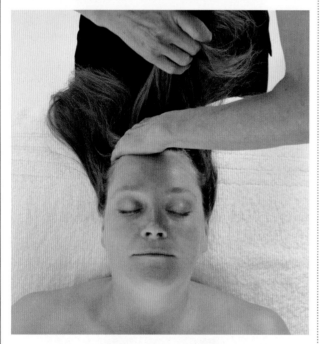

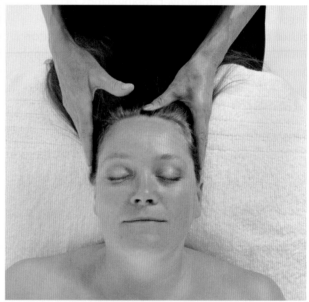

▲ 2. Stroking movements. The right hand works over the left side of the scalp and vice versa. Place the fingers of the right hand on the left side of the scalp at the hairline above the ear. From the hairline slide over the scalp and draw the fingers through the hair, from roots to tips; pull slightly at the roots to stimulate hair growth. As this movement finishes follow with the left hand. Slide fingers through the hair covering the right side of the scalp. Work with alternate hands to cover the scalp

▲ 4. Alternate thumb stroking, working from hairline to crown

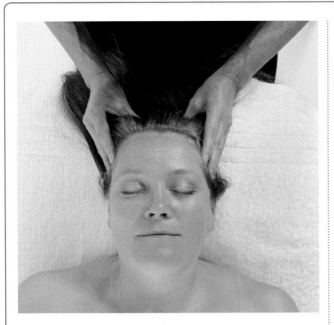

▲ 5. Finger and thumb friction movements to the entire area (digits move the scalp and do not move over the scalp). Use small circular movements

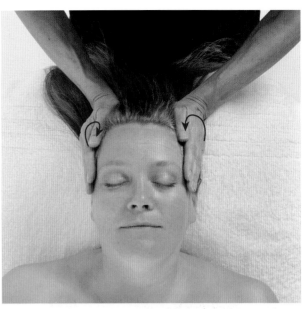

▲ 6. Palmar kneading (static movement). Place hands at each side of the scalp above the ears with fingers covering the temples. Circle the scalp in a clockwise direction twice. Move slightly towards the midline and repeat the movement twice. Place the palms over the crown, thumbs touching, and repeat the movement twice

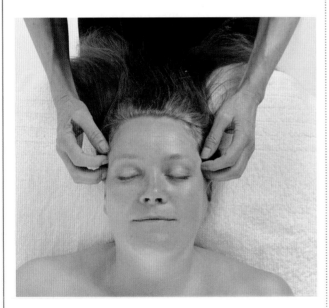

▲ 7. Rake through the hair using fingertips. Place fingers on the hairline above each ear and rake over the scalp from roots to tips. Repeat the movement, each time moving up towards the midline

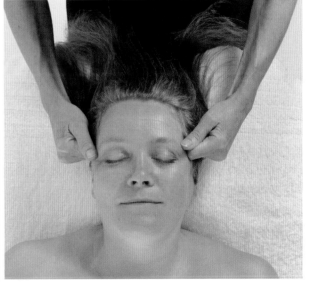

▲ 8. Knuckle and pull. Start above each ear and work towards the midline in lines. Grasp the hair near the roots, turn the knuckles in towards the scalp and hold for a few seconds before releasing and moving on

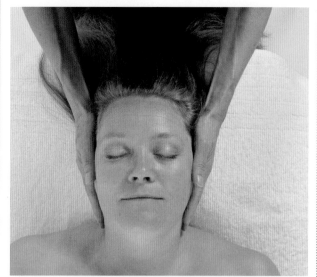

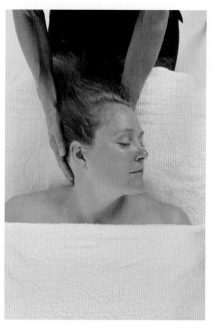

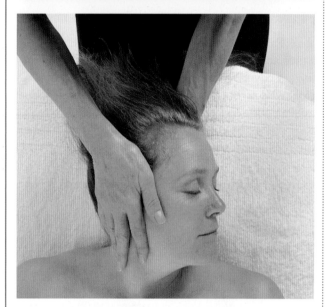

▲ 9. *Turn the head to the left.* Place the hands over the ears with the fingertips pointing downwards towards the shoulders. Gently turn the head to the left. Work the right hand

▲ 10. Stroking. Start at the base of the skull and work medially to laterally in three lines, following the contour of the skull to the crown (each line is similar in shape to a segment of an orange). With the fingers of the right hand, work up the first line contouring the skull and at the crown pull the fingers through the hair from roots to tips. Repeat the movement on the other two lines

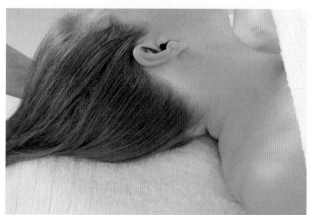

▲ 11. Finger and thumb frictions to the area (see Step 5)

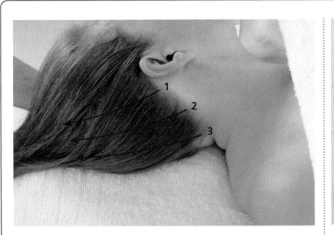

▲ 12. Palmar kneading (static) to the scalp (see Step 6). Contour the right hand over the skull with fingers pointing to the neck. Hand moves the scalp in a clockwise direction. Release move up towards the crown and repeat movement

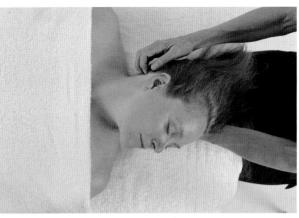

▲ 13. Rake through the hair using the fingertips (see Step 7). Start at the base of the skull and work medially to laterally in three lines following the contour of the skull to the crown

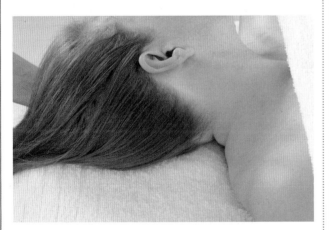

▲ 14. Knuckle and pull (see Step 8). Start at the base of the skull and work medially to laterally in three lines, following the contour of the skull to the crown

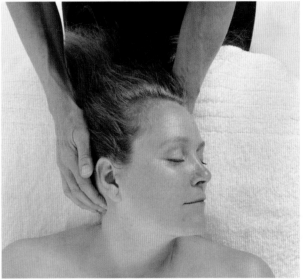

▲ 15. Finger kneading (index and middle fingers). Place fingers in the indentation behind the mastoid process and perform finger kneading following the line beneath the occipital bone

▲ 16. *Turn the head to the right.* Place the right hand over the client's right ear and turn the head back to the centre. Pause before continuing to turn the head over to the right, to prevent the client from feeling disorientated

▲ 17. Repeat Steps 10–15 on the left-hand side

▲ 18. *Turn the head to the centre*

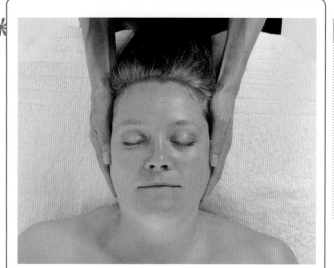

▲ 19. Stroking (repeat Step 1)

Questions

1. The ankle joint is a:

   a. condyloid joint

   b. pivot joint

   c. hinge joint

   d. gliding joint.

2. The action of the sartorius muscle is to:

   a. flex the hip

   b. adduct the thigh

   c. extend the knee joint

   d. abduct the thigh.

3. The lymph node located behind the knee is the:

   a. supratrochlear

   b. inguinal

   c. iliac

   d. popliteal.

4. The vein that transports deoxygenated blood from the leg is the:

   a. cephalic

   b. great saphenous

   c. inferior vena cava

   d. brachial.

5. The interphalangeal joint is a:

   a. pivot joint

   b. hinge joint

   c. saddle joint

   d. condyloid joint.

6. The radius is:

   a. one of the bones that forms part of the wrist

   b. one of the bones that forms the shoulder joint

   c. the long bone of the upper arm

   d. the bone on the lateral aspect of the lower arm.

7. The posterior fibres of the deltoid:

   a. extend the shoulder joint

   b. adduct the shoulder joint

   c. abduct the shoulder joint

   d. flex the shoulder joint.

8. The lymph node that drains the forearm is the:

   a. submandibular

   b. supratrochlear

   c. axillary

   d. supraclavicular.

9. The flexors of the forearm originate from the:
   a. biceps
   b. olecranon process
   c. medial epicondyle
   d. styloid process.

10. Oxygenated blood is carried to the abdomen by the:
    a. subclavian vein
    b. external carotid artery
    c. brachial artery
    d. common iliac artery.

11. The rectus abdominis muscle working on both sides of the body:
    a. rotates the trunk to the opposite side
    b. flexes the trunk
    c. compresses the abdomen
    d. extends the trunk.

12. Which of the following movements should be avoided over the abdomen and chest?
    a. Skin rolling.
    b. Picking up.
    c. Kneading.
    d. Tapotement.

13. The rhomboid muscles are found:
    a. between the scapulae
    b. covering the upper shoulders
    c. covering the lower back
    d. running up either side of the spine.

14. The action of the corrugator muscle is to:
    a. compress the nostrils
    b. wrinkle the forehead
    c. draw the eyebrows inwards and down
    d. form lines on the bridge of the nose.

15. An abnormal curvature of the spine is called:
    a. kyphosis
    b. osteoporosis
    c. scoliosis
    d. lordosis.

16. Which of the following is a cranial bone?
    a. Lacrimal.
    b. Vomer.
    c. Palatine.
    d. Ethmoid.

17. The action of the platysma muscle is to:
    a. depress the angle of the mouth
    b. flex the neck
    c. raise the mandible to close the mouth
    d. draw the teeth together when chewing.

18. An example of a cartilaginous joint is the:
    a. symphysis pubis
    b. shoulder joint
    c. sutures of the skull
    d. atlas and axis vertebrae.

19. The biceps femoris muscle is found:
    a. on the anterior aspect of the upper arm
    b. on the lower back
    c. on the back of the upper leg
    d. covering the abdomen wall.

20. The muscles that abduct the hip joint include:
    a. peroneus longus and gluteus minimus
    b. gluteus medius and tensor fascia lata
    c. rectus femoris and gracilis
    d. gluteus maximus and piriformis.

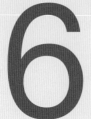

6 Adapting massage for specific conditions

After you have studied this chapter you will be able to:

1. list the problems and conditions that may benefit from massage
2. perform an appropriately adapted massage routine to suit the needs of the client
3. explain how visual and verbal feedback are obtained from the client
4. explain the after-care and home-care advice you would give to the client.

Conditions that benefit from massage

During the initial detailed client consultation you will have established why massage is a suitable treatment for the client. The type of massage will vary depending on the desired outcomes of the treatment and on the age, physical and mental condition of the client. It is important to be flexible and adaptable, and to avoid keeping rigidly to set routines. Manipulations and routines must be adapted to suit each client – some manipulations may be omitted, while others will be used more extensively. Massage is beneficial for a variety of conditions and problems.

Treatment objectives

Relaxation:

- to relieve stress and tension
- to relax very painful, stiff muscles
- to prepare and warm muscles prior to specific activities (pre-performance or event)
- to relieve muscle fatigue, pain and soreness (post-performance or event)
- to relieve stress for clients with certain heart and blood pressure conditions (it may be necessary to seek medical advice)
- to relieve pain and stiffness in specific areas, particularly in the upper and lower back and to treat fibrotic nodules.

Sedation: to relax an overwrought client.

Stimulating:

- for a lethargic client
- for a client who has poor circulation

Learning point
Fibrotic nodules are hardened, lumpy zones, usually painful to touch, lying within superficial muscles or fascia. They are small areas of tense, contracted fibres with restricted circulation. These are treated with pressure techniques.

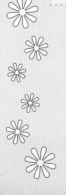

- to improve digestion and relieve constipation
- to improve the condition and tone of the skin.

Aiding weight reduction and combating cellulite:

- stimulating metabolism
- softening areas of excess fat and cellulite
- to promote body awareness during weight loss when used in conjunction with other treatments and diet.

Integrated healthcare:

- following referral from doctor or other healthcare professionals
- to relieve oedema
- to aid recovery from repetitive strain injury
- to relieve musculo-skeletal problems (e.g. trauma and injury, postural problems).

Promoting a sense of well-being:

- to reduce tension and stress resulting from emotional or psychological factors
- to invigorate and promote a positive attitude
- to uplift and instil a sense of optimism.

Client profiles

The client profiles given here are examples of the type of client you may encounter. However, it is important to remember that each individual case is different and you must tailor the treatment to the particular information you obtain from the client during consultation.

Reducing stress and tension

You should adopt a relaxed, unhurried manner, speaking positively, calmly and quietly. The client must be greeted pleasantly and made to feel cared for and cosseted. The procedure should be clearly explained and the client should be encouraged to ask questions, which you must be able to answer immediately, and to discuss any problems or worries that may contribute to stress. A sympathetic but not patronising approach will reduce anxiety and help the client to relax. This is particularly important with new or nervous clients. Relaxation can be further encouraged by suggesting that the client empties the mind or concentrates on some pleasant visual imagery. Keep conversation to a minimum once the massage has started. Although most of these factors apply to most massage treatments, they are particularly important for relaxation and will greatly influence the effectiveness of the treatment.

Treatment technique

The massage must be smooth, slow, deep and rhythmical. The transition between strokes should be continuous and barely perceptible.

Learning point

Where a male therapist is required to give massage to a female client, the chest and abdomen areas may be omitted from the routine. In your professional capacity, you will be able to make a judgement about what is appropriate for each client.

Remember

Before commencing a relaxing massage it is important to prepare the mind as well as the body. The atmosphere created in the working environment must be quiet and calming (see the sections towards the end of Chapter 3 on preparing yourself and the client). The area must be private, warm, well ventilated and free from distracting noises. Lighting should be soft or dimmed. The client must be positioned in a comfortable, well-supported position and they must feel safe and secure.

The tempo must be constant and unhurried. All the effleurage and petrissage movements in the suggested routines may be included. However, percussion must never be included in a relaxing massage, as the movements are too invigorating and stimulating.

You may wish to use more effleurage and kneading manipulations, repeating the movements until you feel the muscles softening and relaxing under your hands. You may need to concentrate and perform more manipulations on specific, identified areas of tension such as around the shoulder region, the upper or lower back or over the large muscle groups of the legs. Slow down each effleurage stroke when completing an area.

Remember that it is very important to work calmly and unhurriedly, with constant, slow rhythm and depth. You must maintain your concentration throughout – you should relax mentally and physically as the massage progresses, but keep concentrating.

> **Be aware** !
>
> If your mind starts to wander onto personal issues the client will sense your lack of concentration through your hands.

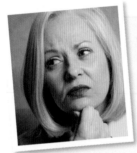

client profile

Rachel is a very nervous, highly strung woman of 50. She has been told that massage would help her to relax and is desperate to give it a try. She is not sleeping well at night and feels that everything is getting on top of her. She is a teacher at a large secondary school and works late into the night hunched over a desk.

Treatment technique

In the case of a nervous client like Rachel, start on the back and spend more time on this area. Repeated manipulations either side of the spine will engage the nerves in this area and help to calm and relax her. Thumb and digital kneading on the upper fibres of the trapezius will help to release tension in this area. The gradual introduction of friction movements on tension nodules and adhesions will be beneficial but should be approached with caution as they are deep movements and can cause discomfort.

> **Remember**
>
> It is important to discuss these movements with Rachel so that she knows what to expect and can let you know if she finds it uncomfortable.

Continue the massage on the backs of the legs then turn Rachel over into a supine position and massage the front of the legs. For a first treatment like this, leave out the abdomen, as it is quite an intimate area to massage and will not address Rachel's stress and tension. Similarly, it is possible to leave out the arms to allow more time for the décolleté, the face and scalp, which will be really relaxing for Rachel.

To conclude the treatment, Rachel should be given the following home-care advice.

- Explain relaxation techniques (see later in this chapter) and advise her to practise them at home.
- Make her aware of correct posture when sitting and standing and give simple pointers that she can practise at home (see later in this chapter).

- Suggest ways of aiding sleep, such as deep-breathing exercises, ensuring the bedroom is comfortably warm but not overheated, taking a warm bath before bed, herbal teas.

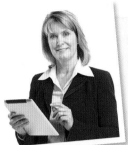

client profile

Cassie is 45. She is a bank manager. She works very long hours in a busy, target-driven office. She is responsible for several demanding clients and regularly has very stressful days. She likes to unwind by going out drinking most nights. She is an occasional gym user and is reasonably fit. She is a 'social smoker', averaging about ten cigarettes a day. She has had a lot of massage treatments in the past.

Treatment technique

For someone like Cassie, who has had many previous treatments, it is important to discuss her preferences before commencing treatment. To address her stress, it would be beneficial to spend a longer time on the back. It would be likely that there will be problem areas on the upper and middle fibres of the trapezius. Cassie would be able to tolerate deep pressure, both because of her previous experience and because of her level of fitness. Many people who suffer from stress carry tension in the lower back, so thumb and digital kneading in this area, as well as of the upper and middle fibres of the trapezius, would be beneficial. Friction movements in these two areas will be required to help release tension and disperse nodules and adhesions.

To conclude the treatment, Cassie should be given the following home-care advice.

Suggest that she:

- considers changing her diet and reducing alcohol consumption and smoking (see later in this chapter for more information). She will feel more alert and notice a definite improvement in her skin and in her sleep patterns
- exercises regularly to reduce secretions of stress hormones (including cortisol) and to increase secretions of endorphins produced by the brain, which promote a feeling of well-being
- follows a course of treatment once or twice a week, for six weeks
- practises breathing and relaxation exercises to help reduce stress levels.

Combating mental and physical fatigue

For a client with mental and physical fatigue it is very important to create a stimulating atmosphere. For example, you could consider using uplifting music and room fragrance to enhance the mood. Although you must be caring and sympathetic, a positive, upbeat attitude is also required.

During the consultation, the client should be encouraged to mention any problems to help to establish reasons for the lethargy or tiredness. There are many factors that may cause the condition: stress at work or in the home; feeling overburdened or overworked; insufficient time for rest, relaxation or enjoyment; feeling unwell, suffering with headaches, migraine, insomnia or heavy and prolonged periods. There may also be psychological problems such as unhappiness, depression, and feelings of low self-esteem or lack of achievement.

Encourage the client to seek solutions to the problems through changes in lifestyle, or to see a doctor if ill health is a cause.

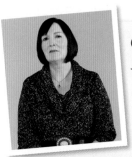

client profile

Jackie is 48 and has a demanding job in social work. Her husband has just left her with two teenage children. She is feeling over-burdened and has lost all motivation. She suffers from headaches and is not sleeping well. Her counsellor has suggested that she might benefit from a course of massage treatment. She has experienced a variety of therapies on holidays and earlier in her life.

Treatment technique

Treatment for Jackie will be similar to that of a general massage. However, certain adaptations should be made. For example, the abdomen could be omitted to allow more time to be spent on the back and on the scalp. The massage movements will again be smooth, deep and rhythmical, but of moderate to brisk speed. The speed of the effleurage strokes may be increased with each movement. This is particularly important at the end of the treatment as it stimulates alertness. (Note the difference from a relaxing or general massage, where the speed slows down towards the last stroke.)

Petrissage movements should be deep and brisk. Tapotement movements should also be included, unless there are contra-indications. These movements are invigorating and may be performed over the quadriceps muscles, calf, hamstrings, buttocks, and very lightly over the top of the shoulders and down each side of the spine. Make sure that the client has a reasonable covering of flesh over the ribs and is not too thin, or tapotement will be painful and contra-indicated. Frictions performed along either side of the spinal column are also very effective, as they stimulate the spinal nerves. Complete the massage with brisk effleurage.

Discuss and plan the strategy for next time. Evaluate the treatment and ask the client whether she found it beneficial or whether she has other preferences.

To conclude the treatment, Jackie should be given the following home-care advice.

- Suggest that she should try to prioritise her workload.
- Suggest changes in her diet that could help raise her energy levels and improve her mood (more fresh fruit and vegetables, less processed food). See later in this chapter for more information on diet.
- Explain the importance of drinking plenty of water to release toxins and hydrate the body.
- Suggest ways of aiding sleep, such as deep-breathing exercises, ensuring the bedroom is comfortably warm but not overheated, taking a warm bath before bed, herbal teas.
- Explain that changes are not always immediate – make sure her expectations are realistic.

Relieving oedema

It is important to understand the structure and function of the lymphatic system before practising this massage (see Chapter 2).

Oedema is swelling of the tissues due to an accumulation and stagnation of tissue fluid in tissue spaces. Normally, this tissue fluid is drained away through the blood vessels or lymphatic vessels. If these systems fail to drain the fluid away, it will remain in the tissue spaces. The amount of swelling can vary from slight puffiness to soft, mobile swelling that yields easily to pressure, or hard, consolidated, unyielding swelling of long standing. There are many possible causes of oedema, including:

- obstruction or blockage of the lymphatic system, such as an infected node
- interference in part of the system following surgery where glands may have been removed
- increase in the permeability of blood vessel walls or pressure within the vessels forcing fluid out. If this excess fluid cannot be removed quickly enough by the lymphatic system it remains in the tissue spaces
- lack of, or poor muscle contraction, which normally acts as a pump and assists blood and lymphatic flow
- standing for long periods so that gravitational pull and lack of muscle contraction slow lymphatic drainage of the leg. Fluid collects around the ankle, which becomes puffy and swollen. The legs will feel tired and heavy.
- systemic problems of the heart, lungs or kidneys (if one of these is the cause of the oedema, advise the client to seek their doctor's advice).

Because massage speeds up the flow of blood in the veins and the flow of lymph in the lymphatic vessels, it is a useful treatment in the prevention and reduction of oedema. A brisk general leg massage will be effective if oedema is recent, soft and due to gravitational effects. However, special techniques must be used if the oedema has been present for a long time, is hard and consolidated, and the covering skin is shiny, thin and stretched. Great care must be taken not to break or damage the skin.

A squeezing movement is used to apply and then release pressure along the path of lymphatic flow. This alternating pressure technique forces the fluid out of the tissue spaces and speeds flow through the lymphatic vessels. It is important to drain and clear the proximal end first (i.e. the part nearest the lymph nodes). This ensures that fluid is not pushed into an already engorged area. The part must be elevated so that gravity assists the flow. Squeezing, kneading, effleurage and vibrations are the manipulations used.

Contra-indications to oedema

There are many causes of oedema and massage will not be suitable in all cases. Massage is contra-indicated if the oedema is due to the following conditions:

- disease of the heart, lungs or kidney
- acute injury
- deep vein thrombosis or phlebitis
- damage to the lymph glands following infection, surgery or radiotherapy.

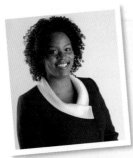

client profile

Caroline is 40 and is currently on a weight reduction diet: she wants to lose around 12.5 kilos. She finds it hard to get motivated to exercise and has got into the habit of finishing her children's meals. She works in a shop, where she is standing for most of the day. Her ankles are puffy and swollen.

Treatment technique

This is a specialised treatment technique and you should follow the step-by-step guide for clients such as Caroline.

Be aware

Note how easily the area 'pits' under pressure and how quickly or slowly it refills. This will give some indication of how much pressure can be applied. If it is hard and unyielding, start with lighter pressure.

Oedematous legs

1. Prepare the client as for a general massage. Make sure that all restrictive clothing is removed and (if underwear is not removed) that there is no tight elastic.
2. Place her in the supine position (face up). Make sure that the legs lie on the elevating end of the couch.
3. Examine the leg carefully before starting the massage. Check the skin and the degree of hardness of the oedema.

4. Elevate the leg to between 30° and 45° from the horizontal – preferably by raising the end of the bed if possible, or by using an arrangement of firm pillows.

5. The legs must be allowed to drain in this position for half to one hour (you may massage other areas during this time). Massaging the abdomen can increase the effectiveness of the following leg massage. This is because lymph flow through the abdominal vessels, iliac nodes and lymphatic ducts is stimulated and drained away, reducing backward pressure.

6. Take up a walk standing stance, level with the client's knee.

7. Imagine that you are pushing fluid through a tube or many tubes. To be effective, pressure must be applied to all the surfaces of the tube.

8. Begin just below the inguinal nodes in the groin. With one hand on the inner leg and the other on the outer side, cover as much of the circumference as possible, then squeeze inward and upward, four to six times.

9. Now place one hand on the front and one on the back and squeeze in an upward direction, four to six times.

10. Repeat this squeezing until the area softens.

11. As you feel the area softening slightly, perform small, circular, palmar kneading movements over the area (both palms pressing together). Cover the sides, front and back thoroughly.

12. Next, effleurage slowly towards the groin.

13. Move the hands down the leg, one hand width only at a time, overlapping the previous area. Repeat the manipulations as described. Work gently and slowly in this way until you reach the knee.

14. Perform palmar kneading, then effleurage over the entire thigh. As the tissues soften, deeper pressure may be applied and larger movements performed.

15. Move below the knee to drain the lower leg into the popliteal nodes. Begin just below the knee.

16. Avoid the anterior border of the tibia (shin bone). Cup the hands around the calf with the heels of the hands on either side of the shin bone. Squeeze in and upwards until the oedema softens. Vibrate the hands in and out. Knead the calf, then effleurage.

17. Work gradually down the leg, one hand width at a time.

18. Work thoroughly around the ankles, as fluid frequently stagnates around the medial and lateral malleoli.

19. Cup one hand behind the ankle joint – the thumb and thenar eminence on one side and the fingers on the other side of the Achilles tendon. Place the other hand across the front of the joint.

20. Squeeze all the areas together in a pumping and upward push manner until the tissues soften. Work around the malleoli with the pads of the index, middle and ring fingers. Make small pressure circles around the bones. Then, with the fingers on either side of the Achilles tendon, push in and up.

Remember
Make sure that the lymphatic nodes in the groin are neither stretched nor compressed.

Learning point
Deep breathing is also beneficial because, as the client breathes in and out, the pressure within the thoracic and abdominal cavities increases and decreases. The alternating high to low pressure acts as a pump, moving fluid along; this also reduces backward pressure.

21. Press and knead the sole and dorsum of the foot with single-handed kneading.
22. Effleurage the lower leg again.
23. Effleurage the entire leg to complete the massage.

After the massage, active muscle contractions should be performed to exert a pumping action:

- Pull foot up and down very slowly.
- Turn foot in and out.
- Circle foot around slowly.
- Tighten the quadriceps by pressing the back of the knee into the pillow and pulling the knee cap towards the groin.
- Repeat these movements 10–15 times.

To conclude the treatment, Caroline should be given the following home-care advice.

- When relaxing, elevate the legs above the heart to improve the flow of lymph.
- Do gentle exercises while standing at work, to help pump fluid from the legs back to the heart.
- Wear support stockings.
- Cut down on the amount of salt in the diet – this will help to reduce fluid retention and swelling.
- Drink plenty of water to flush toxins from the body (6–8 glasses per day).
- Practice deep breathing exercises, which aid flow of blood in the veins and lymph in the lymphatic vessels.

Reducing cellulite

Cellulite is a condition found predominantly in women, where areas of adipose tissue (fat) become hard and lumpy and very difficult to remove.

In women fat is found mainly on the outer thighs, hips and buttocks, abdomen, midriff and back of the arms. In men it is usually distributed around the waist.

The areas of cellulite look dimpled or lumpy, and feel hard and cold to touch. Pushing the flesh between the hands makes the skin very uneven and puckered, similar to the surface of orange peel.

Cellulite is more commonly found in overweight individuals, but is also found in people who are thin and those of ideal weight. In slim people it is present in specific areas, usually the outer thighs, giving the characteristic 'jodhpur' shape. Cellulite is difficult to reduce and remove, even when the individual is on a reducing diet and exercising regularly.

The body stores fat for use as fuel when required. The digestive system breaks down the food we eat to provide energy for bodily functions. If the energy input is greater than the energy output (i.e. if we eat more food than is required for energy), then the excess fuel is stored in the body as fat.

> **Learning point**
> It is more common and more widely distributed in the female because of the greater amount of oestrogen produced. This hormone encourages the laying down of fat.

> **Learning point**
> Research indicates that there is no physiological difference between cellulite and the more easily removed fat, but there are differences in the supporting connective tissue and in the organisation and circulation of the subcutaneous tissues in cellulitic areas.

Fat is stored in specialised cells called **adipocytes**. These form clusters supported by connective tissue, which group together to form adipose tissue. This is found under the skin in the subcutaneous layer, and among muscle fibres around organs such as the kidneys and heart. Complex chemical reactions convert the food eaten into fat for storage, and again from storage to use as fuel for energy. Although fat will be used from areas all over the body when required, it appears to be more difficult to remove from certain areas. These areas of hard, difficult-to-remove fat are called cellulite.

In cellulitic areas there is some alteration of the subcutaneous tissue. The adipocytes become overloaded and develop a tough outer membrane. The supporting connective tissue increases, enmeshing groups of adipocytes together in a lobular structure. This gives the dimpled, uneven appearance of the area.

The overloaded cells and lobules compress the capillary networks and lymphatics. This interferes with the circulation to the area. Stagnation and deficient circulation adversely affect the area: the tissues do not receive the required nutrients and oxygen; waste products (toxins) accumulate in the area as they are not quickly removed; and the temperature of the area will be lowered as warm blood is not circulating normally (hence it feels cold to touch). Fat remains in the overloaded adipocytes as it is not easily removed by the poorly circulating blood for conversion to energy, and the area becomes hard and stagnated. If action is not taken, the condition will become progressively worse, with greater engorgement of the area, degeneration of connective tissue and hardening of the fatty tissue.

The aims of the treatment are:

- to soften and reduce the fatty adipose layer
- to increase the circulation to the area, thus improving nutrition
- to speed up blood and lymphatic drainage from the area, thus removing toxins more quickly
- to improve the condition of the skin.

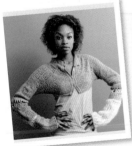

client profile

Colleen is 24, and has a very good figure. She takes a lot of pride in her appearance and is distressed that she has unsightly cellulite around her hips, buttocks and the backs of her thighs. She enjoys going out drinking and partying with her friends and often keeps very irregular hours, not always eating healthily or getting enough sleep. She is due to go on an exotic holiday with her new boyfriend and wants to look good in a bikini.

Treatment technique

Successful treatment will involve combining a variety of treatments into an effective routine, which will include both manual and mechanical massage.

Manual massage

This forms an important part of the treatment. The majority of manipulations will follow the direction of venous return and lymphatic drainage. As the flow in these vessels is speeded up, fluid and metabolites from tissue cells and spaces are removed more efficiently, reducing stagnation (stasis). The arterial circulation will in turn increase, bringing nutrients and oxygen to nourish the tissues, and the metabolic rate will increase. This improves the stagnant area. It may be that fat needed for fuel will be mobilised from this stimulated area, but there is no scientific research evidence to prove this.

The heavier manipulations of kneading, picking up, wringing, hacking, cupping, beating and pounding may be used over the areas of cellulite, according to client needs. The greater the depth and the more consolidated and harder the cellulite, the deeper the manipulations should be, unless the area is sensitive and painful, when manipulations must be within the tolerance of the client. Deep, brisk effleurage along the length of the area should conclude the massage.

Mechanical massage

This produces a deeper effect and more stimulation of the body tissues than manual massage. The skin surface head will stimulate and increase the circulation to the skin, producing an erythema. The increase in the delivery of nutrients and oxygen, the removal of waste products (metabolites), the increase in metabolic rate and the desquamating effect will all improve the condition of the skin. The deep kneading movements, using the four-ball and/or multi-prong heads, will affect the deeper tissues. The pressure of the strokes must be directed upwards to aid venous and lymphatic drainage. This massage warms and softens the area and speeds up the removal of metabolites. Heavy kneading movements should be brisk but not too prolonged, as resulting dilation of capillaries and blood vessels may increase the fluid in the area further, engorging it and increasing compression. (See also Chapter 8 for more on mechanical massage.)

It is important to remember that spot reduction of fat from a specific area is not possible. To reduce body fat, calorie intake must be less than calorie output. Only then is fat removed from body stores and broken down for energy. The client must therefore be given advice on sensible eating and made aware of the factors that are thought to contribute to cellulite (see the sections on home-care and dietary advice, later in this chapter). Although Colleen is not overweight, her irregular eating patterns and the type of foods and drink she consumes all contribute to her cellulite problem.

Be aware !

If galvanic treatment has been used, remember that the area under the pads will be very sensitive. Therefore massage may be given proximal to (above) the area and around the padded areas to conclude the treatment.

As Colleen has very specific areas requiring treatment, a full body massage is not appropriate. Instead, a combination of mechanical massage and manual massage should be targeted on her hips, thighs and buttocks. It is important to make Colleen aware that for best results she will require a course of treatments, two to three times a week over the next six weeks.

Manual massage movements should be deeper, more stimulating movements on the relevant areas. Wringing and skin rolling, beating and pounding are particularly effective to stimulate circulation of blood and lymph and to soften areas of adipose tissue. These should be interspersed with effleurage to increase lymphatic drainage.

As the hips and buttocks are quite intimate areas to massage, Colleen may prefer to wear disposable pants. She should be lying prone with both legs exposed right up to the buttock area. All parts of the procedure should be applied to each leg in turn.

Begin with manual effleurage using a suitable medium, gradually increasing the depth of pressure and working briskly. This should be followed by the gyratory vibrator using the curved sponge and applied in long, sweeping strokes following the direction of venous return. Pressure should be heavier on areas of muscle bulk and adipose tissue.

Manual kneading, wringing and skin rolling movements should follow. Attach suitable kneading head(s) to the gyratory vibrator and use a circular, kneading motion, supporting the tissues with your other hand and lifting them towards the kneading head. Apply pressure and work in the direction of venous return.

Complete the treatment with the curved sponge head, followed by manual effleurage to increase lymphatic drainage.

To conclude the treatment, Colleen should be given the following home-care advice.

- Use the recommended retail body scrub or exfoliation to improve desquamation.
- Use the recommended body brushing or abrasive gloves before or during bath or shower.
- Use the recommended body product to keep skin soft, supple and hydrated.
- Drink plenty of water to hydrate the body.
- Reduce alcohol intake.
- Review diet (see the section on dietary advice later in this chapter).
- Practise regular cardiovascular exercise to help increase metabolic rate, improve circulation and nourish the tissues. If Colleen's energy output is greater than her energy input she will definitely lose weight.

Male clients

The male client must be received with the same polite, caring manner as the female. As always, the highest standards of professionalism apply.

> **Learning point**
> Recommend a preheat treatment, for example infra-red lamp, sauna or steam treatment, to warm and soften the tissues so that they are more receptive to treatment.

> **Be aware** !
> Cellulitic areas can be very sensitive and painful. Check that the depth of pressure is comfortable for the client.

> **Be aware** !
> Heads can be selected according to client needs and preferences. Take note of factors such as erythema and client tolerance.

> **Be aware** !
> You should avoid banter and ignore any suggestive comments or innuendo from clients of either sex.

As a therapist you should be aware of the potentially vulnerable position you are in. Being alone in a treatment room, particularly with a member of the opposite sex, means that you are both open to risks or allegations. To minimise these risks, always give clear instructions about procedures and expectations (e.g. concerning what clothing to keep on) and maintain a calm, professional manner. It is recommended that you leave the room while the client undresses.

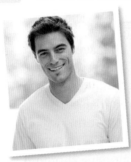

client profile

Brian is 29. He plays a lot of sport, including squash, golf and football. He has been overdoing his training recently, and is complaining of aching muscles in his thighs and his right arm. He has never been for a massage and was dared to come by the lads at the club.

Treatment technique

Because Brian's profile suggests that he may be approaching the treatment in an inappropriate way, take particular note of the points given above on dealing with male clients.

Adaptation of strokes

Men are frequently hairy and massage may be uncomfortable if insufficient oil or talcum powder is used. Talcum powder is often a better medium over hairy areas – apply liberally. If oil is used, ensure that it is not too viscous and apply liberally.

The abdomen may be omitted when massaging male clients because it is sensitive and may arouse a sexual response. As you continue to develop your skills and gain experience after qualifying, you will be confident in dealing with any issues of this kind in a professional manner.

Stroking manipulations may be performed in the direction of hair growth, usually downwards.

Effleurage should be performed in the direction of venous return, using plenty of oil or talcum powder. (If this pulls against the direction of hair growth or is uncomfortable, omit the movement.)

Petrissage manipulations also require care and a liberal amount of the massage medium.

More percussion manipulations may be included unless the client requires a relaxing massage.

Men generally have denser, firmer and larger muscles than women, depending on their degree of fitness. Brian's profile suggests that he has very good muscle tone, so massage manipulations may be deeper and heavier. Client preference will dictate the order of the routine, but in Brian's case, this is his first treatment so you could suggest the following sequence. Starting with the front of the legs will enable you to reassure Brian and take note of his body language to monitor depth of pressure and how he reacts to the massage experience.

Cover the body in the following order, omitting the abdomen:

- **front of legs** – this will focus on Brian's painful quadriceps.
- **arms** – include the side of the chest when massaging each arm. More time would be needed on Brian's right arm.
- **face and scalp** – this depends on client preference, but the scalp massage will definitely help to relax him.
- **back of legs.**
- **back** – by this time Brian should feel more comfortable within this environment and able to enjoy a relaxing back massage.

To conclude the treatment, Brian should be offered the following home-care advice.

- Warm up prior to exercise and cool down afterwards.
- Avoid wearing tight clothing, which can restrict blood circulation.
- Have regular treatments (once a week) for about six weeks.
- Avoid excessive exercise, especially when muscles are fatigued.
- Drink plenty of water to help increase the release of toxins from the body.

> **Learning point**
> You should avoid massaging the sensitive femoral triangle in a male client as this may stimulate in an inappropriate way, causing you both embarrassment.

Contra-actions

Occasionally, a client may experience an adverse reaction during or after treatment. Possible contra-actions should be highlighted during the consultation (see Chapter 3). Any adverse reaction to treatment should be noted on the consultation record for future reference.

Reactions that may occur during treatment:

- an allergic reaction to the medium
- heightened emotional state due to the release of suppressed feelings and emotions
- profuse sweating
- nausea
- headache
- the area becoming very hot and red
- restlessness and irritability
- feeling faint.

Reactions that may occur 24–48 hours after treatment include:

- sore and aching muscles caused by the elimination of carbon dioxide and lactic acid
- an increase in sweat production due to the elimination of toxins
- an increase in lymphatic drainage may result in a feeling of tiredness

- headache, dizziness and nausea as the body starts to cleanse and heal itself
- active bowel movement and frequent urination as the body deals with toxins and waste.

Evaluation of treatment

After each treatment it is important to assess how effective the treatment has been. You must decide whether the treatment has produced the effects that you were expecting, and whether the goals you set at the beginning have been met.

In order to evaluate the treatment you will need to obtain feedback. This means gathering all the information you can that will indicate how effective the treatment has been. Knowledge of the results of the treatment will enable you to make changes or modifications next time, if you feel that you have not achieved your goal.

You will obtain information through touch, i.e. sensing through your hands whether the tissues feel more flexible and pliable and less tense. You will also obtain information by looking at the area to see what changes have been produced. You will acquire more information through asking the client how they feel and whether the treatment met their needs.

As a result of the information you obtain from this feedback you can decide if changes need to be made and formulate a strategy for the next treatment. You have to make a judgement as to whether your selected treatment has been as effective as you hoped.

> **Learning point**
> Evaluating the treatment and your own performance forms the basis of good reflective practice (see Chapter 9). It should become second nature as you become familiar with routines and develop your skills.

> **In the workplace**
> Remember that time is money and your place of work may not allow any extra time between appointments for feedback and preparation of the room for the next client. Use your common sense and allocate time within the treatment.

Through palpating the tissues you will sense whether the tissues feel more relaxed.
- Are the tissues softer?
- Are the tissues more flexible and extensible?
- Have fibrous or fatty nodules disappeared?
- Do the tissues feel warm but not too hot?

By looking at and examining the area you will obtain visual feedback.
- Is there a good even erythema?
- Are there uneven patches of erythema, which would suggest uneven pressure?
- Is the area very red and hot, which would indicate over-treating or a mild allergic reaction to the lubricant?
- Are there red sore spots over bony prominences indicating that these were not avoided?

By questioning the client you will obtain verbal feedback.
- How did that feel?
- Did any part of the massage feel uncomfortable?
- Was it as you expected it to be?
- Was the pressure comfortable?
- Did you feel that you would have liked me to spend a longer time on any area?
- Was there any area that you would prefer me to leave out next time?
- Do you feel entirely satisfied with the treatment?

After-care

When the treatment is completed, the client will need to recover.

- Allow the client time to come around slowly before helping them into a semi-reclining position.
- Offer a glass of water to help hydrate the body.
- Ensure the client is sufficiently alert to leave and continue with their plans for the day.
- Give home-care advice as appropriate.

Home-care advice

Home-care advice is very beneficial for the client, as it involves them in the treatment and encourages them to take control of their condition. It also provides a link between one treatment and the next. The advice given will obviously depend on the client's need and condition, e.g. the overweight client or a client with cellulite will need dietary advice. For the tense, overworked client you may suggest that they try to reduce their workload and plan time to rest, take a relaxing bath and go to bed early.

Each place of work carries a line of retail products available for the client to purchase. It is important that you familiarise yourself with the features and benefits of the range, which may include attending relevant training courses, so that you are able to advise your clients appropriately.

Retail products include:

- body exfoliator/scrub to help to remove dead skin cells and keep skin soft and smooth
- body moisturising lotion to nourish and improve texture of the skin
- body brushing/abrasive glove/loofah to increase blood circulation to the area and remove dead skin cells (particularly good for cellulite).

General home-care advice includes the following:

- Use the recommended retail products in between treatments to help maintain the results achieved.
- Drink 6–8 glasses of water (or suitable alternatives) a day, to help prevent dehydration.
- Take time to relax before continuing with daily tasks.
- Avoid tea and coffee for the rest of the day following treatment, as they contain caffeine.
- Follow a light diet for the rest of the day.
- Avoid smoking, as it produces toxins in the body.
- Avoid drinking alcohol, as it will dehydrate the body.
- Take plenty of exercise and keeping mobile during the day. If in a sedentary occupation, it is advisable to walk around, swing the legs and stretch at regular intervals.

In the workplace

It is likely that you will earn commission from retail sales and thus increase your earning potential. It is important, however, to balance this with meeting the needs of your clients. Always act with integrity.

- Avoid wearing tight clothes that apply pressure and restrict the circulation, such as tight jeans or trousers, belts, underwear and corsets.
- Consult a healthcare practitioner for specific help if appropriate. (This may include doctor, chiropractor, physiotherapist, osteopath etc.)

Discuss with the client any changes that you intend making in their next treatment and explain why they are needed. Note the results of the feedback and the strategy for following treatments on the consultation record. Always refer to these each time the client attends.

Dietary advice

It is important that clients are made aware of the factors that are thought to contribute to the build-up of fat and cellulite. They should be encouraged to follow a daily regime that will increase the efficiency of the treatment. The following advice should be given.

Eat a well-balanced diet, as follows:

- Include all the nutrients necessary for health, i.e., proteins, carbohydrates, vitamins, minerals, water, fibre and a little fat.
- Eat plenty of fresh fruit and vegetables (five portions per day are recommended); do not overcook vegetables, as important nutrients will be lost.
- Eat two portions of fish per week: it is a good source of protein. Include a portion of oily fish such as herring, trout, mackerel and salmon as these contain omega-3 fats, which may help to prevent heart disease.
- Eat wholemeal foods such as wholemeal bread, pasta, rice, cereals, pulses, beans, nuts and seeds.
- Reduce intake of saturated fat (found in butter, dairy products and red meat) as it can increase the amount of cholesterol in the blood, which can result in heart disease.
- Reduce intake of sugar, as it is high in calories; and salt, as it raises blood pressure.
- Reduce intake of alcohol – it dehydrates the skin, increases calorie intake and could damage health.
- Drink 6–8 glasses of water (or suitable alternatives) per day.

Balance energy intake with energy output:

- If the diet provides just enough energy to meet the body's requirements, there is no surplus to be stored, therefore no fat will be deposited. To reduce fatty tissue, energy input must be less than energy output. Only then will fat be utilised from body stores to provide the required fuel.
- Reducing the calorie intake and increasing aerobic activity (e.g. walking, jogging, swimming or cycling) is the best regime for reducing fat. Twenty or thirty minutes of such exercise, twice or three times per week, is extremely beneficial.

Home practice of posture correction

You must ensure that the client is aware of the difference between good and poor posture. Poor posture may be the result of long-term habits. To avoid problems, poor habits must be changed. This can be done through constant practice of the correct positions.

Explain this to the client and give simple pointers for them to practise as often as possible. Good posture will become automatic through constant practice.

- Look straight ahead with the eyes level.
- Pull the chin in, then relax into a neutral position (neither pulled in nor craned forward).
- Feel that the crown of the head is being pulled up towards the ceiling.
- Keep the neck straight but not tense.
- Pull the shoulders back and down; do not hold the chest forward.
- Hold the tummy in and tuck the tail under.
- Balance your weight evenly through the buttocks if sitting, or through the feet when standing.

Common postural problems and corrective exercises

Kyphosis

This is an exaggerated curve of the thoracic region.

The weak, stretched muscles that require strengthening are:
- the middle fibres of trapezius
- the rhomboids
- the middle part of erector spinae.

The tight muscles that require stretching are:
- the pectoralis major
- the neck extensors.

Corrective exercises

Sitting or stride standing – gently drop the head forward pulling chin in, press the head back making a long neck and raise.

Lax stoop sitting – raise the trunk gradually from the base of spine upwards.

Lying, arms at right angles with elbows bent – retract the shoulders pressing back of hand into the floor.

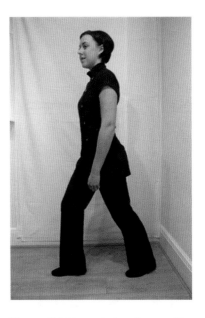

Figure 6.1 Correct standing position

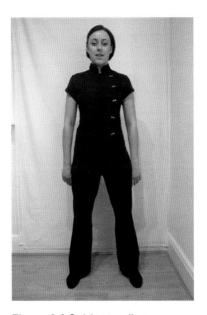

Figure 6.2 Stride standing

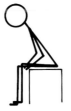

Figure 6.3 Stoop sitting

Prone lying, hands clasped behind back – keep chin in, pull shoulders back and lift head and shoulders off the floor.

Lordosis

This is an exaggerated curve of the lumbar spine, where the pelvis is tilted forwards.

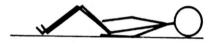

Figure 6.4 Prone lying

The weak stretched muscles that require strengthening are:

- the abdominals – rectus abdominus, internal oblique and external oblique
- the hip extensors – gluteus maximus and the hamstrings.

The tight muscles that require stretching are:

- the trunk extensors – erector spinae and quadratus lumborum
- the hip flexors – ilio-psoas.

Corrective exercises

Crook lying – press small of back into the floor and pull tummy in, tilting the pelvis.

Crook lying – keep chin in and raise head and shoulders to look at the knees; progress to curl up.

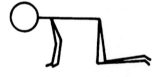

Figure 6.5 Crook lying

Prone kneeling – arch the back to stretch the lumbar spine and return to horizontal.

Prone kneeling – keep the back straight, raise alternate legs out and up, keeping knee bent.

Scoliosis

This is a lateral curvature of the spine, which may be a long C curve or an S curve.

The muscles that will require strengthening will be those on the outside of the curve. The muscles that require stretching will be those on the inside of the curve.

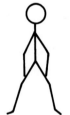

Figure 6.6 Prone kneeling

Corrective exercises

Stride standing – reach up into the air with the arm on the concave side of the curve; reach towards the floor with the other hand. Stretch, hold, and relax.

Stride standing – side flex the trunk towards the convex side, where the muscles are stretched. Slide the hand down the side and return.

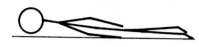

Figure 6.7 Stride standing

Prone lying – stretch the arm on the concave side up above the head along the floor; stretch the other down towards the feet. Hold and relax.

Prone lying – stretch the arm on the concave side up above the head and the opposite leg down along the floor. Hold and relax.

Flat back

This is a condition where there is little or no lumbar curve and the pelvis is tilted backwards. It may be accompanied by kyphosis of the thoracic spine.

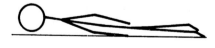

Figure 6.8 Prone lying

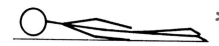

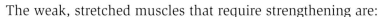

The weak, stretched muscles that require strengthening are:

- the back extensors, namely erector spinae
- in some cases, the abdominals and gluteus maximus are also weak.

The tight muscles that require stretching are the hamstrings on the posterior thigh.

Corrective exercises

Sitting – lean forward, taking the pressure from the buttocks on to the thigh, then extend the back to create a lumbar lordosis. Hold for a count of ten then release.

Prone lying – raise alternate legs.

Prone lying – raise both legs (this exercise is allowed for this condition).

Prone kneeling – arch and hollow the back.

Long sitting – rotate the pelvis forward, then lean backwards to arch lower back.

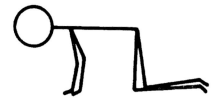

Figure 6.9 Prone lying

Figure 6.10 Prone kneeling

Relaxation

Relaxation means being free from tension and anxiety, which are normally caused by the stresses of life and upset the body balance. It is impossible to remove all the stressors in life and a certain amount of stress is desirable as it can motivate us to get things done and produce feelings of excitement. The ability to relax is extremely important as it prevents stress from building up and reduces its harmful effects, which include fatigue, lethargy, illness and psychological problems. Clients who lead very busy lives, coping with worries and/or dealing with unhappy situations may find it very difficult to relax. Advising them and showing them ways of reducing stress and promoting relaxation can form an important part of treatment. Once they have recognised the difference between the tense state and the relaxed state they can continue to practise at home.

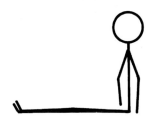

Figure 6.11 Long sitting

Relaxation techniques

The first consideration is to create the right environment to promote the relaxation response: warm, well-ventilated area, away from distracting noise, and with low lighting, a comfortable place to sit or lie down and relaxing music if desired.

There are many techniques that may be used to encourage the client to relax. They may be combined for maximum effect.

The relaxation response involves the client's response to a quiet soothing environment: total concentration on a particular object while trying to let go of all tension. This is sometimes sufficient to promote the relaxed state and can be practised anywhere.

Visualisation or imagining involves visualising pleasantly soothing situations that are conducive to relaxation, e.g. lying on a beach, looking at a tranquil scene.

Progressive relaxation aims to develop an awareness of the difference between feelings of tension and relaxation. Contraction followed by relaxation of all the muscle groups is performed, working around the body. This is a very effective method of promoting relaxation.

Progressive relaxation technique

The client should lie down somewhere comfortable. Suggest that the client takes a few minutes to settle by closing their eyes and concentrating on the sensation of tension and relaxation. They should practise breathing in deeply and letting go of tension on the out breath.

The technique is to contract each muscle group and then to relax it, feeling the tension in the muscles float away. The relaxation (the letting go) should happen on the outward breath.

Repeat each of the following movements three times:

- Pull the feet up hard (dorsi-flexion), then let go.
- Push the feet down hard (plantar flexion), then let go.
- Push the knees down hard against the surface on which you are lying, then let go.
- Push the leg down hard, then let go.
- Tighten the buttock muscles hard, then let go.
- Pull the abdominal muscles in hard, then let go.
- Raise the shoulders, then let go.
- Press the shoulders into the surface on which you are lying, then let go.
- Press the arms into the surface, then let go.
- Curl the fingers to make a fist, then let go.
- Press the head into the surface, then let go.
- Screw up and tighten the face, then let go.
- Tighten all the groups together, then let go.

Breathing exercises

Breathing exercises are given to maintain and improve the expansion of the chest. This increases the amount of oxygen taken into the lungs and increases the amount of carbon dioxide out of the lungs. Breathing in is known as *inspiration*, and breathing out is known as *expiration.*

As explained in Chapter 2, the muscles of respiration are the external intercostal muscles and the internal intercostal muscles (which lie between the ribs) and the diaphragm, which lies horizontally separating the thoracic cavity from the abdominal cavity. The contraction of these muscles will increase the capacity of the thorax from side to side, from front to back and longitudinally from top to bottom.

The effects of breathing exercises

Breathing exercises:

- improve the mobility of the thorax
- increase the intake of the oxygen, which will improve metabolism
- increase the output of carbon dioxide thus eliminating this waste product more quickly
- improve the condition of the lungs
- loosen lung secretions.

In addition, the changing pressure created in the thorax aids the flow of blood in the veins and the flow of lymph in the lymphatic vessels. The increased mobility of the thorax improves posture.

Breathing techniques

Position: sitting on a chair or lying supine (face up). Remove any tight, restricting clothing.

Deep breathing concentrates on three areas of expansion, namely: apical, costal and diaphragmatic.

Apical breathing: Place the hands on the upper chest below the clavicle, breathe in deeply through the nose and expand the chest under the hands. The chest will move up and forward as you breathe in; then breathe out through the mouth and the chest will move back as you breathe out. Try not to allow movement in the other parts of the chest. Repeat three times.

Costal breathing: Place the hands on the side of the ribs, above the waist. Breathe in deeply through the nose and feel the ribs moving out sideways; breathe out through the mouth and the ribs will move back as you breathe out. Repeat three times.

Diaphragmatic breathing: Place the hands in front, above the waist. Breathe in deeply through the nose and feel the lower chest and abdomen moving forward as you breathe in; breathe out through the mouth and pull the abdomen back in as you breathe out. Repeat three times.

Then breathe deeply using all areas of the chest as follows: breathe in deeply through the nose, hold to count of five and breathe out for as long as possible through the mouth. Repeat three times.

> **Learning point**
> Practise yourself before discussing with clients to ensure that you fully understand the movements.

> **Be aware** !
> Deep breathing can make one feel dizzy and faint because the amount of oxygen and carbon dioxide in the body is changing and the balance between these chemicals is disturbed. If this occurs, it is important to rest for a few minutes until the feeling passes and the balance is restored. This must be explained to clients before they are encouraged to practise at home.

Evaluation of own performance

> **Activity** ✳ ✳ ✳
> Carry out an appropriately adapted massage on a client. Then complete an evaluation of your performance, using the questions in the table below. Think about each question carefully and assess how well you think you did and then score each one as follows:
> **RED** — Needs improving
> **AMBER** — Average/OK
> **GREEN** — Good

Name:	Date:			
Questions:	**RED**	**AMBER**	**GREEN**	**Comments**
Did I make sure that everything was in place prior to the client's arrival? i.e. the room (to ensure a suitable, quiet environment), the couch (clean linen, towels and pillows), the trolley (neatly laid out with all commodities to hand).				
Did I abide by the salon's health, safety and hygiene policies?				
Did I adopt a friendly, relaxed, professional, competent manner?				
Did I respect the client's privacy and dignity?				
Did I observe the client's body language?				
Did I adapt my approach to suit the type of client?				
Did I make the client feel at ease?				
Did I communicate well with the client; was I polite, sensitive and supportive?				
Did I carry out a detailed client consultation and note the information on a consultation record and get it signed by the client?				
Did I note all contra-indications and take the required action?				
Did I allow the client the opportunity and time to express her/his needs and expectations?				

Table 6.1 Evaluation of own performance

Name:	Date:			
Questions:	RED	AMBER	GREEN	Comments
Did I listen closely to what they were saying?				
Did I select the most suitable treatment and set long-term goals?				
Did I explain everything clearly to the client and did they understand my explanation?				
Did I agree the treatment plan, cost and timing with the client and obtain her/his written consent?				
Did I maintain eye contact with the client?				
Was I aware of my own body language?				
Did I make the client feel secure, comfortable and cared for?				
Did I select the best possible treatment to suit the client?				
Did I select the most suitable lubricant and make sure I did not waste any?				
Did I wash my hands before treatment?				
Did I adopt the correct posture and position to avoid strain, injury and fatigue?				
Did I use a variety of suitable manipulations at the correct pressure and rhythm?				
Did I check the well-being of the client during the treatment?				

Table 6.1 *Continued*

Name:		Date:		
Questions:	RED	AMBER	GREEN	Comments
Did I evaluate the treatment outcomes?				
Did I offer home-care advice?				
Did I discuss retail products to suit the client's needs?				
Did I review the treatment plan with the client?				
Did I keep within the time constraints for a viable cost-effective treatment?				
Did I dispose of all waste into a lined bin with a lid?				
Did I clean the treatment area and leave it tidy?				

Table 6.1 *Continued*

Learning point

Although this may seem to be a very long list of questions, they should become second nature to you during training, so that this thorough self-evaluation is automatic.

This exercise will also help you to prepare for your massage assessments, as it demonstrates pointers to successful performance.

Additional massage techniques

7

After you have studied this chapter you will be able to:

1. identify the main causes of musculo-skeletal problems
2. recognise abnormalities in the tissues through observation and palpation
3. explain neuromuscular techniques, their uses and effects
4. explain myofascial release techniques, their uses and effects
5. explain passive movement techniques, their uses, effects and contra-indications.

Musculo-skeletal problems

Clients requesting massage frequently complain of pain or stiffness in localised areas of the body, most commonly in the back muscles and the posterior muscles of the neck. Problems may be identified during assessment or when the hands move over the part during a general body massage: these will require further investigation. When the area is palpated, changes may be detected in the tissues that indicate underlying abnormalities of the skin, connective tissue and underlying muscles.

The following changes may be found:

- Muscles may feel hard and tight, indicating increased tension or shortening.
- Tissues may feel thick and unyielding with little or no pliability or flexibility.
- Areas may be tender, painful or hypersensitive to touch, indicating neural (nerve) involvement.
- Fibrous bands, nodules or points of extreme irritability (trigger points) may be felt as the hands move over the part.

A general massage will promote relaxation of these tissues, but deeper and more specific techniques are required to identify the problems and bring about improvement.

The individual components of the musculo-skeletal system must function normally in order to produce full-range, pain-free movement, and any problems or changes in one part will affect the others.

The tissues involved will include:

- the muscles (muscular), which produce movement
- the bones onto which the muscles attach, and the joints where movement occurs (skeletal)
- the connective tissue (fascia), which connects and separates other tissues

- the blood and lymphatic vessels of the area, which deliver nutrients and oxygen and remove the waste products of metabolism (metabolites)
- the nerves (neuro), i.e. the sensory nerves that transmit sensory stimuli to the brain, and motor nerves that transmit impulses from the brain to the muscles to initiate movement and control tension.

Under normal, stress-free conditions the Central Nervous System (CNS) maintains a level of muscle tone that allows normal pain-free movement. Abnormalities such as adhesions entrap nerves and disturb the normal neurological activity between the CNS and the musculo-skeletal system, which will affect muscle tone and normal function.

Stress in any one part of the system will affect all the other adjacent parts as they are all interdependent.

Causes of musculo-skeletal problems

Many factors can contribute to problems of the musculo-skeletal system. The more common causes are:

- trauma and injury
- postural problems
- strain as a result of repetitive movements
- tension produced by psychological or emotional factors
- chilling of the tissues
- a disease of the joints.

Trauma and injury

Injury will result in pain and damage to the joints, bones, muscles, ligaments, tendons or nerves. The extent of the damage and the degree of pain will depend on the severity of the injury. The trauma may result in:

- strains of muscles or tendons, where the fibres may be over-stretched or torn
- sprains of the ligaments that support joints, which may tear or rupture
- extreme forces dislocating joints and/or fracturing bones
- tears or disruption of the connective tissue layers
- increased pressure or damage to nerves
- damage to blood vessels and lymphatic vessels, resulting in bleeding and fluid seeping into the tissues, in turn resulting in swelling of the area
- a protective spasm of the surrounding muscles as the body attempts to prevent further movement, thus limiting and containing the damage. This is an automatic response controlled by the CNS.

The area may be hot, red and swollen, and there may be pain on movement, with loss of function. The heat and redness are due to dilation of the blood vessels, while the swelling is due to fluid seeping out of the blood vessels into the tissues: this fluid is known as **exudate**. The exudate contains cells and plasma proteins, in particular fibrinogen, which forms fine threads of fibrin. As healing progresses, some of the fluid is reabsorbed but some remains in the tissues together with the fibrin threads. This exudate thickens further and the fibres are laid down in a haphazard manner, forming cross-bridges within the tissues.

This binds the tissues together, forming thickenings, tight bands and nodules. The increased tension and pressure will irritate the nerve endings, resulting in areas of tenderness and pain.

The healing of wounds involves the formation of fibrous scar tissue, which contracts and hardens over time. The amount of scar tissue formed will depend on the size of the wound. Scars and fibrous adhesions bind tissue fibres and layers together, preventing smooth movement, and the ability to glide over one another. The tissues lose flexibility and extensibility both lengthways and widthways, and the range of movement is limited. Appropriate massage manipulations can help to loosen these adhesions, realign the tissue fibres and restore their extensibility and pliability, thus increasing the range of movement, relieving pain and restoring full function.

Postural problems

Posture is the term used to describe the alignment of the body. Good posture means that the body is balanced and the muscle work required to maintain it is minimal. Poor posture means that the body is out of balance and certain muscles must contract strongly to maintain the position. Habitual, long-term poor posture will result in some muscles over-contracting and shortening while their **antagonists** (opposite muscle group) lengthen and weaken.

Posture is influenced by many factors, such as a sedentary life style, taking little exercise, poor working conditions, or poor sitting or working postures such as sitting and looking at a computer screen all day, with shoulders rounded and the head craned forward. Back and neck problems are often the result of poor posture.

It is thought that the muscles that maintain the shortened position actually tighten and shorten, and their connective tissue becomes tighter and less flexible. The increased tension in these contracted muscles impedes the circulation, resulting in a decrease in the delivery of nutrients and oxygen and a build up of **metabolites**. This results in stiffness, pain and greater tension.

Nodules and thickened areas may develop in these muscles as a few fibres exhibit extreme tension. The causes of postural problems will need to be identified and rectified through exercise and improved postural habits.

Massage will help by promoting relaxation of the tightened muscles. In addition, stretching techniques and flexibility exercises may be used to restore length to shortened muscle fibres, and mobility to connective tissue.

Learning point
Exudate is defined as a mass of cells and fluid that has seeped out of blood vessels or organs, especially where there is inflammation.

Be aware
Massage must be avoided in the acute stage of injury and the initial stages of healing as it may cause further damage. It should only be considered when healing is complete.

Learning point
Acute pain is short-term, severe pain. Chronic pain is continuous, long-term pain.

Learning point
The antagonists are the opposing muscle group.

Remember
Metabolites are the waste products of metabolism.

255

Strain as a result of repetitive movements

Individuals who perform repetitive movements over a long period of time may be over-loading and over-using their muscles. Tendons and their sheaths may become inflamed, producing pain on movement. Some muscles may be constantly working in shortened positions, resulting in increased tension and adaptive shortening. Joints may be forced to the extreme end of their range. This will alter the stresses and forces on the supporting ligaments and on connective tissue, which contracts and tightens. The circulation will be restricted resulting in fatigue, pain and stiffness.

Clearly, the cause of the problem must be identified, rectified and eliminated if possible. Specific massage techniques are used to stretch connective tissue and free ligaments and tendons around the affected joints. Flexibility exercises and stretching techniques are also given to increase joint movement and aid full function.

Tension produced by psychological or emotional factors

Certain psychological and emotional states can produce increased tension in the muscles. Fear, anxiety and stress can cause the muscles to be held in a rigid state, which produces tenderness and pain. People who are sad, upset or timid are likely to exhibit poor posture, which may result in problems already described if the emotional state persists. Tension exhibited over a period of time may result in adaptive shortening of the tissues, restricted circulation and increased pressure on nerve endings, resulting in pain and stiffness.

General body massage will help to relieve general stress but specific techniques are required to improve areas of extreme tension and to elongate the tissues.

Chilling of the tissues

Cold will increase tension in the tissues, the muscles contract, and the circulation is restricted. Low temperature will also cause vasoconstriction, which further reduces the blood supply. If the chilling is of short duration then the tissues recover quickly but some stiffness will remain. Longer-term cooling, such as sitting in a draught for a period of time, can decrease the pliability of connective tissue, resulting in pain and stiffness.

Massage is used to aid relaxation of the tissues, to produce vasodilation and increase the blood flow to the area. This increased blood flow, together with the heat produced through hand contact with the part, will warm the area, increasing the pliability of the tissues. Stretch techniques are used to improve flexibility and extensibility of the tissues.

Disease of the joints

The most common diseases are inflammatory and degenerative arthritis, but there are many others that cause primary changes in the joints and secondary changes to the surrounding soft tissues.

During the chronic stage, when pain has subsided, gentle massage may be used to soothe and relax the tissues, and aid the absorption of any swelling. When the disease has completely 'burnt out', localised massage techniques performed around the joints will help to reduce swelling, and loosen the ligaments and tendons. This may be followed by gentle passive and active movements.

Palpation of the tissues to identify any abnormalities

When abnormalities are present in the tissues, they are detected through the palms of the hands or the pads of the fingers, as these have large numbers of sensory receptors. This probing and feeling for changes and abnormalities is known as **palpating** the tissues. The ability to palpate the tissue layers accurately and identify abnormalities is extremely important, as selection of the appropriate treatment is based on these findings. This skill requires a great deal of practice and experience.

Problems may be identified during consultation, during a general massage while performing effleurage or stroking movements or during specific exploratory movements. Palpation is best carried out on dry skin without any lubricant, although this is not always possible, as a lubricant may already have been applied before the problem was identified. In this case, it is better to continue the massage and return to the localised area towards the end, when the lubricant will have been absorbed.

Remember that you are looking for abnormalities: explore the tissues under the hand and feel for thickened areas or nodules. Then move the tissues around, and sense the pliability and stretch in the tissues. Note anything that feels different from the surrounding areas, and compare it with the other side for guidance. Are there areas of tenderness or pain that produce a reaction from the client? When conditions are identified, appropriate techniques can be selected to improve and normalise the tissues.

> **Learning point**
>
> Palpation is mostly done with the pads of the fingers or thumb, as these are the more sensitive areas of the hand, but sometimes the whole palm is involved, 'feeling and sensing' the tissues as it moves along. Pressure is adjusted depending on the depth of the tissue being palpated. Light pressure is required for palpating the skin and superficial fascia, becoming heavier for muscle and bone.

Abnormalities

Any of the following abnormalities may be encountered as you palpate the tissues:

- pain
- muscle tension
- oedema
- fibrous adhesions
- fibrotic nodules
- fatty nodules
- trigger points
- crepitus.

Pain

Contact with the part may elicit pain: it is important to obtain verbal and non-verbal responses. The client will be able to describe the pain but always be aware of the client's reaction when and as you touch them. If you can see the client's face, note if they grimace with pain. If they are lying prone, watch for a body reaction. If they are feeling discomfort or pain they will twitch and move away from your touch. Ask them to describe the pain: is it sharp or dull? How severe is it? On a scale of 1–10 when 1 equals no pain and 10 equals intense pain, where does the pain lie?

Pain is a symptom of some underlying cause or stress: when pain is present the underlying cause must be identified. Pain may be **acute**, i.e. sharp and of sudden onset, indicating the acute stages of injury or disease, when massage is contra-indicated; or it may be **chronic**, i.e. deep, dull pain, which may be the symptom of a long-standing chronic condition. The pain may come on gradually and develop slowly, it may be fairly static or may steadily increase or it may be intermittent or constant and difficult to relieve. It may radiate over a large area or be localised to small points within muscles or fascia, which may be extremely painful when touched.

Pain is not always felt in the immediate vicinity of the problem: it may radiate away from the exact site. It may be referred to another area some distance away that has the same nerve supply, e.g. tension in the neck muscles can refer pain to the head. Malfunction of internal organs can refer pain and produce changes in superficial tissues that share the same nerve root, e.g. problems in the liver may refer pain to the skin area below the right scapula.

Muscle tension

A mild degree of tension is present in healthy skeletal muscle at all times and is known as muscle tone. It ensures that the muscle can contract quickly in response to a stimulus. This tension may increase in response to many factors such as pain, injury, postural or psychological problems, as previously outlined. As tension increases, pain increases due to pressure on, and reflex activity of the nerves. More pain results in greater tension, setting up a tension/pain cycle.

Over a period of time tension will result in physiological changes within the tissues. There will be circulatory changes, due to increased pressure on the blood vessels. The blood supply to the area will be limited, oxygen and nutrient supply will be reduced, and metabolites will build up. At this stage there will be aching and soreness in the muscles, and they will feel hard and unyielding when palpated. If tension is prolonged, the muscles and fascia will shorten and contract and will feel tight and rigid.

This will result in loss of elasticity and flexibility: the muscles resist sideways movement and efforts to lift them from underlying structures. All these factors limit function and produce further pain.

General massage routines will help to relieve tension and improve the circulation. However, localised and more specific

Be aware !

Intractable pain must always be medically investigated. This is any pain (whether it be dull, throbbing, sharp, severe etc.) that never diminishes and is not relieved by rest. There may be a serious underlying cause, and massage should not be carried out.

Remember

Increased *tension* produces *pain*, which results in *further tension*, which produces *more pain*.

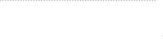

techniques will be required if the pain is chronic, with thickened hypersensitive areas in the tissues.

Oedema

This is swelling of the tissues, which can often be seen without the need to palpate. The skin and underlying tissues will appear tight with loss of pliability.

Any swollen area should be palpated very gently, as the skin will be stretched and may break down easily. If it is not too severe, the swelling will feel soft and spongy. Severe swelling will feel hard and unyielding. Chronic oedema of long standing feels dense and firm to touch: **pitting** will occur when pressed with the thumb, i.e. the indentation made by the thumb will remain in the flesh for some time but will eventually refill with fluid.

The build-up of fluid will increase the pressure within the tissues, which presses on the nerves and stimulates the pain receptors, resulting in pain.

Massage can aid the removal of fluid from the tissues but it is very important to establish the cause of the oedema, as massage does not help all cases. (Treatment of oedema is explained in Chapter 6.)

Fibrous adhesions

As explained previously, the healing processes following injury or inflammation may result in the fluid exudate and fibrin forming fibrous adhesions among the tissues. These are laid down in a haphazard manner and limit the flexibility and extensibility of the area. Adhesions may form within the muscles following micro tears of the fibres, or they may develop within the superficial and deep layers of fascia as a result of stress or trauma. They may also form around ligaments and tendons, binding them down to underlying bone. Adhesions form cross-bridges or bonds within the tissues, preventing the smooth glide of the tissues over each other during movement. They restrict the lengthening and sideways movement of the fibres. The tissues feel dense, stiff and less pliable and movement is limited in all directions.

Fibrous adhesions within a muscle or in the connective tissue layers surrounding the muscle will restrict the elasticity and full lengthening of the muscles. This will limit full-range movement and may produce pain on movement.

Massage manipulations such as stroking and myofascial release techniques are used to stretch the fibrous adhesions in all directions and also to realign them. Flexibility and extensibility are increased, and normal movement of the tissues is restored.

Fibrotic nodules

These are hardened, lumpy zones, usually painful to touch, lying within superficial muscles or fascia. They are small areas of tense, contracted fibres with restricted circulation. The tight, hardened nodule may be mobile, i.e. it moves within the tissues when gently pushed around; or it may adhere to the underlying tissues when there is little movement. They tend to be painful in the area of the nodule but do not refer pain to other areas. Nodules are treated with pressure techniques: the degree of pressure used is dictated by the amount of pain produced, which must be within the tolerance of the client. Pressure may be increased as the pain subsides. Nodules frequently disappear when the pressure is applied.

Fatty nodules

These are lumps of fatty tissue within the fascia: they feel softer than fibrous nodules and can be moved around more easily. They are usually less painful and disperse more easily with pressure. They are treated with pressure techniques.

Trigger points

These are small areas of hypersensitive contracted tissue. They may produce pain over the exact location of the trigger point, which may radiate over the surrounding area, or the pain may be referred to another area known as the target zone. The pain in these areas increases with pressure. They are treated with pressure techniques (see later in this chapter).

Crepitus

This sounds and feels like fine crackling among the tissues. It results from changes arising from inflammation within the tissues. When acute inflammation subsides, it may leave a chronic thickening and dryness in the tissues.

Neuromuscular-skeletal techniques

These techniques should not be viewed as apart from general massage movements, but rather as additional skills that may be used to relieve pain and restore function to localised conditions. They may be incorporated into a general body massage, or may form part of the routine for a specific part of the body, such as the neck or back. Localised tissue abnormalities may be identified during consultation or during the course of a body massage. The appropriate techniques must then be selected and extra time spent on these areas to bring about improvement.

These techniques are sometimes referred to as bodywork techniques, soft tissue manipulation or neuromuscular treatments. They all use pressure and/or stretch manipulations to reduce tension, ease pain and stiffness, and to restore full function. Specific manipulations are used to target the following conditions:

- increased tension within muscles (hypertension)
- thickening or fibrous adhesions within the tissues (muscles or connective tissue)
- contracted fascia; small areas of hypersensitive tissue (known as trigger points)
- fibrotic or fatty nodules.

The techniques included in this text are:

- neuromuscular stroking technique
- trigger point therapy
- myofascial stretch/release techniques.

Deep effleurage and frictions can also be used (see Chapter 4).

You must adopt a sensitive, caring and gentle approach, bearing in mind that these manipulations are aimed at releasing abnormal tension within the muscles. Through reducing and normalising neural (nerve) activity, relieving hypersensitive areas, stretching contracted tissue, realigning fibres, and restoring flexibility and pliability to the tissues, the continuing cycle of *pain–tension–more pain* is interrupted and normal function is restored. Contra-indications are the same as those for general massage (listed in Chapter 3).

Neuromuscular stroking

This involves sensitively searching through the tissues for abnormalities such as areas of increased tension, dense thickened areas, loss of pliability, and manipulating them. The area is explored in all directions using stroking movements with the thumb or fingers. Superficial pressure is used for assessing and treating superficial tissues but deeper pressure is required for assessing and treating the deeper tissues.

The aims of this treatment are to:

- release areas of hypertension and contracted tissue
- loosen adhesions and realign tissue fibres
- increase the pliability of thickened tissue
- reduce pain and restore normal function.

Uses of neuromuscular stroking

Neuromuscular stroking is used to:

- identify abnormalities in the tissues
- stretch contracted thickened tissue
- realign tissue fibres
- reduce reflex activity through the nervous system
- reduce tension
- relieve pain
- restore full function.

Best practice

Anatomical knowledge of the area is essential, in particular, knowledge of muscle shape and fibre direction. If you are unsure, refer to a muscle chart or detailed diagram before commencing the treatment. This is extremely important because, as you palpate through the area, some strokes are performed across the fibres to loosen adhesions and reduce thickenings but other strokes are performed along the fibres to release tension and realign the fibres.

Effects of neuromuscular stroking

Superficial manipulations will produce the following effects:

- The skin and superficial fascia are loosened and mobilised.
- The elasticity of the skin and superficial fascia is improved.
- Adhesions are stretched and mobilised, thus improving the glide between the superficial and deep fascial layers.
- The circulation of blood and lymph is increased to the superficial tissues, improving their condition.

Deeper manipulations will produce the following effects:

- Stretching of the deep fascia will improve its flexibility.
- When the fascia is stretched and separated, the glide and movement between the deep fascial layers, and between the fascia and the muscles, is improved, thus smooth movement of the tissues is facilitated. Mobility increases and the tension decreases.
- The movement and the heat generated by the hand on the part increases the pliability of the fascia.
- Stretching and mobilising of any fibrotic adhesions within muscles or fascia will reduce tissue tension and restore flexibility.
- The tissue fibres that have become distorted by stress or the pull of adhesions are realigned along their normal lines of stress. Muscles are then more able to withstand stresses applied to them. This will limit damage such as micro tears of the fibres.
- Decreased tension within the muscles reduces the pressure on sensory nerve endings, thus reducing pain.
- The pressure manipulations and relaxation of the tissues decrease neural reflex activity, hence the pain cycle is interrupted.
- Blood and lymph are able to circulate more freely through the tissues, therefore the delivery of oxygen and nutrients is increased and the removal of irritating chemical metabolites is accelerated. The physiological functioning of the whole area improves.

Treatment technique for neuromuscular stroking

To palpate the tissues, proceed as follows:

- Move the pads of the fingers or thumb superficially over the tissues and search carefully for any areas that feel harder and less pliable than normal. These will be areas of increased tension, thickening, fibrotic adhesions or nodules.
- Continue moving deeper into the tissues with increased pressure to locate the exact site of the problem.
- When abnormalities are identified, the area should first of all be warmed with general manipulations such as effleurage and kneading and then treated with the deeper stroking movements.

- The treatment is completed with more effleurage.

How to apply pressure:

- When the thumb is used, contact is made with the lateral border of the ball of the thumb while the fingers rest lightly on the part.
- For greater pressure, both thumbs may be used, positioned one behind the other with the fingers of both hands resting on the part.
- Alternatively, the pads of the fingers may be used. On small areas, contact is made with the middle finger supported by the index and ring fingers. On larger areas, the three fingers may make contact reinforced by the same fingers of the other hand.

> **Learning point**
> For neuromuscular stroking, strokes may be long or short, depending on the size of the area. Short strokes are used for small areas of tension but longer strokes are used on larger areas. Strokes may be applied with the fingers, the thumb, and sometimes with the elbow when deeper pressure is required.

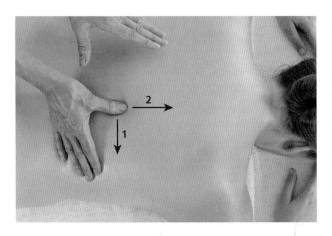

Figure 7.1 Neuromuscular stroking on erector spinae

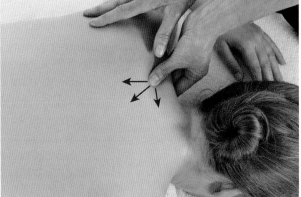

Figure 7.2 Neuromuscular stroking to trapezius

Technique:

- stroke over the area in all directions to stretch the tissues and loosen any adhesions
- stroke in the direction of the muscle fibres until the tissues yield or give slightly: this will elongate and realign the tissues
- repeat several times until any pain is reduced and the area feels softer and more pliable
- effleurage the area to complete the treatment.

> **Learning point**
> Neuromuscular stroking can also be used to treat fibrotic and fatty nodules.

Trigger point pressure

Trigger points are small, taut areas of extreme irritability, usually located within a muscle but can also be found in the fascia. They are often tender and painful: the degree of pain can vary from mild discomfort to severe pain. When palpated they feel like short, thick, tight bands of contracted fibres, which produce a 'twitch' when directly palpated. The muscles in which trigger points are located may be tense and shortened, their elasticity is limited and they are unable to extend to their normal length. Pain is usually produced when the muscles contract or are stretched or manipulated.

> **Learning point**
> Active trigger points can often emit a 'twitch-like' response when directly palpated.

263

Trigger points may be described as **latent** or **active**. Latent trigger points are painful only when direct pressure is applied. Active trigger points are tender, radiate pain, and may also refer pain to another area known as the target zone, or target area. This occurs because the trigger point and the target zone are innervated by the same spinal nerve or are linked by the autonomic system.

Trigger points develop in muscles and fascia following repetitive microtrauma, or when extreme tension develops and the tissues are held in a shortened position over a period of time. This increased tension increases pressure on nerve endings, resulting in pain. It also restricts the blood circulating through the area. The supply of nutrients and oxygen is reduced, metabolites, including chemical irritants, build up in the muscle and the normal physiological functioning of the area is disturbed. The chemicals irritate the sensory receptors in the tissues, resulting in more pain.

Identifying trigger points

Trigger points may be found as the hands move over the part during a general massage or during palpation to identify the cause of pain or tenderness in an area.

The pads of the fingers are more sensitive at detecting changes in the tissues but the whole palm may also be used. Light to moderate pressure is applied depending on the degree of pain. The hands move very slowly and gently over the area until a very tender spot is encountered.

The following signs can indicate the presence of a trigger point:

- Pain is produced or increased in the exact location of the trigger point when pressure is applied and/or pain may be referred in the target zone.
- A tight, rope-like band can be felt in the tissues.
- A twitch response occurs when the finger slides over the area.
- The client describes the pain as extremely tender and attempts to move away from the pressure.

Uses of pressure techniques and stretching

Pressure techniques and stretching are used to:

- deactivate the trigger point and relieve pain
- relieve the tightness/spasm of the muscle fibres
- improve the circulation and return normal physiological function
- stretch and mobilise the muscles and return to full-range movement.

Effects of pressure techniques and stretching on trigger points

Pressure techniques and stretching on trigger points will produce the following effects:

- The initial pressure applied will increase the pain. However, as the pressure is maintained or increased, the pain will decrease. This is due to factors that reduce the activity of the nervous system:
  - The nervous system adapts to the pressure, and sensitivity of nerve endings is reduced.
  - The chemical metabolites that irritate the nerve endings are reduced.
  - The release of endorphins (the body's natural analgesic), which suppress pain, is possible.
- When pressure is applied into the trigger point, the underlying blood vessels are compressed and the blood is squeezed out; when the pressure is released, the blood vessels dilate and fill with fresh blood. This flushes the area with fresh blood, which will remove the build-up of metabolites, including chemical irritants, and also bring oxygen and nutrients to the tissues, thus aiding return to normal physiological function.
- As pain is relieved during the treatment then the degree of tension in the muscle decreases because it breaks the pain cycle (*pain–tension–pain*).
- The stretching techniques that are applied after the pressure treatment also reduce spasm in the muscle fibres. In addition, they loosen and realign the fibres, which improves extensibility and lengthening of the muscle.

Treatment technique for trigger points

In an attempt to deactivate a trigger point, do the following:

- Apply direct pressure *at 90° to the fibres*. Pressure can be applied through the pads of the thumb or fingers, or through the elbow.
- As the pressure is applied it must activate the trigger point: consequently the pain may initially increase. The client may feel the pain at the exact point of pressure only, or the pain may also be referred to a target zone but it should be just bearable for the client.
- If the pressure is too great, it will make the client tense up: this is obviously counter-productive.
- If the trigger point is extremely sensitive, treatment should commence with light pressure, deepening as pain diminishes, but it must always be within client tolerance.
- The pressure is sustained for 30–90 seconds until the pain diminishes. If necessary massage the area before applying the pressure again.
- The client should be instructed and encouraged to relax into the pain. This helps to break the pain–tension cycle.

Be aware

When treating trigger points, if the pain continues to increase and does not ease, release the pressure and stop the treatment, as there may be an underlying inflammatory condition that is a contra-indication.

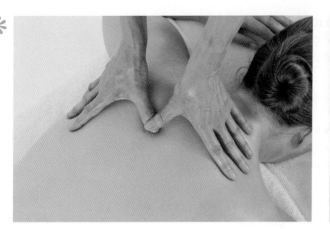

Figure 7.3 Thumb pressure to trigger point at medial border of scapula

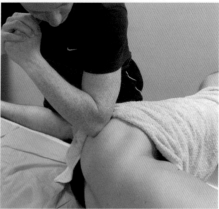

Figure 7.4 Elbow pressure to trigger point in gluteal muscles

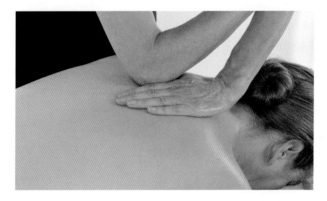

Figure 7.5 Elbow pressure to trigger point in trapezius

Following the direct pressure technique, the shortened muscles should be stretched (using the stretch techniques already described) and every attempt made to restore elasticity and full length.

Myofascial-release techniques

These techniques work on the muscles and the fascial layers of the body. Fascia is areolar tissue: it is an irregular connective tissue composed of a loose arrangement of collagen and elastin fibres in a viscous ground substance. It is the most widespread tissue in the body: it connects and supports tissues and organs.

It is laid down in large sheets throughout the body, which:

- connect skin to muscle
- wrap around muscle bundles
- connect muscles to each other and to bone
- support organs and line body cavities.

There are *three types,* located in different areas of the body, as follows:

- *Subcutaneous fascia* lies beneath the skin and is a continuous layer all over the body. It connects the skin to the underlying tissues and in the normal state allows smooth movement between the two.

- *Deep fascia* lies in sheets and bands around and between muscles. It binds muscle fibres into bundles, and muscle bundles together; it surrounds the entire muscle and also lies in layers between muscles, linking them together and attaching them to the bones. Pliability and flexibility of this deep fascia is therefore essential to facilitate smooth movement during contraction and relaxation of the muscle. When conditions are normal the connective tissue is pliable and allows full movement of the muscle but under abnormal conditions, when the fascia becomes thickened, tight and inflexible, full-range movement will be limited.

- *Subserous fascia* lies between the deep fascia and the serous membrane that lines the body cavities. It supports organs and facilitates movement between them (these techniques will not reach or affect this layer).

Connective tissue is capable of change: it becomes more pliable with movement and temperature increases, but becomes tight and inflexible with tension and cold. Following trauma or when abnormal postures are held over a period of time, the connective tissue in the area thickens and becomes more fibrous. It becomes less pliable and may cause distortion of the tissues. These sheets of fascia interconnect throughout the body and any tightness or distortion in one area may cause problems in another.

Any of the causes mentioned can result in tightening of the connective tissue with distortion and limited function of adjacent tissues, e.g. injury, postural or psychological problems.

Identifying myofascial problems

The skin and the superficial tissues will feel less mobile. There will be a general thickening and loss of pliability in the area. The movement of the skin over the underlying tissues will be restricted and the tissues feel less flexible. The client may complain of stiffness or/and a dull ache.

Assessment of the posture will indicate any areas held in shortened positions, e.g. a chin protrusion will result in shortened cervical tissues and posterior neck muscles. Lordosis will result in shortening of the tissues and muscles of the lumbar region, e.g. psoas major.

Uses of myofascial techniques

Myofascial techniques are used to:

- restore mobility to the fascia
- release the subcutaneous layer from the skin

> **Remember**
> The aim of myofascial techniques is to realign fibres, to soften and increase the mobility and pliability of the fascia and restore full function.

- release deep fascia from the muscle
- soften thickened fibrous areas
- restore pliability and flexibility
- correct any distortion of the tissues
- restore normal movement and function
- relieve stiffness and pain.

Effects of myofascial techniques

Myofascial techniques will produce the following effects:

- The skin and superficial fascia are lifted away from the underlying tissues: this loosens and improves the flexibility of the skin and fascia.
- The deeper techniques stretch the deep fascia, realign the collagen fibres and release any cross-bridges.
- The flexibility of the fascia is improved, therefore adjacent muscles are able to function normally.
- The circulation to the area is increased, partly due to the alternate pressure and release on the vessels, but also because the tightness between the fascial layers, which restricts blood and lymphatic circulation to the tissues, is released. When fascial tension is released, blood and lymph flow improve, and tissue fluid passes more freely through the fascia. The tissues receive more nutrients and oxygen, and the rate of removal of waste products is increased, therefore condition and function of the tissues improve.
- When tension in the tissues is released, extensibility improves, which aids the return to full function.

Myofascial treatment techniques

These techniques are used to stretch the tissues. Skin rolling and vertical lifting are used to stretch the skin and superficial fascia. Muscle rolling and stretch-release are aimed at the deeper fascial layers. These techniques are applied without any lubricant because the skin must not slide under the hands.

Skin rolling

This may be used to release superficial fascia, and is frequently performed on the back, over the ribs, as follows:

- Place the hands on the part with the thumb abducted.
- Lift and push the flesh with the fingers towards the thumbs.
- Roll this flesh with the thumbs, back towards the fingers.
- Repeat three or four times as needed, then move on to an adjacent area.

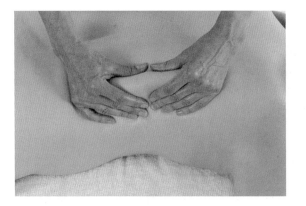

Figure 7.6 Skin rolling over the ribs

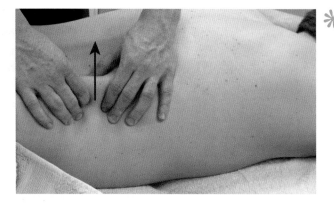

Figure 7.7 Vertical lifting technique on back

Vertical lifting technique

This may be used to lift the skin and superficial fascia away from underlying tissues, as follows:

- The hands are positioned vertically above the part, and fingers and thumb are held straight and pointing towards the tissues.
- The skin and superficial fascia are grasped between the fingers and thumb, and lifted directly upwards, held for a few seconds and then released.
- This is repeated three or four times in one area and then the hands move along to the adjacent area.
- Take care not to pinch the flesh: the effort is directed towards the lift.

Muscle rolling technique

This is usually used on the long-limb muscles, as follows:

- Place the muscles in their shortened, relaxed position.
- Grasp the muscle between the fingers and thumb: the larger muscles will fill the palm.
- Lift the muscle if possible, then push it away from you and then pull towards you.
- Pull and push the muscle transversely in this way several times, to stretch and release the fascia.
- On long muscles, it will be necessary to move along the muscle, and repeat the lift and pull/push again.

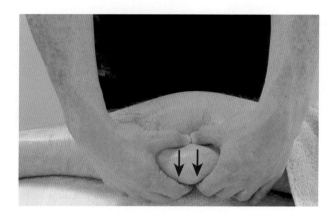

Figure 7.8 Muscle rolling to gastronemius

Stretch–release

This is a technique that targets the muscles and deeper fascial layers, as follows:

- The stretch must be applied in the direction of the muscle fibres.
- It is performed slowly and requires great concentration and ability to feel the resistance, and then the yield, in the tissue.
- With the arms crossed, one hand anchors the skin while the other hand applies movement in the opposite direction, pushing the skin and fascia horizontally until the point of resistance is felt.
- This point is held until the tissues release and yield slightly.
- Repeat the stretch until there is no further release.
- The hand then moves on to another area.
- Take care not to slip and chafe the skin.

> **Learning point**
> A similar **stretch–release** technique involves placing the crossed hands on the skin and moving them **apart**. Pressure is applied through the ulnar border of the hands as they move away from each other. Stretch is applied to the underlying tissues, held for a few seconds at the end of the stroke and then released.

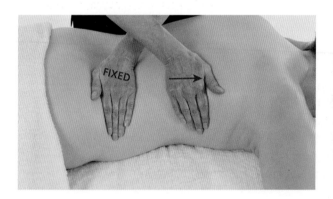

Figure 7.9 Stretch-release applied by one hand to the back

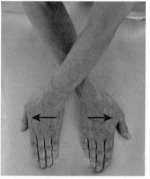

Figure 7.10 Stretch-release applied by both hands to the back

Passive movements

Passive movements may be incorporated into massage routines to aid client relaxation. These movements carefully move the client's joints through the physiological range. Normally, our movements are the result of muscle contraction. Muscles contract in response to impulses/stimuli from the brain and spinal cord transmitted via motor nerves to the muscles. As the muscles contract, they pull on the bones at the point of attachment, and movement occurs at the joints over which they pass. This is known as **active movement**.

Movement at joints can also be produced by an external force, such as another person moving the joint when the muscles are relaxed, that is, not contracting.

This is known as **passive movement**.

Active movement is controlled by the nervous system, which stimulates the muscles to contract and produce movement at the joints. It may be *voluntary* movement, which is under the conscious control of the client, such as moving the arm; or *involuntary*, which is not willed by the client but is a reflex movement, such as blinking.

Passive movement is performed by an external force while the muscles are relaxed, usually one person moving another person's joints.

There are three grades of passive movements: *relaxed, forced* and *manipulative*, depending on the degree of force used.

This text relates to relaxed passive movements. Forced and manipulative movements are medical procedures.

You should perform relaxed passive movements while the client's muscles are relaxed. The joints are moved through the existing range by you: that means the fullest pain-free range possible without applying force.

It is very important to assess accurately the possible range at each joint and work to this limit, offering only slight over-pressure.

Joint structure

The classification, structure and factors that affect the range of movement of joints are explained earlier (see Chapter 2). You must revise and understand these facts before performing passive movements. The different types of synovial joint have different movements. These movements include the following:

- **flexion:** the bringing together of two surfaces (a bending movement), e.g. bending the elbow or knee
- **extension:** movement in the opposite direction to flexion (a straightening movement), e.g. straightening the elbow or knee
- **abduction:** movement away from the mid-line, e.g. taking the arm from the body
- **adduction:** movement towards the mid-line, e.g. taking the arm back to the body
- **rotation:** movement around a long axis, which may be medial rotation, e.g. turning the arm in; or lateral rotation, e.g. turning the arm out

> **Be aware** !
> The range of movement may be restricted if the joint has been affected by disease or prolonged poor posture conditioning etc. Any damage or erosion of the bone surfaces or residual adhesions will produce tightness and eventually contractures of the soft tissues around the joint, which will limit the movement.

> **Be aware** !
> If the disease or injury is acute then passive movements are contra-indicated.

- **circumduction:** movement where the limb describes a cone whose apex lies in the joint: a combination of flexion, extension, abduction and adduction, e.g. circling the shoulder joint or hip joint round and round.

Movements that occur between the radius and ulna:

- **supination:** turns the hand forwards or upwards
- **pronation:** turns the hand backwards or downwards.

Movements of the ankle joint:

- **dorsi-flexion:** pulling the foot upwards
- **plantar flexion:** pointing the foot downwards.

Movements of the foot occurring between the tarsal joints:

- **inversion:** turning the sole of the foot inwards
- **eversion:** turning the sole of the foot outwards.

> ## Activity
>
> Perform all the movements of each of the joints on yourself until you are confident of each movement, its direction and its range. Familiarise yourself with all the terms.

Relaxed, passive movements are performed on synovial joints, which are the moveable joints of the body. For full range of movement to occur, all the component structures of the joint must function normally.

Common conditions that affect joints

Two common conditions that affect the structure and function of joints are rheumatoid arthritis and osteoarthritis. Although differing in pathology, they both result in damage to the hyaline cartilage that lines the bones, inflammation of the synovial membrane and an increase in synovial fluid entering the joint space. These factors produce heat, swelling and pain around the joint, which limit movement.

Inflammation may spread to other structures surrounding the joint such as the capsule, ligaments and tendons. The inflammatory exudate (fluid) tends to thicken and solidify, forming adhesions among the tissues. At the same time, the muscles around the joint will contract and shorten in response to pain (this is the body's protective mechanism to resist movement, thus protecting the body from further pain).

Changes and shortening of the soft tissues initially produce tightness of the joint, which can be rectified by giving passive movements and flexibility exercises. However, if no treatment is given, the tissues will continue to shorten and become bound down resulting in fixed permanent contractures.

Tightness will limit the movement. However, this can be rectified and a return to full-range movement is possible, but when

Learning point

Study the parts of a synovial joint: it will help you to understand the following common conditions that affect joints.

Learning point

Injuries and other conditions involving the joint may also result in degeneration, adhesions and shortening of the soft tissues (i.e. the capsule, ligaments, tendons and muscles around the joint). These factors will result in stiffness, tightness and contractures, which will limit the range of movement.

contractures develop, the problem can only be rectified by forced passive movements or surgical manipulative procedures.

Consultation

Passive movements are usually integrated into a massage treatment, therefore a full client consultation and assessment will have been carried out. During the consultation it is important to ask specific questions relating to joints, as follows:

- Do you have any pain in any of your joints?
- Have you suffered from joint pain in the past?
- Have you ever injured any joints or fractured a bone near a joint?
- Have you had surgery for any joint problems recently?
- Do you suffer from stiffness in any joint?
- Have you had any bone- or joint-related illness, either lately or as a child?
- Do you ever have swelling of any joints?
- Have you noticed any bony growths around any joint (will indicate that changes have taken place in the joint, produced by arthritis or past trauma)?

Positive answers to any one of these questions will mean that great care must be taken during treatment. If the condition is severe, the treatment must not be carried out.

Contra-indications to passive movements

Examine the joints carefully and ask appropriate questions. If any of the following conditions are present, the treatment should not be carried out:

- bone fractures. Avoid working on the affected limb until healing is complete. The unaffected limbs can be treated.
- bruising around the joint. There is a risk of further bleeding: healing must be complete before commencing treatment.
- dysfunction or disorders of the nervous system, such as multiple sclerosis, strokes, Parkinson's disease. These conditions should be treated by therapists who specialise in the particular field.
- hot or painful joints. These signs indicate that pathological changes are occurring in the joint.
- metal pins or plates within a joint or within the bones forming the joint. These will have been inserted to stabilise the joint or bone following trauma. There is the risk of displacing or loosening these pins.
- open wounds, cuts and abrasions near the joint. There is a risk of increasing the bleeding; risk of infection and blood contamination.

- recent or active arthritic conditions. The joint will usually be hot, stiff and swollen.
- recent scar tissue. There is a danger of breaking down scar tissue. However, when the scar is completely healed (after about six months) passive movements may help to stretch it.
- recent sprains of the joint. Healing must be complete before commencing treatment.
- recent strains of any muscle around the joint. Healing must be complete before commencing treatment.
- skin infections and very fragile skin. There is a risk of spreading an infection and also of cross-infection. If the skin is very thin and fragile, great care must be taken to avoid splitting or causing open sores.
- spasticity in the muscles, i.e. muscles with increased tone. Pulling against spastic muscles may increase the spasticity.
- swelling of the joint. Swelling may indicate some damage to the joint and passive movements are contra-indicated. However, if there is no damage, swelling around the ankles may be due to an accumulation of tissue fluid: passive movements combined with massage can then be carried out to improve this condition.
- thrombosis or phlebitis. These conditions are explained in Chapter 3. Although the muscles are not actively contracting during passive movements, the alternate stretch and release of the muscles acting on the joint may be sufficient to dislodge a blood clot from the vein wall, releasing it into the blood stream. The clot may then be carried to a vital organ such as the lungs where it may cause a blockage of the blood supply with potentially fatal consequences.

Uses of passive movements

Passive movements are used to:

- maintain and slightly improve the existing range of movement
- prevent the formation of adhesions
- prevent stiffness of the joint
- aid relaxation.

Passive movements in a massage routine should move each joint smoothly and rhythmically through all its movements. The client is relaxed and neither assists nor resists the movement. Passive movements will have an effect on all the structures inside and outside the joint.

Effects of passive movements

Passive movements:

- maintain the present range of movement (Moving the joint as far as possible each time and giving slight overpressure will ensure that the range is maintained.)

- prevent tightness or stiffness of the joints
- maintain the extensibility of the soft tissues around the joint
- prevent the formation of adhesions
- stimulate the production of synovial fluid and lubrication of the joint
- may slightly assist venous and lymphatic flow as the muscles are stretched and relaxed over the moving joint
- have a soothing and relaxing effect if done slowly and rhythmically.

Technique of passive movements

Ensure that you know the anatomy and direction of movement of each joint. Remember that the movements vary according to the type of joint. The hinge joints of the knee and elbow can move to flexion and extension only, while the ball and socket joints of the shoulder and hip can move through flexion, extension, abduction, adduction, medial and lateral rotation and circumduction.

Explain the procedure to the client, as follows:

- Ask if they have any questions.
- Encourage them to relax.
- If you are including passive movements in your massage routine do not interrupt the flow and continuity to explain the procedure, but include this in the initial explanation and discussion with the client.

Maintain the highest standard of client care and hygiene throughout:

- Check that the client is comfortable.
- Check that all areas not being treated are covered and supported.

Adopt the correct stance and maintain good posture throughout:

- Stride standing is the most common position but some movements require a change to walk standing.

Fix the joint:

- Movement should only occur at the joint being worked on.
- The joints above and below should be fixed.
- This is done either by your hand support or by positioning the limb on the plinth for support.

Movements:

- Grasp above and below the joint firmly but gently.
- Pressure should be even and constant.
- Do not pinch or dig in to the client.
- Avoid bony points.
- Apply slight traction. When you have a firm hold on either end of the joint, apply a slight, gentle pull, giving traction to the joint surfaces.

> **Learning point**
> Explain all movements should be pain free or conducted in a pain-free range.

- Move the joint smoothly, slowly and rhythmically to the end of the range, giving slight overpressure, then move back in the opposite direction.
- Complete the movements of one joint before moving smoothly on to the next.
- Move each joint through the fullest pain-free range possible without applying any force.
- Consider the speed, which must be moderately slow, even and rhythmical.

You should decide on the joints to be treated and the number of movements performed when the treatment begins and should be the same for each joint and for each side of the body. This will depend on the purpose of the treatment and the time constraints when these movements form only part of the whole treatment plan.

Repeat the movements between four and six times.

Passive movements to joints of the upper limb

This is done with the client lying supine. If passive movements are used for relaxation only, it is usual to limit hand movements to flexion and extension or to omit them altogether and begin at the wrist joint. They are included here for those who may require them for mobilisation treatments.

Hand

With the interphalangeal joints, i.e. joints of the fingers, the movements are flexion, extension of the fingers.

With the metacarpo-phalangeal joints, i.e. the knuckle joints, the movements are flexion and extension, abduction, adduction.

Procedure for finger joints(interphalangeal joints):

- Fix the client's finger by gripping with your fingers, leaving only the joint to be passively moved.
- With the opposite hand, use finger and thumb to grip above the isolated joint.
- Move the joint through full range flexion and extension.
- Repeat with each joint.

Procedure for the knuckle joints (metacarpophalangeal joints):

- Fix the client's hand with the palm facing upwards.
- Place both thumbs underneath the dorsal aspect of the base of the finger.
- With the hand fixed and the joint isolated, apply direct pressure with both thumbs to passively flex the metacarpophalangeal joint through its range.
- For extension, turn the hand over so the palm is facing downwards, fix the hand and isolate the joint. Grip above the joint to be mobilised and extend the joint.

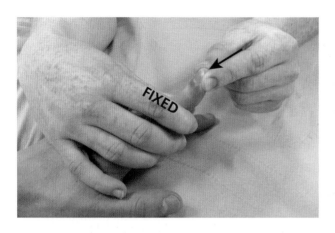

Figure 7.11 Passive extension of the second distal interphalangeal joint (N.B. for photographic purposes the right hand is placed slightly lower)

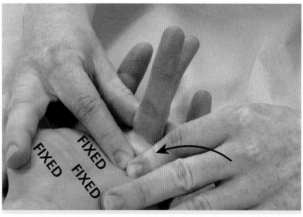

Figure 7.12 Passive flexion of the fourth metacarpophalangeal joint

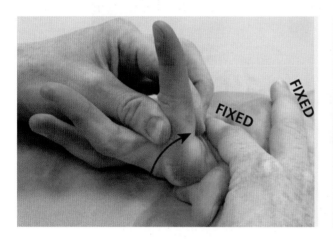

Figure 7.13 Passive flexion of the second metacarpophalangeal joint (knuckle joint)

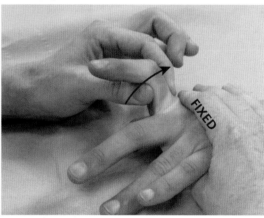

Figure 7.14 Passive extension of the second metacarpophalangeal joint (knuckle joint)

The thumb can be omitted unless there is a particular reason for mobilisation.

The two inter-phalangeal joints should be individually flexed and extended by holding below and above the joint.

The saddle joint at the base of the thumb (near the wrist) has the following movements: flexion, extension, abduction, adduction, circumduction and opposition.

Place your hand across the wrist to fix it and use the other hand to move the thumb: take care not to overstretch, as the saddle joint is susceptible to stiffness and pain.

Wrist joint

The movements are flexion, extension, abduction, adduction and circumduction.

Proceed as follows:

- Place one hand around the forearm about two inches proximal to the wrist.
- Rest the upper arm on the couch and flex the elbow to 90°.
- Fix in this position.
- Hold the client's hand firmly above the joint and move the wrist into flexion and extension. To further extend, you can also turn the arm over and apply a passive force (see Figure 7.16).
- Move into abduction and adduction.
- Move into circumduction.

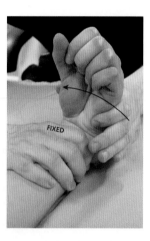

Figure 7.15 Passive flexion of the wrist joint

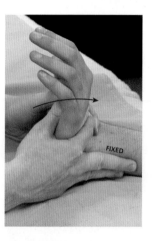

Figure 7.16 Passive extension of the wrist joint

Radio-ulnar joints (superior and inferior)

The movements are **supination** and **pronation.**

Proceed as follows:

- With the client's arm extended, hold firmly with one hand just above the elbow to fix it.
- With your other hand, hold the client's hand, as for a handshake.
- Keep the wrist in mid-position and turn the forearm into pronation and supination.

Elbow joint

The movements are flexion and extension.

Proceed as follows:

- Cup the client's arm above the elbow to isolate the joint.
- Hold the client's wrist with your other hand preventing movement at this joint.

- Flex the elbow until the flexor surfaces make contact preventing further movement.
- Extend the elbow taking care not to hyperextend, i.e. extending beyond the normal limit.
- Use the hand that is cupped around the elbow to feel or sense the end of range and to give support at this point.

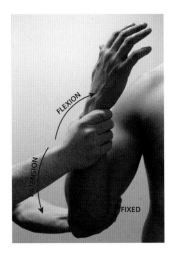

Figure 7.17 Passive flexion and extension of the elbow joint

Shoulder joint

The movements are flexion, extension, abduction, adduction, medial rotation, lateral rotation and circumduction.

This is a complex ball and socket joint with many planes of movement. The arm can be taken through flexion into elevation, i.e. taken above the head. It may also be taken from abduction across the body into horizontal flexion. When including passive movements for relaxation purposes it is easier to maintain rhythm and continuity by limiting shoulder movements to abduction, adduction, flexion/elevation and extension. However, for mobilisation all movements must be included.

Procedure for abduction and adduction:

- Hold the arm behind the elbow, place the other hand over the scapula to stabilise it, using the thumb and fingers.
- Keep the arm level with the body and move it away from the body into abduction.
- Return it to the side of the body into adduction.

Procedure for flexion of the shoulder joint:

- Hold the client's arm just above the elbow, placing the other hand over the scapula to stabilise it.
- Rotate the arm laterally and lift it upwards above the client's head.
- Bring it down and behind into extension. You will need to have your client standing to perform these movements effectively.

Best practice

For elevation through flexion and extension of the shoulder, it is not desirable to move the client if these movements are part of a treatment when limited extension is acceptable. However, if the purpose is mobilisation the client should be moved.

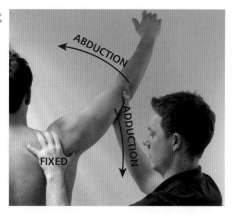

Figure 7.18 Passive abduction and adduction of the shoulder joint

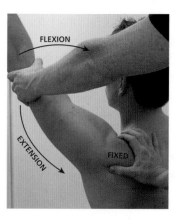

Figure 7.19 Passive flexion of the shoulder joint (glenohumeral joint)

Procedure for horizontal flexion and extension:

- Hold the client's arm just above the elbow and fix the scapula with the other hand.
- Abduct the arm to 90°.
- Take it across the body (at chest level) into flexion.
- Bring it back as far as possible into extension (in the abducted position).

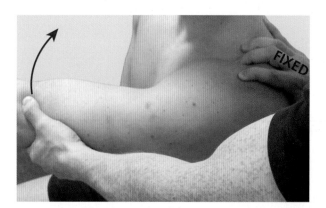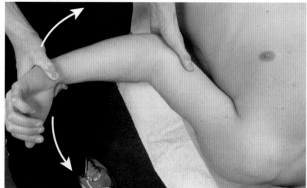

Figure 7.20 Passive horizontal flexion of the shoulder joint (glenohumeral joint)

Procedure for medial and lateral rotation of the shoulder joint:

- Grasp the client's arm just above the elbow with one hand and hold the wrist with the other hand.
- The upper arm can rest on the couch.
- Rotate it outwards into lateral rotation.
- Rotate it inwards into medial rotation.

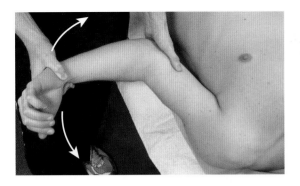

Figure 7.21 Passive medial and lateral rotation of the shoulder joint

Passive movements to the joints of the lower limb

This is done with the client lying supine. If passive movements are given for relaxation only, the toe joints can be omitted. These movements are, however, important if the objective is to mobilise the joints, because contractures and curling of the toes affect gait and can be disabling.

Toe joints

With the interphalangeal joints, the movements are flexion and extension.

With the metatarso-phalangeal joints, the movements are flexion, extension, abduction and adduction.

Proceed as follows:

- Hold the foot firmly at the head of the metatarsal joints with one hand.
- Place the other hand over the toes, then flex and extend them all together or one at a time.
- Abduction and adduction is then performed individually at the metatarso-phalangeal joints.

Ankle joint

The movements are **plantar flexion** (pointing the toes down) and **dorsi flexion** (pulling the foot up).

Proceed as follows:

Plantar flexion

- Place one hand behind the heel, cupping it in your palm, (or alternatively grasp the metatarsals with your thumbs and place fingers under the foot like pistols).
- Move the foot downwards into plantar flexion.

Dorsi flexion

- Fix the joint by grasping the distal aspects of the tibia and fibula.
- Move the foot into dorsi flexion with the assistance of your forearm if necessary.

Be aware

Pay particular care and attention to the big toe, as movement at this joint may be painful and restricted due to deformity and a bunion.

Be aware

For the ankle joint, ensure that you push beyond the 'soft end feel' of each movement, especially dorsi flexion, as it is important to maintain the stretch on the Achilles tendon that passes down the back of the leg to insert into the calcaneum. Greater stretch of this tendon can be produced by holding the heel in the palm of your hand with the foot lying along your forearm. The other hand holds above the ankle and the foot is pushed up by the forearm into dorsi flexion.

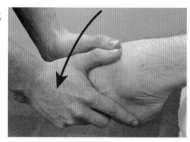

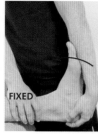

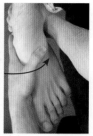

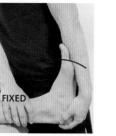

Figure 7.22 Passive plantar flexion of the ankle joint

Figure 7.23 Passive inversion and eversion of the ankle joint

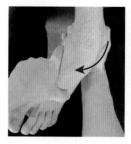

Learning point
Flexion and extension of the knee can also be performed with the client in the prone lying position with the foot over the edge of the bed. One hand is placed on the lower thigh while the other hand grasps above the ankle. The knee is then flexed and extended.

The mid-tarsal joints
The movements are **inversion** and **eversion**.

- Fix the ankle with one hand and hold the foot at the instep and turn it inwards and outwards. A combination of these inward and outward movements will produce circumduction, i.e. circling the foot.

The knee joint
The movements are **flexion** and **extension**.

Proceed as follows:

- Client seated on the couch or supine.
- Grasp above the knee joint (distal thigh) with one hand to stabilise the joint.
- With the other hand grasp the distal aspects of the tibia and fibula.
- Place knee through its range of flexion.
- Move the knee into extension, sliding the hand that grips the thigh to the popliteal fossa for support.

End range extension:

- Fix the femur onto the couch with one hand on the distal femur.
- Cup the heel of the foot with the other and gently move the knee to end range extension.

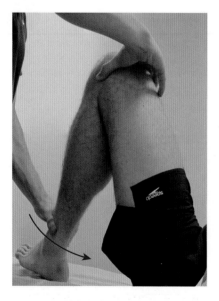

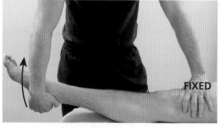

Figure 7.24 Passive flexion of the knee joint

Figure 7.25 Passive end range extension of the knee joint

The hip joint

The movements are flexion, extension, abduction, adduction, medial and lateral rotation and circumduction.

Procedure for flexion and extension:

Hip flexion

Client lies supine:

- Grasp the client's proximal tibia and passively move the knee joint towards the client's shoulder (note, knee flexion will occur simultaneously to hip extension).

Hip extension

Client lies prone:

- Stand to the side of the hip to be extended and place overpressure to the opposing buttock and base of the lumbar spine to isolate the joint.
- Flex the client's knee to 90° and grasp underneath the anterior thigh (supporting the lower leg with your forearm).
- Take the weight of the leg before moving the hip through its range of extension.

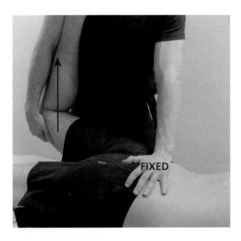

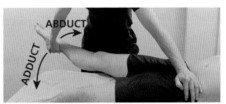

Figure 7.27 Passive abduction and adduction of the hip joint

Figure 7.26 Passive extension of the hip joint

Procedure for abduction and adduction:

- Place the leg not being worked on into abduction.
- Support the moving leg by cupping under the ankle with one hand, while the other hand is placed over the opposing pelvis to help isolate the moving joint.
- Keep the leg in line with the body and take it out sideways into abduction and back across mid-line into adduction.

Procedure for medial (internal) and lateral (external) rotation:

- With the legs slightly apart but supported on the couch throughout, place one hand on the thigh and the other on the lower leg.
- Grasp the leg gently and turn it inwards and outwards.

Be aware

For continuity, it is suggested that hip joint flexion is carried out with knee joint flexion: this is then followed by abduction, adduction, medial and lateral rotation, with the client in the supine position. Then ask the client to turn over into the prone position. From here you can carry out extension of the hip.

Short-answer questions

1. Name two changes in muscle tissue that indicate increased tension.

2. List four causes of musculo-skeletal problems.

3. State why massage should not be used in the acute stage of injury.

4. Give two non-verbal responses that will indicate to you that the client is in pain.

5. Briefly explain the physiological changes that occur as a result of prolonged increase in muscle tension.

6. Give two ways in which you would differentiate between fibrous nodules and fatty nodules.

7. Complete the following sentences:

    (a) Superficial pressure is used to palpate .... tissues.

    (b) .... pressure is used to palpate deeper tissues.

8. Give two signs that will indicate the presence of a trigger point.

9. Briefly explain why knowledge of muscle shape and fibre direction is important while performing neuromuscular stroking techniques.

10. List the four techniques that may be used for myofascial release.

11. Define the term 'passive movement'.

12. List any six questions that you would ask the client during consultation to ensure that there are no joint problems, before performing passive movement.

13. List six contra-indications to passive movement.

14. Explain briefly why thrombosis or phlebitis are contra-indications to passive movement.

15. List six effects of passive movement.

16. State why it is important to know the anatomy and direction of movement of each joint.

17. Complete the following:

    Each joint should be moved through .... without applying force.

18. Name the movements possible at the elbow joint.

19. Name one other joint that has the same movements as the elbow joint.

20. Give two examples of a ball and socket joint.

Mechanical massage and infra-red treatments

8

After you have studied this chapter you will be able to:

1. explain the different types of equipment, the physiological effects, benefits and contra-indications
2. select the appropriate equipment to suit the needs of the client
3. treat the client, paying due consideration to maximum efficiency, comfort, safety and hygiene.

Mechanical massage

Mechanical massage is the manipulation of body tissues using machines. Generally, mechanical massage is used in conjunction with other treatments to relieve muscle tension and muscle pain, to improve the circulation and to improve certain skin conditions. Also, provided the client is on a reducing diet, the heavier vibrations of the gyratory vibrator and hand-held vibrator may help to disperse fatty deposits from specific areas of the body.

Many different types of appliance are manufactured to produce effects similar to those of a manual massage. They vary from the small, hand-held, audio-sonic equipment designed to treat small, localised areas, to the large, heavy, gyratory vibrators used for deeper effects on large areas of the body. Although the effects are similar to those of manual massage, the sensation felt by the client is very different. The treatment is rather impersonal and the use of a machine rather than the touch of hands less intimate, so it can be useful in treating male clients.

In practice, most mechanical vibratory treatments should be combined with some manual massage, thus gaining the more personal aspects of manual massage as well as the depth and power of vibratory equipment. Using mechanical massage equipment is certainly less tiring for the therapist than performing a long, vigorous manual massage. The effects produced are similar with all types of massage equipment, but are deeper and greater with the heavier machines. The treatment is very popular with clients, as they feel invigorated and consider that the desired results will be achieved.

Gyratory vibrator

Massage with this type of appliance is much heavier than with an audio-sonic machine. It is therefore more suitable for heavier work on large and bulky areas of the body.

There are two main types of appliance: the hand-held vibrator and the floor-standing vibrator.

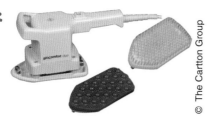

Figure 8.1 Hand-held vibrator and applicators

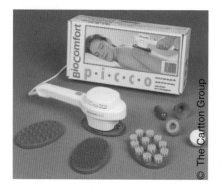

Figure 8.2 Portable machine and heads

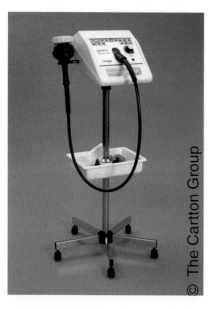

Figure 8.3
Floor-standing gyratory vibrator

Be aware !

If the applicators are made of silicone you can use oil. However, do not use oil with the rubber or sponge applicators as it may cause them to deteriorate.

The hand-held vibrator

The hand-held vibrator is versatile and has a variety of attachments. It produces simultaneous horizontal and vertical vibrations. As this machine is portable it is useful for the mobile therapist.

The floor-standing vibrator

The floor-standing vibrator is a very popular treatment. All the electrical components are housed in the main body of the machine, which is supported by a stand, and only the moving head is held in the hand. This machine uses a rotary electric motor to turn a crank, which is attached to the head. The head is driven to turn in gyratory motion, moving round and round, up and down and side to side with pressure, providing a deep massage. A variety of attachments are available, which screw onto the head. These are stored in and easily accessed from the tray on the stand.

As with manual massage, a massage medium is first applied to the skin.

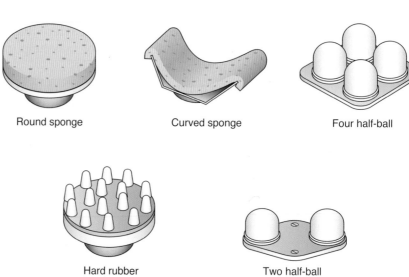

Round sponge   Curved sponge   Four half-ball

Hard rubber multiple prong

Two half-ball

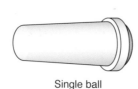

Single ball

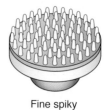

Fine spiky

Figure 8.4 Different applicators for the gyratory vibrator

When these machines were first developed, they were designed to simulate manual massage movements. The different applicators are employed to attempt to replicate the effects of these movements. Because the massage is delivered by machine, greater depth and intensity is possible. For example:

- Effleurage can be simulated by the curved and round sponges.
- Petrissage can be simulated by the multiple-prong, four-ball, two-ball and blunt-tip applicators.

New developments and technologies are constantly coming onto the market, with new applicators and methods of operation, replicating a growing range of massage effects. The net result of this is that gyratory vibrator treatment has become a treatment in its own right, and while this book gives an overview of technique, it is vital that you keep abreast of developments and always refer to your manufacturer's manual.

Gyratory vibrator treatment technique

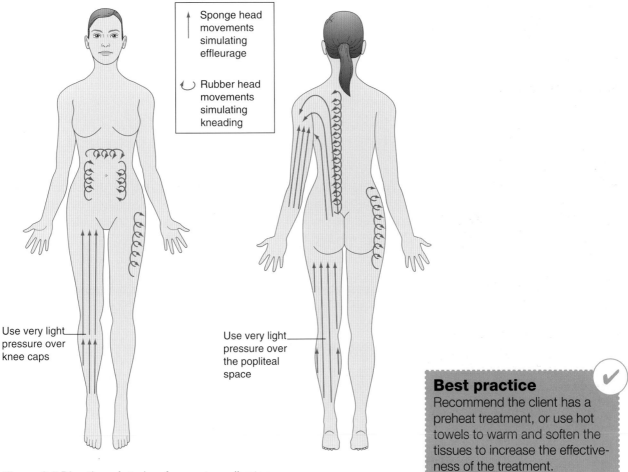

Figure 8.5 Direction of strokes for gyratory vibrator

Best practice
Recommend the client has a preheat treatment, or use hot towels to warm and soften the tissues to increase the effectiveness of the treatment.

Body Massage

Check for contra-indications.

↓

Check that all jewellery has been removed.

↓

Place the client in a well-supported, comfortable position.

↓

Explain the treatment to the client.

↓

Clean the skin with a suitable product.

↓

Select the appropriate applicators to suit the needs of the client for this treatment.

↓

Apply an appropriate medium to the area, using manual effleurage strokes.

↓

Use the curved sponge on limbs and the round sponge on other areas, to introduce the gyratory vibrator and to continue to warm the tissues.

↓

Apply in long, sweeping strokes following the direction of venous return and natural contours of the body. The stroke should be smooth and of a pressure suited to the tissues being worked on.

↓

At the end of the stroke break contact or return with superficial strokes.

↓

Reapply medium if necessary, using manual massage.

↓

Change the applicator to one that simulates petrissage movements. Use a circular kneading motion, using the other hand to support the tissues and lift them towards the applicator. Again, apply upward pressure and work with venous return. Intersperse use of the applicators with manual massage movements.

↓

Use the curved or round sponge head to complete the treatment.

↓

Wash the applicators according to manufacturer's instructions.

Be aware

If using talcum powder, apply sparingly and with care. Airborne particles can cause respiratory problems.

Learning point

The short prong (spiky) applicator is ideal for a desquamating effect and for increasing the circulation, producing erythema.

Be aware

The degree of erythema and client tolerance dictates the length of the treatment.

In the workplace

The client expects maximum treatment time, so avoid changing the applicators too often as this breaks the continuity of the treatment. For example, prepare both legs and use chosen applicator on both legs before changing it.

Best practice

To maintain high standards of hygiene, the applicators can be placed in a disposable cover, which should be changed for each client.

Be aware

When you switch on the machine, hold the head below the level of the couch. This is a safety precaution: if the applicator is insecure and flies off it will not hit the client.

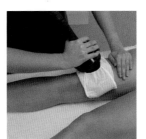
Figure 8.6 Effleurage on the upper leg

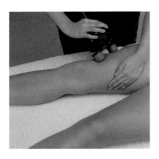
Figure 8.7 Kneading on the upper leg

> **Be aware** !
>
> Keep the surface of the attachment parallel to the surface of the body at all times. If one side lifts off the body, there is a danger of damaging the tissues with the hard edge of the applicator.

When massaging the abdomen, particular care should be taken when selecting applicators. Abdominal organs have no bony framework for protection – their only protection is provided by the muscles and tissues of the abdominal wall. Overstretched muscles with poor tone offer less protection.

Physiological effects and the resulting benefits

- As with manual massage, the main effect is stimulation of the circulation. The movements speed up the flow of blood in the veins, removing deoxygenated blood and waste products more rapidly. This affects the arterial circulation, bringing oxygenated blood and nutrients to the area. Lymph drainage via the lymphatic vessels is also increased. This helps to remove stagnation of fluid in areas of cellulite.
- Increased blood supply will increase the metabolic rate in the tissues. This will improve the condition of the tissues and aid poor circulation.
- Increased blood supply and friction of the applicators will raise the temperature of the area and therefore aid muscle relaxation.
- Rapid removal of waste products such as lactic acid will help relieve pain in muscles.
- Surface capillaries dilate giving an erythema. This improves skin tone.
- The desquamating effect of the applicators helps to improve the texture of the skin.
- The continuous heavy pressure on adipose tissue and increased circulation to the area may aid the dispersal of fatty deposits if the client is on a reducing diet.

Benefits of the gyratory vibrator

Benefits include:

- improving poor circulation
- relieving muscular tension
- reducing muscular aches and pains
- improving skin tone

- improving the texture of dry, flaky, rough skin
- spot reduction of fatty deposits (in conjunction with other treatments and reduced food intake).

Contra-indications

The contra-indications are:

- abrasions – risk of cross-infection and aggravating the condition
- acute back and spinal problems (e.g. disc trouble) – may aggravate the condition
- bruises – may be uncomfortable for the client and could worsen the condition
- extremely hairy areas – the applicators will pull on the hairs
- lymphangitis (a bacterial infection of the lymphatic vessels) – risk of cross-infection and also the disease can spread via the blood-stream with fatal consequences
- malignant lesions – risk of spreading the disease via the blood and lymphatic circulation
- menstruation – may cause heavier blood flow especially during the first three days, so avoid abdomen
- pacemaker – the mechanical vibrations may interfere with the rhythm of the pacemaker
- phlebitis – may aggravate the condition
- pregnancy – risk to foetus
- recent operations and scar tissue – danger of breaking down recently formed scar tissue
- skin diseases – risk of cross-infection
- skin tags, warts or pigmented moles – applicator may pull on them causing discomfort
- thin, crêpy skin or lack of subcutaneous fat – may be uncomfortable
- thrombosis – the increase in circulation could cause the blood clot to be transported in the blood stream to the lungs and heart with fatal consequences
- varicose veins – may worsen the condition, especially if the pressure is too heavy.

Be aware

Heavy and prolonged treatments can cause bruising and dilated capillaries.

Audio-sonic vibrator

The audio-sonic vibrator is a hand-held appliance. Its name is derived from the fact that the machine produces sound waves (which can be heard as a humming sound). This vibrator generates sound waves using an electromagnet. When the current is passing one way, the coil moves forward; as the current reverses, the coil moves back. The speed of the movement is measured in Hertz and is referred to as frequency (the number of oscillations per second).

Sound waves can be divided into three groups:

- Infrasonic waves have a frequency of less than 16Hz (too low to be heard).
- Intrasonic waves have a frequency between 16Hz and 20,000Hz. This is the frequency band which the human ear can hear.
- Ultrasonic waves have a frequency above 20,000Hz (too high to be heard).

Audio-sonic vibrators use part of the **intrasonic** frequency band. When the applicator is placed on the area, the sound waves penetrate the tissues causing the oscillation of molecules making up the cells. Different molecules oscillate at different inherent frequencies; when they are made to oscillate at a frequency close to their own inherent frequency they resonate more strongly, producing a beneficial effect.

Because the applicator does not physically move forward and backward, this appliance has a gentle action. It penetrates more deeply into the tissues, but is less stimulating on the surface of the skin.

There are two applicators:

- flat-disc applicator
- ball-type sound applicator.

In both cases, refer to the manufacturer's instructions for use.

Treatment technique

Check for contra-indications.

↓

Check that all jewellery has been removed.

↓

Place the client in a well-supported, comfortable position.

↓

Explain the treatment to the client.

↓

Clean the skin with a suitable product.

↓

Select the appropriate applicator to suit the needs of the client for this treatment.

↓

Apply an appropriate medium to the area according to manufacturer's instructions.

↓

Be aware

Audio sonic should not be confused with ultrasound therapy, which is quite different and has various medical uses.

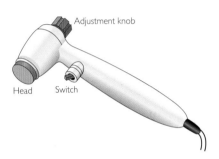

Figure 8.8 Audio sonic machine

Be aware

Avoid the delicate area around the eyes, as the skin is thin. Also avoid prominent cheek bones as the sound waves will be too intense.

Be aware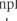

Use minimum intensity on the head, face and neck.

Learning point

Do not use directly over bony areas. Cover the area with your hand to absorb some of the sound wave.

Commence the treatment using straight lines or a circular motion, ensuring coverage of all the area. Keep the applicator moving and parallel to the surface for maximum benefit.

↓

The skin reaction indicates the length of the treatment time. When an even erythema is produced, the treatment should stop. It may take 5–15 minutes to achieve this effect.

↓

Remove the medium and complete the treatment.

↓

Clean the applicators according to manufacturer's instructions.

Physiological effects and the resulting benefits

The treatment produces an increase in circulation to the treated area, bringing nutrients and oxygen and removing waste products. This is especially beneficial around aching and painful joints as it will help the healing process.

The increase in circulation and the friction of the applicators raise the temperature of the area. This promotes relaxation of muscle fibres and relieves pain. It is particularly effective over localised tension nodules.

It produces vasodilation, giving hyperaemia and erythema, improving tone of the skin.

The friction of the applicators aids desquamation: this removes the surface layer of cells, improving the texture of the skin.

It increases the metabolic rate, thus improving the condition of the tissues.

Benefits

Benefits include:

- helping to disperse aches and pain around joints
- helping to relieve cramp, pain and muscle spasms
- relieving tension nodules
- improving tone and texture of the skin.

Learning point

Because the sound waves penetrate all body tissues at a cellular level (lymph, cartilage, muscle and especially bone all conduct the sound waves), the benefits are at a particularly deep level, which is hard to achieve through manual massage alone.

Contra-indications

The contra-indications are:

- metal or plastic plates – could cause discomfort or damage the implant
- pacemaker – the frequency of the sound waves can interfere with the function of the pacemaker

- pregnancy – risk to foetus
- skin diseases – risk of cross-infection
- thrombosis – the increase in circulation could cause the blood clot to be transported in the blood stream to the lungs and heart, with fatal consequences.

Wavelength A to B

Figure 8.9 Wavelength

The electromagnetic spectrum

The electromagnetic spectrum is made up of bands of radiation with differing wavelengths and frequencies, each of which will have different physiological effects on body tissues. It is thought that all electromagnetic rays are similar in form, being particles in motion. They are transverse waves, which travel through space without the need of a conductor. The speed or velocity, at which they travel is the same for all bands, being 300,000 km/sec (the speed of sound).

The bands of the electromagnetic spectrum have different wavelengths. The **wavelength** is the distance between a point on one wave and the same point on the next wave.

The distance from **A** to **B** is the wavelength.

Wavelengths are measured in **nanometres**. One nanometre is a very small unit of measurement, being one millionth of a millimetre. It is written as nm. The following table gives the wavelength of each band emitted from the spectrum.

Cosmic	Up to 0.002 nm
Gamma	0.002 nm to 0.14 nm
X-rays	0.14 nm to 13.4 nm
Ultraviolet	10 nm to 400 nm
Visible	400 nm to 770 nm
Infra-red	770 nm to 400,000 nm
Radio	100,000 nm upwards

Table 8.1 Wavelength of each band emitted from the spectrum

The shortest wavelength rays are **cosmic** rays and the longest are **radio** waves. There is overlap between some of the bands.

The bands of the spectrum also have different frequencies. **Frequency** is the number of complete waves that pass a point in one second. Many more waves of short wavelength will pass the point in one second than those of long wavelength. The rays of shorter wavelength will have a higher frequency than the rays of longer wavelength. In other words, as the *wavelength increases*, the *frequency decreases*.

Units of frequency

Frequency is measured in **Hertz** (**Hz**). The number of waves past a point in one second is the number of Hertz, for example

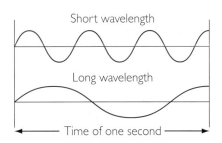

Figure 8.10 Rays of different wavelengths will have different frequencies

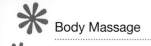
50 waves passing a point per second = 50 Hz. For higher frequencies the units become

> 1 kilohertz (kHz) = 1000Hz
>
> 1 megahertz (mHz) = 1000 kHz (= 1,000,000 Hz)

Properties and laws of radiation

In order to give the most effective and safe treatment, you should be aware of certain laws and principles, which govern the behaviour of rays/waves. Both infra-red (IR), visible light and ultraviolet (UV) rays will travel in straight lines until they meet a new medium, where they may be **refracted**, **reflected** or **absorbed**.

Refraction

This is the bending of rays when they meet a new medium. A good example is looking at a stick held in water – it appears to bend. Refraction occurs when rays pass from one medium to another, for example from air through glass or water.

Reflection

This is the reflection of rays when they meet a surface. Shiny or white surfaces reflect more rays than dark surfaces, which absorb rays; a greater proportion of light rays will be reflected by snow than by soil. A mirror is designed to reflect rays.

The law of reflection states the *angle of incidence* is *equal* to the *angle of reflection*. To measure these angles, an imaginary line is drawn perpendicular to the surface struck by the rays: this is the *normal*.

- The angle of incidence lies between the ray of incidence and the normal.
- The angle of reflection lies between the ray of reflection and the normal. In Figure 8.11, X is the angle of incidence. Y is the angle of reflection. These are always equal.

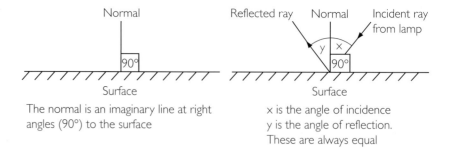

Figure 8.11 Reflection

The angle of incidence is *one* of the factors governing the proportion of rays absorbed by the medium that the rays strike. This is an important consideration when giving IR and UV treatments, as the effectiveness of the treatments will depend on the number of rays absorbed.

Absorption

The law of Grotthus states that: *'rays must be absorbed to produce an effect'*. The amount of absorption and consequently the effect depends on the following:

the wavelength and frequency of the rays (infra-red is absorbed by body tissues to a depth of 3mm approximately)

the type of medium (in this case, body tissues)

the angle at which the rays strike the part also affects absorption. The cosine law governs the way intensity, hence absorption, is affected by the angle of incidence.

Cosine law

The cosine law states that the intensity of radiation at a surface varies with the cosine of the angle of incidence (i.e. the angle between the incident ray and the normal).

If the incident rays strike the part at 90°, there will be no angle between the incident ray and the normal (it is 0°). Here, there is maximum intensity and absorption.

For example, when the sun is at its highest at noon, it is shining directly onto the earth at 90°, so it is at its most intense. At 4pm the sun is lower in the sky, therefore the angle of incidence of the sun's rays is increased and the incident ray is reflected, rather than all the rays being absorbed. This means that the sun is less intense and so a person sunbathing would be much less likely to burn at 4pm than at noon if sunbathing for the same length of time.

In order to ensure the most effective treatment, the rays of the lamp must strike the part at 90°; this will ensure maximum intensity, absorption and effect.

> **Learning point**
>
> The law of inverse squares states that the intensity from a point source varies inversely with the square of the distance from the point source. The further away the lamp is from the part, the less intense the rays are at the part.

> **Be aware** !
>
> Because the lamp's rays are more intense when it is closer, the time the client can spend under the lamp is less, so if the intensity is quadrupled, the time must be halved. If the intensity is quartered, the time spent under the lamp can be doubled, but check manufacturer's instructions for guidance.

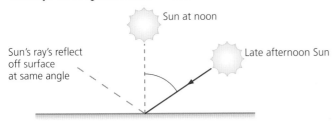

Figure 8.12 Cosine law

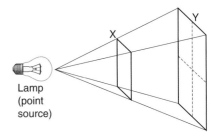

Figure 8.13 Radiation from a point source illustrating the law of inverse squares. The distance from the lamp to y is twice the distance from the lamp to x. The area covered by the light rays is four times greater at y than at x, therefore the intensity of the rays is four times less at y than at x.

Law of inverse squares

The intensity of rays from an infra-red lamp is also impacted by the distance the lamp is placed from the part being treated. The *law of inverse squares* governs this. In simple terms, this means that if the distance of the lamp from the part is doubled (i.e. twice as far away), then the intensity is quartered. If the distance is halved (i.e. the lamp is nearer), the intensity is quadrupled.

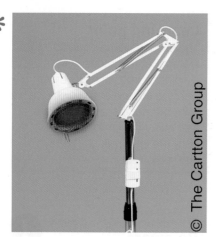

Figure 8.14 An infra-red lamp

© The Cartton Group

Treatment lamps

Infra-red lamp

Infra-red rays are electromagnetic waves with wavelengths between 700 nm and 400,000 nm. They are given off by the sun and by any hot object, for example electric fires, gas and coal fires, hot packs and various types of lamps.

The lamps that produce infra-red rays can be divided into two main types:

- The non-luminous type called infra-red lamps
- The luminous type are called radiant heat lamps.

Both these types of lamp emit infra-red rays. The difference lies in their wave-length. The non-luminous type emits rays of longer wavelength, while the luminous type emits rays of shorter wave and include waves from the visible spectrum and ultraviolet rays. The differing wavelengths produce slightly different effects when absorbed by body tissues.

The non-luminous lamps – infra-red lamps

Many types of non-luminous lamps are produced but they all have a *non-glowing* source that emits infra-red rays. A common type uses a coil of wire embedded in fireclay, which is placed in the centre of a reflector. When the lamp is switched on, the wire gets hot and heats the fireclay; the rays are then emitted from the hot fireclay, they pass through the air and are absorbed by a body placed in their path.

The rays from non-luminous lamps are:

- of longer wavelength
- invisible
- less irritating
- less penetrating (approximately 1mm of the epidermis) than the shorter rays from luminous lamps.

The luminous lamps – radiant heat lamps

These lamps give off infra-red rays from *glowing* or incandescent sources, such as hot wires or powerful bulbs. These are also placed in the centre of a reflector. When the lamp is switched on, the wire glows, giving off infra-red and small amounts of ultraviolet rays. Some bulbs have filters to cut out some visible rays and ultraviolet rays; these bulbs are usually red in colour.

The rays produced by these lamps:

- have a shorter wavelength
- include some visible rays
- are more penetrating (approximately 3mm down to the dermis/subcutaneous layer)
- are more irritating than the rays from non-luminous lamps.

Non-luminous (infra-red)	Luminous (radiant heat)
Rays emitted from a heated wire embedded in fireclay	Rays emitted from glowing wires and bulbs
Long wavelength	Shorter wavelength
Includes no visible rays	Includes some visible rays and a small amount of UVL
Penetrates approximately 1mm of skin to the epidermis	Penetrates approximately 3mm of tissue to the dermis/subcutaneous layer
Less irritating	More irritating
May feel hotter at equal power and distance	Will feel less hot at equal power and distance
Takes 10–15 minutes to heat up	Heats up quickly, approximately 2 minutes

Table 8.2 Comparisons of infra-red and radiant heat lamps

Intensity of radiation

The intensity of radiation will depend on three factors:

- The *intensity* of the lamp
- The *distance* between the lamp and the skin
- The *angle* at which the rays strike the part.

The intensity of the lamp

This can be controlled manually by the dials. Check manufacturer's instructions for recommended levels and timing of treatment.

The distance between the lamp and the skin

The *law of inverse squares* governs intensity in relation to distance.

The lamp should generally be placed between 45 and 90 cm from the part, but check manufacturer's instructions.

The angle at which the rays strike the part

When giving an infra-red treatment the lamp should be positioned so that the rays strike the part at 90°. This will ensure maximum intensity, absorption and effect (cosine law). By ensuring that the surface of the lamp is parallel to the part being treated, this will mean that the rays will strike at 90°.

If you are giving infra-red treatment to the back, for example, it is important to consider exactly where you place and point the lamp. Putting the lamp at 90° does not mean that you place it over the client's prone body; if you do this there is a risk of the lamp falling on the part and burning it. If you simply point the lamp in the general direction of the part from the side of the body, the rays are not going to hit the part at 90°. *You must*, therefore, ensure that you place the client either in the *recovery position*, or *side-lying*, supported by pillows so that a lamp placed at the side of the body can be directed at 90° onto the part being treated.

In the workplace

The majority of lamps used in salons are the radiant heat type, as opposed to infra-red lamps. This is because they heat up more quickly and it is easy to tell by looking whether or not they are on, which aids safety.

Remember

If you double the distance that the lamp is placed from the part, the intensity is quartered; if you reduce the distance by half, the intensity will increase four times (quadruple).

Be aware

It is important to explain to the client that they must remain in this position for the duration of the treatment, so make sure that they are comfortable before commencing treatment.

Be aware **!**

Check the reflector for dents as these could cause hot spots and burn the client.

Remember

Infra-red lamps take 10–15 minutes to reach maximum output. Radiant heat lamps take around 2 minutes.

Be aware **!**

Always ensure that the angle-poise joints are tight so that there is no risk of the lamp collapsing onto the client.

Remember

When treating areas of the back, use side lying or the recovery position, well supported by pillows. For any body part, ensure that the rays from a lamp placed at the side of the couch, will strike the part at 90°, and use appropriate support.

Learning point

Carry out a sensitivity test using two test tubes, one filled with hot water and the other filled with cold water. Instruct the client to close their eyes. Carry out the test all over the area to be irradiated. Touch the client with either the hot test tube or the cold test tube at random over the area. Ask the client if they feel hot or cold. If the client cannot tell the difference between the hot and the cold, they have defective sensation, and the treatment should not be carried out.

If you are giving infra-red treatment to the face, again, it is unsafe to place the lamp over the supine client because of risk of the lamp falling and burning the client. Instead, position the client half lying with their head turned towards the lamp, which is placed at the side of the client, so that rays hit the face at 90°. It is vital that the eyes are protected by damp cotton wool secured.

Infra-red treatment technique

Switch it on to warm up according to manufacturer's instructions, making sure the lamp is away from all surfaces and directed at the floor for safety.

↓

Check for contra-indications.

↓

Check that all jewellery has been removed.

↓

Place the client in a well-supported comfortable position.

↓

Explain the treatment to the client.

↓

Clean the skin with a suitable product.

↓

Cover the areas not receiving treatment.

↓

Position the lamp ensuring stability.

↓

Make sure that the face of the lamp is parallel with the part so that the rays strike the part at 90° for maximum penetration, absorption and effect. Do *not* place the lamp directly above the client.

↓

Select an appropriate distance, between 45 and 90 cm. The selected distance depends on two factors:
- the intensity of the lamp
- the client's tolerance: 60 cm is a good average, but check manufacturer's instructions.

↓

Observe the client throughout the treatment.

↓

Treatment time is 15–20 minutes (check manufacturer's instructions), until the desired effect is obtained.

The treatment may be followed by massage.

Physiological effects

Heating of body tissues

When infra-red rays are absorbed by the tissues, heat is produced in the area. The rays from luminous generators penetrate more deeply than those from non-luminous lamps. Penetration is approximately 3mm of tissue, therefore superficial and deeper tissues are heated directly.

With non-luminous lamps (which have infra-red rays only) the top 1mm of skin is heated directly, but the deeper tissues are heated by conduction.

Increased metabolic rate

Van't Hoff's law states that a chemical reaction capable of being accelerated will be accelerated by heat.

Metabolism is a chemical change that will be accelerated by heat. The increase in metabolic rate will be greatest where the heating is greatest, i.e. in the superficial tissues, therefore more oxygen and nutrients are required and more waste products and metabolites are produced.

Vasodilation with increase in circulation

Heat has a direct effect on the blood vessels, producing vasodilation and an increase in blood flow in an attempt to cool the area. Vasodilation is also produced by stimulation of sensory nerve endings, which causes reflex dilation of arterioles.

Fall in blood pressure

If the superficial blood vessels dilate, the peripheral resistance is reduced and this will result in a fall in blood pressure. (When blood flows through vessels with small lumen, it exerts a certain pressure on the walls. If the lumen is increased by the vessels dilating, the pressure on the walls will be reduced.)

Increase in heart rate

The increased metabolism and circulation mean that the heart must beat faster to meet the demand: therefore the heart rate increases.

General rise in body temperature

When one area of the body is heated for a prolonged time, there is a general rise in body temperature by **conduction** and **convection**. The heat will spread through surrounding tissues and will be carried by the blood circulating through the area.

Increased activity of sweat glands

As the body temperature rises, the heat-regulating centres in the brain are affected and the sweat glands are then stimulated to produce more sweat in order to lose body heat. This increases the elimination of waste products.

Be aware

Warn the client that warmth should be comfortable and to alert you if the heat becomes too intense. The client should also be instructed not to touch the lamp or move closer to it.

Be aware

If the lamp has three feet, place the head of the lamp over one of the feet, ensuring that the angle joints are secure.

Be aware

The head of the lamp will be hot. Use a towel to protect your hands when moving or adjusting the position of the lamp.

Be aware

Do not use infra-red before using tanning equipment as the reaction to UVL will be intensified. Infra-red may, however, be used after over-exposure to UVL to reduce the reaction.

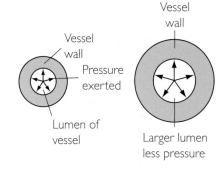

Figure 8.15 Pressure on vessel walls

Be aware

The client should not rise suddenly after infra-red treatment, as the blood pressure is lowered and the client may feel faint.

Effects on muscle tissue

Muscle tissue is affected in two ways:

- The rise in temperature produces muscle relaxation and relieves tension and pain.
- The increase in circulation provides the nutrients and oxygen necessary for muscle contraction, and the removal of waste is speeded up.

When muscles are warm, they contract more efficiently than when cold.

Effects on sensory nerves

Mild heat has a soothing effect on sensory nerve endings. However, intense heat has an irritating effect.

Benefits of infra-red treatment

The treatment can be used in the following ways to produce a variety of benefits:

- as a general heating treatment to promote relaxation
- as a localised treatment for relief of pain and tension in muscles and joints
- as a preheating treatment, either generally or locally, to increase the circulation and thus make subsequent treatments more effective.

Contra-indications

Contra-indications include:

- any area where liniments or ointments have been applied. They may contain products which heat more rapidly (such as oil or alcohol), and so cause skin to burn
- areas of defective skin sensation and hypersensitive skin – the skin could burn
- areas of deficient circulation – could cause overheating or burning of the area
- diabetes – skin sensitivity may be impaired
- extensive bruising – may slow down the healing process
- heart conditions and blood pressure disorders (high or low) – may have an adverse effect
- heavy colds and fevers – may aggravate the condition
- menstruation – avoid the first two to three days as it may increase the blood flow
- migraines and headaches – may aggravate the condition further
- phlebitis – may aggravate the condition
- pregnancy (avoid the last four months) – risk to the foetus
- recent scar tissue – defective sensitivity

- recent soft tissue injury – this requires treatment with ice applications to constrict the capillaries and reduce tissue swelling
- skin diseases – risk of cross-infection
- thrombosis – the increase in circulation could cause the blood clot to be transported in the blood stream to the lungs and heart, with fatal consequences.

Dangers

Burns may be caused if the:

- heat is too intense
- client is too near the lamp and fails to report overheating
- skin sensation is defective and the client may not be aware of overheating
- client touches the lamp
- lamp should fall and touch the client, or the bedding. Overheating of pillows and blankets can cause fire and burns.

Other dangers include:

- electric shock from faulty apparatus or from water near the treatment area, which may produce a short circuit
- headache due to irradiating the back of the neck and head or overheating by prolonged exposure
- faintness due to overheating or extensive irradiation, which may cause a fall in blood pressure, making the client feel faint
- damage to the eyes: infra-red exposure of the eyes can cause cataracts. The client should close their eyes and turn away from the lamp, wear goggles or have cotton wool over their eyes
- catching a chill from going out into the cold too quickly after exposure. Clients should dress appropriately.

Questions

GYRATORY VIBRATOR

1. Which of the following gyratory vibrator applicators is suitable for tension nodules on the upper fibres of the trapezius?

   a. Four ball.

   b. Multiple prong.

   c. Sponge.

   d. Blunt tip.

2. Why is it important to keep the applicator parallel to the surface?

   a. To avoid damaging the tissues.

   b. For maximum absorption.

   c. For deeper penetration.

   d. To avoid over-stretching muscles.

3. The short prong (spiky) applicator is used to help:

   a. spread the medium

   b. desquamate

   c. soften adipose tissue

   d. vasoconstriction.

4. Removal of lactic acid will improve:

   a. the condition of muscles

   b. oedema

   c. poor circulation

   d. osteoporosis.

5. Lymphangitis is:

  a. a malignant lesion

  b. a bacterial infection of the lymph vessels

  c. an inflammation of the veins

  d. a clot in the lymphatic vessels.

6. How should you clean the applicators?

  a. With surgical spirit.

  b. Wash in warm soapy water.

  c. According to manufacturer's instructions.

  d. Wipe with diluted disinfectant.

AUDIO-SONIC

7. What type of medium should you use?

  a. Oil.

  b. According to client preference.

  c. Talc.

  d. According to manufacturer's instructions.

8. Audio-sonic is suitable for:

  a. oedema due to acute injury

  b. dislodging blood clots

  c. aching joints

  d. softening adipose tissue.

9. Hertz refers to:

  a. the number of beats per second

  b. the number of oscillations per second

  c. wavelength

  d. depth of penetration.

10. Which of the following frequency bands does the audio-sonic use?

  a. Ultrasonic.

  b. Infrasonic and intrasonic.

  c. Intrasonic.

  d. Infrasonic.

INFRA-RED

11. Which of the following has the longer wavelength?

  a. Visible light.

  b. Radio waves.

  c. Infra-red rays.

  d. Ultraviolet rays.

12. The rays with the higher frequency are:

  a. visible light

  b. radio waves

  c. infra-red rays

  d. ultraviolet rays.

13. Which of the following surfaces will reflect rays the most?

  a. Water.

  b. Soil.

  c. Snow.

  d. Dark colours.

14. The cosine law dictates that for maximum benefit the angle infra-red rays strike the body should be at:

  a. 45°

  b. 50°

  c. 60°

  d. 90°

15. The law of inverse squares is concerned with the:

  a. distance of the lamp from the part being treated

  b. wavelength of infra-red rays

  c. type of infra-red lamp being used

  d. frequency of the wavelengths.

16. Which of the following statements is associated with radiant heat lamps?

  a. Less irritating, superficial penetration.

  b. Longer wavelength, contains visible light.

  c. Penetrates deeper, contains ultraviolet rays.

  d. Rays embedded in clay, more irritating.

17. When carrying out an infra-red treatment to the back place the client in:

  a. prone position

  b. recovery position

  c. supine position

  d. half-reclining position.

18. Carrying out a sensitivity test will confirm if the client has:

a. diabetes

b. an allergy to the medium

c. defective sensation

d. poor blood circulation.

19. An infra-red treatment can be used:

a. after an ultraviolet treatment to reduce the reaction

b. before an ultraviolet treatment to intensify the tanning process

c. to reduce the client's blood pressure

d. on recent scar tissue to promote the healing process.

20. A radiant heat treatment:

a. increases the amount of melanin produced in the skin

b. constricts the superficial blood vessels resulting in a rise in blood pressure

c. irritates the sensory nerve endings

d. soothes sensory nerve endings.

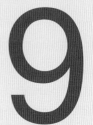

9 Reflection, evaluation and continuing professional development

After you have studied this chapter you will be able to:

1. use effective reflection practices to maximise your skills during training
2. recognise the importance of Continuing Professional Development (CPD)
3. use effective reflection to evidence ongoing lifelong learning
4. use tools to evaluate your own performance
5. record evidence of CPD.

Remember
All registered therapists are required to do CPD to certify that their knowledge is current, thereby ensuring public safety.

Introduction

Reflective practice is now included as part of professional and personal development during training and, once qualified, therapists can, and should, use reflective practice to evidence continuing professional development (CPD).

Using good, effective reflective practices can re-affirm your commitment to your studies and to your chosen career path. It can help clarify what you are trying to achieve in both your personal and your professional life. Good reflective practice underpins good professional practice and should be viewed as an opportunity to evaluate and review your progress. This is not only useful and necessary as you study for your qualification, but also as you go on to work as a professional therapist.

Identifying areas of practice that you need to develop further and those that you have already developed successfully is a route to continuing enhancement of your skills. This will benefit both you and your clients.

For reflective activity to be effective it is essential that you are prepared to be honest in self appraisal, and to learn from mistakes or areas of weakness. By reviewing behaviour and skills honestly, we are able to identify weaknesses and find suitable solutions and opportunities for development. Reflection without action is not sufficient. Student and practitioner alike must always strive for ways to improve.

What is reflection?

Reflection is a process of reviewing your working practice in order to be able to describe, analyse and, most importantly, evaluate that work so as to inform your learning about practice.

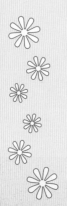

This allows you to consider ways of improving in order to develop into a better and more effective practitioner. It should be a continuous, lifelong process, as each client consultation and treatment provides a new opportunity to grow in your role as therapist.

Reflective practice uses each new situation as a learning opportunity so that you are learning through the work you do. It is important to constantly review, update and renew your attitudes to and methods of working, building on your experience in order to keep a fresh outlook. Anyone working in a customer-centred industry must keep the needs of their clients at the forefront of all that they do. It is always apparent to the client when a therapist is just 'going through the motions'.

In the workplace
Always think about what you are doing and why you are doing it; regardless of how many times you have done it.

The basic elements of a reflective process

Reflection is essentially a personal and individual activity. However, it also benefits from the input of others.

Features of effective reflective practice include:

- being open-minded about what you do and how you do it
- questioning what you do and why and how you do it
- considering what others do, and how they do things
- considering a range of possible options and working practices
- analysing and comparing results of different working practices
- asking for and accepting feedback; both positive and negative
- considering how others perceive you and what you are doing
- being able to adapt processes rather than sticking rigidly to proscribed methods
- being prepared to try new things and to analyse and review new experiences
- learning from mistakes and negative experiences and building on the positive.

Activity

Make a list of your skills and positive traits. Then make a list of aspects of your personality or behaviour and attitudes you feel you need to work on. How do you think others perceive you? Share your results with a partner or group. Give each other sensitive feedback. How accurate was your idea of how you are seen by others?

You can only learn from feedback if you are open-minded and able to accept criticism. As a student you need to practise giving and receiving feedback from each other. Helpful feedback should not be taken personally, but it should be taken seriously.

Be aware

As you learn each new technique, try to become aware of the learning process: from apprehension ('I don't think I can do this'), through growing confidence as you make links between the theory and practice, to familiarity ('I can do this'). However, beware of becoming complacent; always keep in mind the first stage, so that each time you practise the technique you are striving to do it better.

In the workplace

You will be accustomed to review and evaluation at the end of each lecture or practical lesson when feedback may be from your tutor, your peers, your clients. Consider applying the process in the workplace. Who else could give you useful feedback?

What constitutes specific and useful feedback? 'Ouch!' is certainly a response to a painful massage, but does not help the therapist to improve her technique. 'I feel a sharp pain in my shoulder when you press there with your thumb,' is both specific and useful.

By practising massage techniques on each other, you will gain awareness of the client's perspective as well as that of the therapist. Try commentating on how the massage feels when you are in the role of the client. Describe any discomfort or any particularly effective strokes. Pinpoint areas of pain or discomfort and try to explain what is causing them. Keep your feedback specific.

The reflective therapist is an adaptive therapist; able to think on their feet and respond quickly, confidently and competently to any new situation. The more you practise reflection, the more flexible you will become to meet the needs of different clients.

Your training course requires you to think on your feet all the time and to adapt routines and techniques to different hypothetical situations. In the workplace this would be *Reflection in action*: the ability to respond appropriately to each new situation. In order to be able to do this, develop the habit of retrospective *Reflection on action*, i.e. looking back on what you have done and applying the elements of reflection to your work.

It is sometimes useful to write up your experiences for future reference, or for evidence of ongoing personal professional development. This writing might take the form of part of the client consultation notes; including feedback from the client may be part of your assessment activities while studying.

Both as a learner and as a practitioner, part of *Reflection on action* should involve relevant research. Use the internet. Use libraries. Keep in touch with fellow students. Don't be afraid to ask for help or advice.

As a professional therapist, you may feel you don't have enough time to bother with reflective activity, either during or after practice. As a student, you may feel that you have enough to do! However, it is important to recognise that the process of reflection need not be burdensome or time-consuming and can in fact become almost enjoyable. It should not be seen as a chore, but something that you do automatically as part of the routine of delivering an effective treatment. As thinking beings, we evaluate situations and experiences almost constantly, without being aware that we are doing it. Taking a few extra moments to organise your thoughts on paper is not difficult and is a useful tool to develop for all aspects of your life. The long-term impact in relation to your studies is that it will help to prove to yourself and others that you are competent and capable of development. Once you are qualified, your written notes will provide evidence of CPD.

Continuing Professional Development (CPD)

The industry is constantly evolving and updating: so too must good practitioners. It is vital to keep in touch with developments and new ideas. It is a good idea to maintain a **portfolio** of evidence of your qualifications and ongoing training. You can also include positive feedback from clients as well as self evaluation and an annual (or regular) review of your career development (see Figure 9.1).

Sample career and CPD review sheet

Name:

CPD for year ending:

Time period: from: to:

My current position: ....

Areas for development: ....

Aims and objectives: ....

Training and/or support needs: ....

Realistic timescale: ....

Additional comments: (*How am I doing? Do I need some support? Who could I contact?*)

    ....

    ....

Figure 9.1 Sample career and CPD review sheet

Continuing your professional development does not mean constantly having to pore over books after a tiring day at work, although new publications will give some insight into current working practices.

There are other important ways of keeping up to date, including:

- regular staff meetings in the workplace to compare notes and share ideas
- visiting exhibitions and trade shows
- networking with other practitioners
- keeping up to date with new product lines and reading manufacturers' information
- using the internet to research international trends

- reading industry-linked publications
- attending training courses for new skills and forms of treatment
- attending training sessions for particular product lines
- attending conferences
- reviewing any of the above for publication
- visiting other practices as a client to help you keep client perspective in mind.

Keep a written record in your portfolio of your responses to these events, courses and programmes of research, including how you are going to incorporate them into your working practice. This could be in the form of notes, a diary entry or filling in a form as in Figure 9.2, below.

Sample activity review sheet

Name: ……………………………

CPD for year: …………………..

CPD activity undertaken:

……………………………………………………………………………………………………

Date of activity: ………………………………………

Provider: ………………………………………………

Number of hours for this activity: …………………………

Why I undertook this activity:

……………………………………………………………………………………………………

……………………………………………………………………………………………………

……………………………………………………………………………………………………

How I benefited from the activity: ………………………………………………………

……………………………………………………………………………………………………

……………………………………………………………………………………………………

Activity reviewed with: (*Organiser/Supervisor/Colleague etc. where applicable*)

Signed: …………………………………………………

Name: …………………………………………………………

Date: …………………………………………

Figure 9.2 Sample activity review sheet

How to reflect effectively

After each treatment, analyse your performance. Did the treatment go well? Be specific in your analysis.

Ask yourself the following questions:

- Was I polite? Neat? Welcoming? Did I put client at ease?
- Was the work station appropriately prepared?
- Did client know what to expect? Was the client comfortable?
- Did I go through appropriate consultation and take note of client responses?
- Did I check my posture and positioning relative to the client?
- Did I plan my routine with the needs of the client in mind?
- Were my massage strokes and movements correct?
- Did I manage to work rhythmically and with appropriate pressure?
- Did I focus on appropriate areas for the client's needs?
- How do I feel, both physically and emotionally?

Did you find any aspects of the routine or the encounter with the client difficult or uncomfortable? If so why? And what can you do to change that next time?

This may seem like a lot of questions. However, asking them will become second nature to you, so that you are analysing each experience automatically. Just as medical practitioners carry out numerous routine checks before, during and after any surgical procedure, so too should the good therapist; no matter how many times you have performed the treatment.

Be aware

Feeling something to be really easy might indicate a lack of awareness or sensitivity on your part or perhaps highlight the fact that you are not delivering all aspects of the treatment effectively.

Question your client

Clearly, no client wants to be badgered throughout what is supposed to be a relaxing massage with questions about your technique. After all, the client wants to feel that you are the expert and you know what you are doing! However, you do need to create an atmosphere where the client feels able to tell you if something you are doing is uncomfortable or painful. Simply suggesting before you start the massage that they should tell you at once of any discomfort should achieve this.

Similarly, it is not appropriate to finish your massage routine by immediately asking for feedback. Allow the client to provide feedback in their own time, maybe on a section of the consultation form or on a separate feedback form, after they have had time to relax and get dressed. Allow them time and privacy to do this so that they feel able to give honest feedback.

Be aware

It may help to let the client know how certain techniques should feel. I know of a very slim lady who endured numerous painful massages because she mistakenly believed that it should hurt in order to be beneficial! Don't assume your client will know what to expect.

Consider the responses to your questions.

The next step of the reflective process is to think about what could have been done differently to make the treatment better.

Compare your own review with that of the client. Any differences in response need to be addressed. If you thought you were polite but the client has noted that you were abrupt, then you need to re-evaluate your understanding of what constitutes politeness.

Consider how you could improve

Don't be satisfied with an 'average' performance. Do you need to practise particular techniques, change your attitude or research a particular area? Where you have been particularly successful, is there scope for further development? Which aspects of the treatment did you find most fulfilling? Is there scope to take those aspects further?

Focus on the positive elements; don't be weighed down by the negative. Your practice can be developed and improved as long as you are prepared to learn from your experience and use it as a catalyst for change.

During your studies to achieve your massage qualification you will have plenty of opportunity to share experiences, ideas and knowledge with your peers and your tutors. Much time will be given to group reflection and to self- and peer-assessment. It is equally important in the workplace, to carry on this process of shared experience. Try to maintain the curiosity and excitement you felt when you first embarked on this course of study and it will give you a strong basis on which to build a strong portfolio of continued professional development.

Consider what interests you about the industry. Are there techniques or product lines you would like to know more about? Do your research – use the internet and ask other therapists and manufacturers for information.

Many companies offer training courses for their equipment or products. Put any certificates or proof of attendance records into your CPD folder. You could also write brief notes from your course to remind you of key points and as evidence that you attended.

The evidence will be useful for planning your career, preparing for interviews and marketing your skills to different organisations. It can highlight your strengths and indicate which career areas need development. Evidence also provides a document on which to base performance reviews in the workplace. It can enhance your self-esteem and make your career goals more attainable.

> **Be aware** !
> Check that sources of information that you find on the internet are reliable. Don't accept everything you read at face value.

> **Activity** ✳ ✳ ✳
> Take some time to make a career plan. Where would you like to be in 10 years' time? Include plans for career breaks where applicable. List the ways you could achieve your goal, and the possible barriers to achieving it. Set out a plan to overcome the barriers, with an appropriate timescale. (It is important to do this exercise at intervals when you are a qualified practitioner, not only when you are a student. Continue to regularly reassess your aims throughout your career.)

Answers to multiple-choice questions

Chapter 1
1. b   2. c   3. a   4. d   5. c   6. a   7. a   8. b
9. d   10. c

Chapter 2
Cells and tissues
1. b   2. d   3. c   4. d   5. a   6. b   7. a   8. c
9. a   10. b

Integumentary system
1. d   2. b   3. a   4. b   5. d   6. a   7. c   8. b
9. a   10. c

Skeletal system
1. b   2. c   3. d   4. a   5. c   6. d   7. b   8. a
9. d   10. a

Muscular system
1. c   2. a   3. b   4. d   5. b   6. d   7. b   8. c
9. a   10. c

Cardiovascular system
1. b   2. a   3. d   4. c   5. d   6. b   7. c   8. a
9. b   10. c

Lymphatic system
1. b   2. a   3. d   4. c   5. a   6. d   7. b   8. a
9. c   10. d

Respiratory system
1. b   2. c   3. d   4. a   5. d   6. b   7. c   8. c
9. d   10. a

Digestive system
1. a   2. c   3. d   4. b   5. c   6. d   7. c   8. b
9. b   10. a

Nervous system
1. a   2. d   3. c   4. b   5. b   6. a   7. c   8. b
9. c   10. d

Urinary system
1. b   2. c   3. a   4. d   5. d   6. a   7. b   8. a
9. c   10. b

Endocrine system
1. c   2. c   3. d   4. b   5. c   6. a   7. d   8. b
9. c   10. a

Reproductive system
1. a   2. c   3. b   4. c   5. d   6. b   7. a   8. c
9. d   10. b

Chapter 3
1. b   2. c   3. d   4. a   5. c   6. b   7. a   8. d
9. b   10. a   11. d   12. b   13. c   14. b   15. a
16. d   17. c   18. d   19. a   20. c

Chapter 4
Effleurage group
1. b   2. d   3. d   4. c   5. c   6. b   7. a   8. b
9. a   10. c

Petrissage group
1. c   2. b   3. d   4. c   5. d   6. a   7. b   8. b
9. a   10. c

Percussion group
1. d   2. a   3. c   4. b   5. d   6. a   7. c   8. a
9. b   10. d

Vibrations and frictions
1. d   2. c   3. a   4. d   5. a   6. c   7. c   8. a
9. b   10. b

Chapter 5
1. c   2. a   3. d   4. b   5. b   6. d   7. a   8. b
9. c   10. d   11. b   12. d   13. a   14. c   15. c
16. d   17. a   18. a   19. c   20. b

Chapter 8
1. d   2. a   3. b   4. a   5. b   6. c   7. d   8. c
9. b   10. c   11. b   12. d   13. c   14. d   15. a
16. c   17. b   18. c   19. a   20. c

Glossary

Acetycholine neurotransmitter that facilitates the passage of an impulse.

Acid mantle a mixture of sweat and sebum that forms a coating on the skin.

Actin protein found in muscle that is involved in muscle contraction.

Adenosine triphosphate (ATP) energy-carrying molecule found in cells.

Adhesions fibrous tissue strands which join two surfaces that are normally separate. They form as a result of inflammation.

Alveoli the air sacs of the lungs.

Anatomy the study of the structure of the body.

Aponeurosis a flat sheet of connective tissue, which attaches muscles along the length of bones.

Appendicular skeleton bones that form the upper and lower limbs and their girdles.

Axial skeleton the bones that form the core/centre of the body.

Cancellous bone spongy inner mass of bone.

Centrosome an organelle involved in cell division.

Compact bone hard outer layer of bone.

Connective tissue many different types of tissue that connect and hold other tissues together.

Contra-action a condition that develops during or after a treatment.

Contra-indication a condition that may prevent or restrict treatment.

Crepitus a condition that results from inflammatory changes within the tissues.

Cytoplasm jelly-like substance within a cell membrane.

Deoxyribonucleic acid (DNA) genetic material of the cell.

Desquamation the removal of the dry, scaly surface cells of the stratum corneum of the skin.

Digestion the breaking down of food.

Electromagnetic spectrum bands of radiation with differing wavelengths and frequencies.

Endoplasmic reticulum a series of channels for transporting substances within a cell.

Epithelium/epithelial tissue layers of cells that form the covering (skin) and linings of the body (mouth, digestive tract).

Erythema reddening of the skin produced by dilation of the blood vessels and an increase in blood flow.

Erythrocytes red blood cells; contain haemoglobin which transports oxygen around the body.

Expiration expelling air out of the lungs.

Exudate fluid seeping into the tissues from the blood vessels.

Fasciculi muscle bundles.

Fibrotic nodules hardened, lumpy zones lying within superficial muscles or fascia.

Flagella whip-like projections on the surface of some live cells that provide them with the ability to move.

Golgi apparatus involved with the production of membrane and protein lipids and lipoproteins.

Hazard anything that can cause harm.

Homeostasis the body's inner balanced state.

Hyaline cartilage a hard connective tissue that covers the ends of bones: it reduces friction at the joints.

Hygiene the precautions and procedures necessary for maintaining health and preventing the spread of disease.

Hygiene requirements the hygiene standards specified by an organisation or laid down by law.

Hyperaemia increase in blood flow to an area.

Hypertonic muscles muscles with greater than the normal degree of tone.

Hypotonic muscles muscles with less than the normal degree of tone.

Inclusions chemical substances produced by cells.

Ingestion taking food into the body.

Inspiration taking air into the lungs.

Interstitial fluid fills the spaces between the cells of the body, also known as tissue fluid.

Joint where two or more bones join or articulate.

Keratin a protein found in the skin cells that protects the skin from injury, from invasion by micro-organisms and also makes the skin waterproof.

Kyphosis an exaggerated curve of the thoracic spine.

Lactic acid waste product of muscle.

Law of Grotthus states rays must be absorbed to produce an effect.

Law of reflection states the angle of incidence is equal to the angle of reflection.

Leucocytes destroy foreign material and protect the body against micro-organisms.

Lordosis an exaggerated curve of the lumbar spine.

Lymphocytes type of white blood cell involved in immunity.

Lysosomes a type of organelle which digest and deal with waste.

Macrophages circulate in the blood and engulf and destroy bacteria.

Mast cells release histamine following injury or reaction to an allergen.

Melanin pigment found in the skin that protects against ultra-violet rays.

Melanocytes cells in the skin that produce melanin.

Membranes cover or line body parts.

Merkel's discs nerve endings sensitive to touch.

Metabolites waste products of metabolism.

Micturition urination.

Mitochondria organelles which generate adenosine triphosphate (ATP) energy.

Mitosis the process of cell division into two identical cells.

Muscle hypertension greater than normal degree of tension in muscles.

Muscle tone slight degree of tension always present in muscles, enabling them to react quickly to stimuli.

Myosin protein found in muscle that is involved in muscle contraction.

Naevus an abnormality in the pigmentation of the skin.

Nephron functional unit of a kidney involved in filtration.

Neural referring to the nervous system.

Neurotransmitter chemical that transports impulses across synapses to other nerves.

Nucleus controls the activities of the cell and contains DNA.

Oedema swelling of the tissues caused by an excess of tissue fluid.

Organelles mini-organs that carry out the functions of a cell.

Osseous tissue bone tissue which is a type of connective tissue.

Osteology the study of the structure and function of bones.

Palpation the examination of the tissues through touch and feeling.

Periosteum tough fibrous tissue that covers bones into which the tendons of attachment blend.

Peristalsis involuntary wave-like contractions that push the contents through the gastro-intestinal tract.

Physiology the study of how the body functions.

Plasma proteins the protein substances suspended in the plasma of the blood, such as fibrinogen, albumin and globulin.

Plasma membrane outer layer or boundary of the cell. It gives shape to the cell and protects it.

Reflex action a rapid involuntary response to a stimulus.

Refraction bending of rays when they meet a new medium.

Repetitive strain injury (RSI) performing repetitive movements that overload or over-use specific muscles.

Ribonucleic acid (RNA) required for the manufacture of protein in the cell.

Ribosomes organelles that synthesise protein.

Risk the chance – great or small – that someone will be harmed by the hazard.

Scoliosis an abnormal curve of the spine, a 'C' or 'S' shape.

Sensory receptors sensory nerve endings that relay sensations to the brain and spinal cord.

Skin tone the colour of the skin, which varies from person to person and race to race.

Sphygmomanometer measures blood pressure.

Stasis an area of stagnation due to poor circulation.

Synapse a connection between two neurones or between a neurone and its muscle fibre.

Tendons tough cord-like structures of connective tissue, which attach muscles to bones.

Tension nodules areas within a muscle where fibres show abnormal increase in tone.

Thrombocytes type of white blood cell involved in blood clotting.

Tissue fluid provides a medium for substances to move across from the blood to the cells and from the cells to the blood.

Trauma injury or damage to a part.

Trigger points areas of extreme pain within the tissues, which may radiate around the area *or* may refer pain to an area some distance away.

Urea waste product of protein metabolism.

Uric acid waste product of protein metabolism.

Vasoconstriction constriction of the blood vessels: the lumen becomes smaller.

Vasodilation dilation of blood vessels: the lumen becomes larger.

Villi finger-like projections that line the walls of the small intestine that greatly increase the surface area, for absorption to take place.

Workplace legislation all the laws and regulations governing all the activities in the workplace.

Index